? HOW the Chinese Eat Potatoes

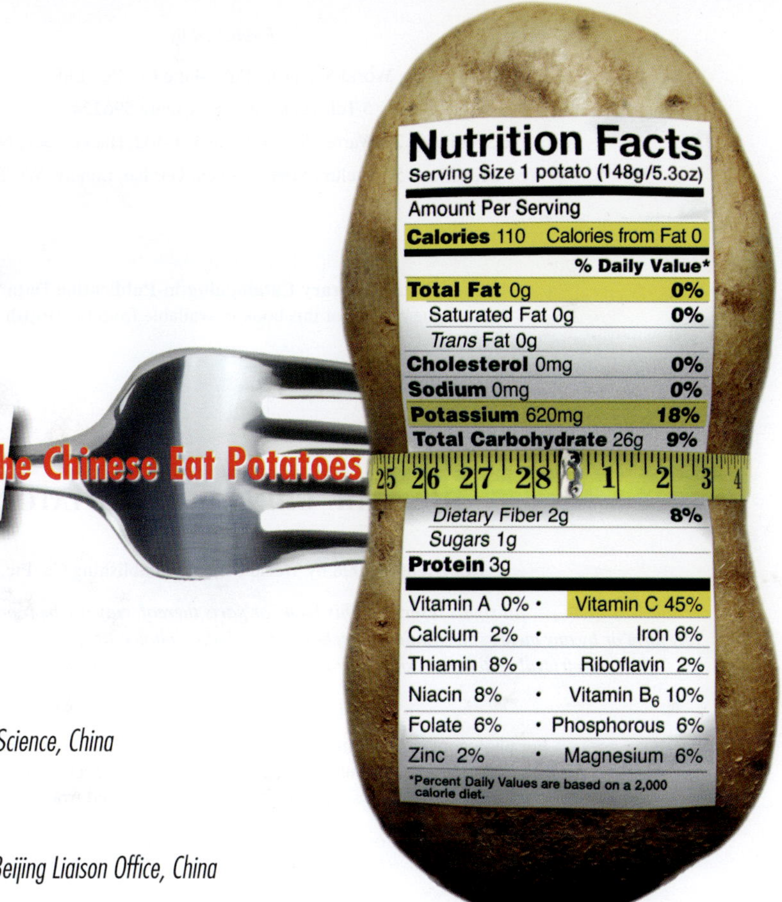

editors

Dongyu Qu

Chinese Academy of Agricultural Science, China

Kaiyun Xie

International Potato Center, CIP Beijing Liaison Office, China

World Scientific

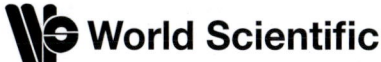

NEW JERSEY • LONDON • SINGAPORE • BEIJING • SHANGHAI • HONG KONG • TAIPEI • CHENNAI

Published by

World Scientific Publishing Co. Pte. Ltd.
5 Toh Tuck Link, Singapore 596224
USA office: 27 Warren Street, Suite 401-402, Hackensack, NJ 07601
UK office: 57 Shelton Street, Covent Garden, London WC2H 9HE

British Library Cataloguing-in-Publication Data
A catalogue record for this book is available from the British Library.

Agriculture and Food — Vol. 1
HOW THE CHINESE EAT POTATOES

Copyright © 2008 by World Scientific Publishing Co. Pte. Ltd.

All rights reserved. This book, or parts thereof, may not be reproduced in any form or by any means, electronic or mechanical, including photocopying, recording or any information storage and retrieval system now known or to be invented, without written permission from the Publisher.

For photocopying of material in this volume, please pay a copying fee through the Copyright Clearance Center, Inc., 222 Rosewood Drive, Danvers, MA 01923, USA. In this case permission to photocopy is not required from the publisher.

ISBN-13: 978-981-283-291-7
ISBN-10: 981-283-291-2

Design by **LAB Creations** (A Unit of WorldScientific Publishing Co. Pte. Ltd.)
Printed in Singapore.

This book is dedicated to
International Year of the Potato 2008

How the Chinese Eat Potatoes

Editors-in-Chief

Dongyu Qu and Kaiyun Xie

Contributors

Liping Jin • Yili Chen • Fengyi Wang • Wanmin Sheng • Ying Shi
Ruofang Zhang • Yuhe Yin • Jiang Yin • Hui Ma • Zhen Du
Leru Zhang • Di Wang • Junlian Zhang • Yong Chang • Min Fan
Wei He • Qijun Sui • Shanyun Li • Zuoyi Liu • Zunguo Lei • Zhenlin Huang
Conghua Xie • Jun Liu • Hao Tang • Peilun Wang • Guangcun Li
Zhanwang Gao • Jingli Jia • Mingya Ding • Zhiqian Guo • Jiandong He
Xiaoxue Wang • Jianmiao Gu

The Potato: A World-saving Treasure (Preface)	21
The Biology of the Potato	26
Potato morphology	27
The potato's nutrition value	33
Special nutritional and medicine functions of potatoes	37
Chinese Potato Recipes	42
Potato Recipes from Northeast China	45
Braised potato with goose (Da E Men Tudou)	47
Cooked potato chips (Peng Tudou Pian)	48
Flavored mashed potatoes (Fengwei Tudou Ni)	49
Fried lichen and potato chips (Dipi Tudou Pian)	50
Fried potato cake I (Jian Tudou Bing)	51
Fried potato chips with green pepper (Chao Tudou Pian Qingjiao)	52
Fried potato chips with spicy cabbage (La Baicai Chao Tudou Pian)	53
Fried potato strips with garlic bolt (Zha Tudou Tiao Chao Suantai)	54
Fried shredded potato (Suchao Tudou Si)	55
Golden fried potato balls (Zha Huangjin Tudou Qiu)	56
Mashed potatoes with sauce (Jiaozhi Tudou Ni)	57

Mixed shredded potatoes (Ban Tudou Song)	58
Potato and cabbage soup (Hongcai Tang)	59
Potato balls (Tudou Li Wanzi)	60
Potato cake I (Tudou Bing I)	61
Potato salad with green vegetables (Qingcai Tudou Shala)	62
Seasoned potato strings and noodles (Qiang Tudou Si, Fensi)	63
Shredded potato and bean salad (San Si Bao Dou)	64
Steamed potato and eggplant served with soy sauce (Nongjia Dajiang Zheng Tudou Qiezi)	65
Stewed potato chips with goose (Tudou Gan Dun Da E)	66
Stewed potatoes with cowpeas (Tudou dun Doujiao)	67
Stewed potatoes with curry chicken (Tudou Dun Gali Ji Kuai)	68
Stewed potatoes with eggplant in thick sauce (Tudou Jiang Dun Qiezi)	69
Stewed potatoes with yellow sturgeon (Xunhuangyu Men Tudou)	70
Stewed small potatoes I (Youmen Xiao Tudou I)	71
Stir-fried potato, green pepper and eggplant (Di Sanxian)	73

Potato Recipes from North China 75

Bag-shaped oat potato pie (Malingshu Tuntun)	77
Baked potato cake (Lao Malinghshu Yangzi)	78
Black soy sauce potatoes (Jiangyou Malingshu Tiao)	79
Braised beef with potato (Malingshu Shao Niurou)	80
Braised potato pieces (Hongshao Shukuai)	81
Braised potato, cabbage and tofu (Malingshu Baicai Tofu)	82

Braised potatoes (Malingshu Dahuicai)	83
Braised potatoes and cabbage (Malingshu Baicai Hui Fenkuai)	84
Braised potatoes and tofu with spareribs (Malingshu tofu Dun Paigu)	85
Braised potatoes with cowpeas and spareribs (Malingshu Doujiao Dun Paigu)	86
Braised potatoes with fish-shaped oat noodles (Malingshu Hui Youmian Yu)	87
Braised sheep entrails with noodles (Guozai Fentiao Yangza)	88
Braised side pork and rape with potatoes (Wuhuarou Youcai Hui Malingshu)	89
Braised sirloin with potatoes (Malingshu Dun Niunan)	90
Braised small potato balls with oxtail (Xiao Tudou Shao Niuwei)	91
Camel palm encircled with shredded potato (Tuozhang Tudou Si)	92
Chinese chess fun (Qi Qu)	93
Cold potato strings in oil, vinegar and spices (Liangban Malingshu Si)	94
Countryside tricolor potatoes (Nongjia Tianyuan Sanse)	95
Deep-fried potato doughnuts (Youzha Malingshu Guozi)	96
Deep-fried potato strips with tomato sauce (Mizhi Shasi Tudou Tiao)	97
Drunk potato (Zuijiu Malingshu)	98
Egg, shredded bottle gourd and potato cake (Jidan Hulusi Malingshu Bing)	99
Elegant taste (Ya Qu)	100
Fish-shaped potato (Malingshu Yu)	101
Fish-shaped potato with fried pork fillet (Guoyourou Malingshu Yu)	102
Fish-shaped potato-oat flour noodles (Tudou Yuzi)	103
Flavored potato balls (Fengwei Tudou Qiu)	104

Fried chicken-flavored potato (Youzha Malingshu)	105
Fried Chinese sauerkraut and noodles (Suancai Chao Fentiao)	106
Fried Chinese sauerkraut and potato chips (Suancai Malingshu Tiao)	107
Fried Chinese sauerkraut and potato slices (Suancai Malinghsu Ni)	108
Fried mashed potatoes, carrots and mushrooms (Jinsha Fengguang)	109
Fried potato balls (Youzha Malingshu Wanzi)	110
Fried potato cake II (Xiangjian Tudou Bing I)	111
Fried potato slices I (Youzha Malingshu Pian)	112
Fried potato strings (Youzha Malingshu Si)	113
Fried potato strings with pickled celery cabbage and mutton fat (Yangyou Suancai Malingshu Si)	114
Fried potato strips coated with sugar (Liuli Shutiao)	115
Fried potato strips with chili (Ganbian Tudou Tiao)	116
Fried potato strips with pork (Youbailuo Chao Malingshu Tiao)	117
Fried potatoes with egg (Tudou Jian Dan)	118
Fried potatoes with soybean sprouts (Tudou Chao Huangdou Ya)	119
Fried shredded potato cake I (Xiang Jian Tudou Pai)	120
Fried shredded potato with Chinese chives and egg (served with cake) (Malingshu Si Jiucai Jidan Dai Bing)	121
Fried side pork with potato (Wuhuarou Jian Malingshu)	122
Handmade noodles with potatoes in an earthen pot (Shaguo Malingshu Shouganmian)	123
Hotpot potato pieces (Malingshu Huoguo Pian)	124
Hunyuan cold potato jelly (Hunyuan Liangfen)	125

Mashed garlic scallop with potato noodles (Suanrong Fensi Zheng Shanbei)   126

Min Bagu (Min Bagu)   127

Mini embroidered potato balls (Mini Xiuqiu Wan)   128

Noodles with potato and spinach (Malingshu Bocai Gangsimian)   129

Oat dumplings with potato filling (Malingshu Youmian Jiaozi)   130

Oat flour-wrapped shredded potato (Youmian Tuntun)   131

Pepper oil-flavored shredded potato (Jiaoyou Tudou Si)   132

Pickled Chinese cabbage with mashed potatoes (Suancai Tudou Ni)   133

Potato and millet porridge (Qiangguo Malingshu Xifan)   134

Potato and oat pancake (Tudou Bing II)   135

Potato cake II (Malingshu Bing)   136

Potato chips with fried pork fillet (Guoyourou Malingshu Pian)   137

Potato egg cake with sesame seeds (Malingshu Jidan Zhima Bing)   138

Potato Kuilei (Tudou Kuilei)   139

Potato lambsquarter goosefoot salad in vinegar sauce (Malingshu Ban Huicai)   140

Potato noodles mixed with sauce (Jiachang Ban Fen)   141

Potato noodles with needle mushrooms (Malingshu Fensi Jinzhengu)   142

Potato pie (Malingshu Gao)   143

Potato pot-stickers (Malingshu Guotie)   144

Potato strings with lichen (Dipicai Malingshu Si)   145

Potato strips with Japanese rhodea (Wannianqing malingshu Tiao)   146

Potato-oat flour made fishlike noodles (Xiangjian Tudou Roujuan)   147

Roasted potato (Kao Malingshu)	148
Roasted potato slices (Kao Malingshu Pian)	149
Shredded potato and wild vegetables in vinegar and spices (Malingshu Si Ban Yan Kucai)	150
Shredded potato with sow thistle (Malingshu Si Ban Kucai)	151
Silver boat carries the valuables (Yinzhou Zaibao)	152
Soft-shell turtle encircled with small potatoes (Xiao Tudou Jiayu)	153
Spareribs with Chinese sauerkraut and mashed potatoes (Paigu Suancai Malingshu Ni)	154
Spicy diced potatoes I (Xiangla Malingshu Ding)	155
Spicy shredded potatoes (Xiangla Tudou Si)	156
Steamed abalone-shaped potato pie (Su Bao Pai Fan)	157
Steamed buns with potato and Chinese chive filling (Tudou Jiucai Baozi)	158
Steamed dumplings (Zheng Jiao)	159
Steamed fish-shaped oat noodles (Youmian zheng Yu)	160
Steamed fish-shaped potatoes with Chinese sauerkraut (Suancai Malingshu Yu)	161
Steamed oat rolls with potato and eggplant (Malingshu Men Qiezi)	162
Steamed potato balls (Tudou Wanzi)	163
Steamed potato cake (Zheng Malingshu Yangzi)	164
Steamed potatoes and pork balls (Jing Wan Wan)	165
Steamed potatoes I (Zheng Malingshu)	166
Stewed chicken with potato (Malingshu Dun Xiaoji)	167
Stewed chicken with potato and tofu (Malingshu Tofu Dun Jiaji)	168
Stewed pork bones with potato and squash (Malingshu Wogua Dun Gutou)	169

Stewed pork ribs with potato and squash (Malingshu Wogua Dun Paigu)	170
Stewed potatoes with chicken (Xiaoji Dun Tudou)	171
Stewed potatoes with eggplant (Malingshu Men Qiezi)	172
Stewed potatoes with pumpkin I (Malingshu Dun Wogua)	173
Stewed spareribs with potato and frozen tofu (Malingshu Paigu Dong Tofu)	174
Stir-fried knife-sliced noodles with potato chips and fried pork fillet (Guoyourou Malingshu Pian Chao Daoxiaomian)	175
Stir-fried mashed potatoes (Chao Malingshu Kuailei)	176
Stir-fried potato strips and shredded carrot (Malingshu Tiao Chao Huluobo Si)	177
Swan playing with water (Tian E Xishui)	178
Tired bird returns to the nest (Juan Niao Gui Chao)	179
Tofu soup with potato and cabbage (Malingshu Baicai Tofu Tang)	180
Translucent dumplings (Boli Jiaozi)	181
Tricolor mashed potatoes (Sanse Tudou Ni)	183

Potato Recipes from Northwest China   185

Baked potatoes (Kao Tudou)	187
Baked potato cake with red bean filling (Tudou Dousha Bing)	188
Black beauty potato slices (Hei Meiren Yangyu)	189
Braised assorted dishes, Yulin style (Yu Lin Da Huicai)	190
Braised chicken with potato and green pepper (Da Pan Ji)	191
Braised potatoes with mutton rack (Tudou Wei Yangpai)	192
Braised potatoes with pumpkin (Dun Nangua Tudou)	193

Braised spareribs with potatoes (Tudou Dun Paigu)	194
Braised tofu with pakchoi (Xiao Baicai Hui Tofu)	195
Crisp potato balls coated with sugar (Yinzhuang Suguo)	196
Crystal mashed potato roll (Yuni Shuijing Juan)	197
Cucumber with potato noodles (Huanggua Fenpi)	198
Dark steamed potato balls (Heilengleng)	199
Deep-fried potato balls covered in sesame seeds (Tudou Matuan)	200
Dongxiang county potato chips (Dongxiang Tudou Pian)	201
Fried meatballs (Zha Ge Wanzi)	202
Fried pork liver with potato (Zhugan Tudou Tiao)	203
Fried pork slices with potato (Tudou Chao Rou Pian)	204
Fried potato cake III (Tudou Jianbing)	205
Fried shredded potato cake II (Tudou Tanbing III)	206
Fried shredded potatoes with vinegar (Culiu Yangyu Si)	207
Fried stick-shaped mutton-potato mash (Tu Yang Jiehe Bang)	208
Fried tofu and potatoes with green and red Pepper (Jin Yu Man Tang)	209
Golden shredded potato nest (Jin Quechao)	210
Golden thread with lotus (Jinsi Wang Lian)	211
Goulash with potato (Tudou Shao Niurou)	212
Grape-shaped potato dish (Fengshou Putao)	213
Mashed potatoes with pakchoi (Hua Cai)	214
Pear-shaped potato (Xiang Sheng Li)	215

Potato and buckwheat pancakes (Malingshu Jianbing)	216
Potato and oat pancakes (Tudou Bing IV)	217
Potato and pumpkin sandwich (Baihua Tudou He)	218
Potato and shiitake mushroom cake (Tudou Xianggu Bing)	219
Potato bula (Yangyu Bula)	220
Potato cake III (Tudou Gao)	221
Potato chicken egg soup (Tudou Jidan Geng)	222
Potato noodles (Yangyu Mian)	223
Potato nut cake (Malingshu Ganguo Gao)	224
Potato salad (Tudou Shala)	225
Potato starch jelly (Malingshu Liangfen)	226
Potato-wrapped beef rolls (Tudou Niurou Juan)	227
Rolls with potato and beef filling (Tudou Niurou Bing)	228
San zha wu pin (San Zha Wu Pin)	229
Shredded potatoes with sweet and sour sauce (Yuxiang Tudou Si)	230
Soft potato cake (Yangyu Langao)	231
Steamed potato and lichen dumplings (Tudou Diruan Baozi)	232
Steamed potato flakes mixed with flour (Yangyu Caca)	233
Steamed potato jelly (Yangyu Jinjin)	234
Steamed potatoes II (Zheng Tudou)	235
Steamed potatoes with chicken (Tudou Zheng Ji)	236
Stewed potatoes (Men Tudou)	237

Stewed sheep entrails with potato noodles (Yu Lin Yang Zasui)	238
Stir-fried beef with potato noodles (Niurou Chao Fen)	239
Stir-fried pork with potato noodles (Zhurou Qiao Ban Fen)	240
Strawberry-filled mashed potato cake (Caomei Yuni Su)	241
Sweet fried potato chips (Huanying Tudou Pian)	242
Three kinds of stewed vegetable balls (Shao San Yuan)	243
Xinjiang chicken and potato dish (Xinjiang Da Pan Ji)	244
Yulin three fresh delicacies (Yulin Pin Sanxian)	245

Potato Recipes from Southwest China — 247

Baked shredded potatoes (Gan Bei Yangyu Si)	249
Birds nest-shaped shredded potatoes (Niaochao Shu Si)	250
Braised potato balls with black soy sauce (Hongshao Tudouqiu)	251
Braised potatoes with duck (Tudou Huang Men Ya)	252
Braised potatoes with rice (Tudou Men Fan)	253
Braised side pork with potatoes in soy sauce (Tudou Hongshao Rou)	254
Charcoal-roasted potatoes (Tanhuo Kao Tudou)	255
Chinese date-filled potato balls with honey (Mizhi Nuoxiang Tudou Zao)	256
Colorful shredded potatoes (Qicai Tudou Si)	257
Crisp potato strips I (Xiangsu Shu Tiao I)	258
Crisp potato strips II (Xiangsu Shu Tiao II)	259
Deep-fried fat pork and diced potatoes (Cuishao Tudou li)	260
Deep-fried potato chips (Youzha Tudou Pian)	261

Dish	Page
Deep-fried potato chips with peanuts and chili (Youzha San Pin)	262
Diced potatoes with salted egg yolk (Yan Danhuang Tudou Li)	263
Finely shredded potatoes with ginger (Jiangwei Longxu Si)	264
Fried dried potato slices (Zha Gan Yangyupian)	265
Fried green pepper and shredded potato (Qingjiao Tudou Si)	266
Fried potato chips (Su Chao Tudou Pian)	267
Fried potato chips with soy sauce (Jiang Bao Tudou Pian)	268
Fried potato pancake (Qiaoshou Tuanyuanbing)	269
Fried potato pie (Youzha Shu Bing)	270
Fried potato slices with dried pickles (Gan Yancai Chao Shu Pian)	271
Fried potato slices with sour bamboo shoots (Suan Sun Chao Shupian)	272
Fried potato strips coated with yolk (Jinsha Tudou Tiao)	273
Fried potatoes and chicken with pickled pepper (Paojiao Tudou Ji)	274
Fried potatoes and pork with pickled pepper (Jiang Rou Tudou Ding)	275
Fried potatoes with four treasures (Jin Shu Hui Sibao)	276
Fried prawn coated with fine potato strings (Jinsi Fengwei Xia)	277
Golden potato string cake (Jinhuang Dousi Bing)	278
Green onion-flavored potato chips (Conghua Shu Pian)	279
Ham-flavored potato strings (Huotui Fengwei Tudou Si)	280
Honeycomb-shaped potatoes (Fengwo Tudou)	281
Hot and spicy diced potatoes I (Mala Tudou Ding)	282
Hot and spicy diced potatoes II (Xiangma Tudou Ding)	283

Hotpot potatoes with preserved ham and radish (Yi Guo Hui)	284
Long life shredded potatoes (Changshou Tudou Si)	285
Mashed potatoes fried with fennel (Huixiang Tudou Ni)	286
Mashed potatoes in lotus leaf (Heye Tudou Ni)	287
Mashed potatoes with pine nuts (Songren Tudou Ni)	288
Mashed potatoes wrapped in sticky rice pancakes (Zhibao Tudou Ni)	289
Megranate-shaped fried chicken (Fugui Shiliu Ji)	290
Minced beef in potato bowls (Yi Wan Chi)	291
Pan-fried potato pastry (Xiangjian Tudou Bing II)	292
Potato and chicken with chili powder (Yangyu Lazi Ji)	293
Potato chips served with Yunnan ham (Yuntui Tudou Pian)	294
Potato pancake with salted vegetables (Xuecai Tudou Bing)	295
Potato shoot salad in vinegar (Liangban Shumiao)	296
Potato shoot soup with sour bamboo shoots (Suan Sun Shumiao Tang)	297
Potato soup with pickled cabbage (Suancai Tudoupian Tang)	298
Potato string cake with five spices (Wuxiang Tudou Si Bing)	299
Potato with laver (Zi Cai Tudou Bing)	300
Potato with twice-cooked pork (Tudou Huiguo Rou)	301
Potatoes cooked in tin foil (Xizhi Tudou)	302
Potatoes in soy sauce (Jiang Xiang Tudou)	303
Potatoes in soybean milk (Hezha Yangyu)	304
Roasted potatoes (Kang Yangyu)	305

Salted meat with colored potatoes (Yanrou Caiyangyu)	306
Shredded potato salad in vinegar (Liangban Shu Si)	307
Shredded potatoes with beef jerky (Ganba Yanyu Si)	308
Shredded potatoes with pickles (Yangyu Si Xiancai)	309
Silver thread noodles and potato strings (Yinsi Tudou Chuan)	310
Sizzling Potato (Tieban Tudou)	311
Soft-fried sliced potatoes (Ruanzha Tudoupian)	312
Sour and spicy potato chips (Suanla Tudou Pian)	313
Sour and spicy shredded potato soup (Suanla Tudou Si Tang)	314
Sour diced potato soup (Shu Kuai Suan Tang)	315
Sour pickle and chive flower potato soup (Suanyancai Tudou Tang)	316
Sour pickle and potato chip soup (Suanyancai Tudou Pian Tang)	317
Spicy and hot potatoes (Xiangla Tudou)	318
Spicy diced potatoes II (Xiangla Shu Kuai)	319
Spicy potato chips (Xiangla Tudou Pian II)	320
Spicy potato slices (Xiangla Tudou Pian I)	321
Spicy Sichuan-style potato strings (Ganbian Tudou Si)	322
Steamed potatoes and spareribs (Fen Zheng Tudou Paigu)	323
Steamed potatoes with pickled chili (Culajiao Zheng Tudou)	324
Stewed potatoes and pork ribs with spices (Xiangla Paigu Men Tudou)	325
Stewed potatoes served in wok (Ganguo Tudou)	326
Stewed potatoes with cucurbit (Xiao Gua Men Yangyu)	327

Stewed potatoes with pumpkin II (Nangua Dun Tudou)	328
Stewed potatoes with rice (Yangyu Kongganfan)	329
Stewed silver carp soup (Guiyu Zahui Tang)	330
Stewed small potatoes II (Youmen Xiao Tudou II)	331
Stir-fried potato shoots (Su Chao Shumiao)	332
Stir-fried shredded vegetables (Chao San Si)	333
Street potato snacks from Yunnan (Jie Bian Xiao Chi)	334
Sweet and sour potato sandwiches (Tangcu Tudou Jia)	335
Toothpick potato diamonds (Yaqian Tudoukuai)	336
Tree tomato-flavored potatoes (Shu Fanqie Fenwei Tudou Si)	337
Western-style mashed potatoes (Xi Shi Tudou Ni)	339

Western Style Potato Dishes and those from Other Regions   341

Curry potatoes (Gali Malingshu)	343
Deep-fried potato balls (Cuizha Tudou Qiu)	344
French-style mushroom and potato salad (Fashi Xianggu Malingshu Shalazi)	345
Fried country-style potato balls (Shancun Zha Malingshu Wanzi)	346
Fried diced potatoes and lettuce stems (Chao Malingshu Wosunding)	347
Fried egg and potato string cake (Jianjidan Malingshusi Bing)	348
Fried potato cake IV (Cui Zha Tudou Bing)	349
Fried potato slices II (Zha Malingshu Pian)	350
Fried potato strips (Zha Malingshu Tiao)	351

Fried potato strips with spicy peanuts (Xiang Su Shutiao)	352
Fried potato with jellyfish (Tudou Bao Zhetou)	353
Honey potatoes (Mizhi Malingshu)	354
Pagoda-shaped mashed potatoes with shiitake mushroom (Xianggu Malingshu Ni Ta)	355
Potato and egg soup (Tudou Danhua Tang)	356
Potato and vegetable salad (Qingcai Malingshu Shalazi)	357
Potato balls with ham (Huotui Malingshu Wanzi)	358
Potato dumplings (Shu Jiao)	359
Potato rolls wrapped in dried tofu (Fupi Malingshu Juan)	360
Potato sandwich with pork (You Su Tudou He)	361
Potato strings with sea cucumber (Tudou Si Ban Haishen)	362
Potatoes in hot caramel (Basi Tudou)	363
Roasted potatoes with jam (Guojiang Malingshu Pai)	364
Steamed potato strings with mashed garlic (Suan Ni Tudou Si)	365
Stewed beef with potato (Tudou Shao Niunan)	366
Stir-fried potato strips with celery (Shan Qin Chao Tudou)	367
Three earthly delights (JiaoDong Di Sanxian)	369

The Development and Role of the Potato in China   370

Introduction of the Potato to China   371

Development of the Potato Industry in China after the 20th Century	373
Potato Production in China	**382**
Huge planting area and low yield	382
Achievements in the breeding and extension of new potato varieties	385
Incomplete seed system and the shortage of high quality seed potatoes	386
The majority of farms are small-scale	388
The frequent occurrences of potato pests and diseases	389
Main Roles of the Potato in China	**390**
Food safety	391
Energy security	395
Poverty elimination	397
Potato processing and value-added	398
The potato and natural disaster relief	405
Appendix 1: Index of all dishes	**407**
Appendix 2: Index of the dishes for vegetarians	**418**
Appendix 3: Index of the dishes for Muslims	**424**

The Potato: A World-Saving Treasure

The 20th century was rife with war and famine. The world population quadrupled, from 1.6 billion in 1900 to 6 billion in 2000; the Chinese population alone increased more than threefold—from 0.426 billion in 1900 to 1.275 billion in 2000. The advancement of agricultural technologies, supported by industry and coupled with the fortitude of humans, resulted in all kinds of disasters. Entering the 21st century, the world continues to be faced with a rapidly increasing world population and a serious food shortage problem. According to data from the Population Division of the United Nations, the world population will have increased to 9.5–10 billion in 2050; that is, 3.5–4 billion more people than there are now. Based on predictions from demographers, the global population will be over 12 billion by the end of the 21st century, double that in 2000. Thus, the pressing issues of food supply and food safety will continue to be key concerns for scientists and governments.

China's rapidly increasing population trend was held back by family planning policies, which were successfully implemented for the past 30 years. The total fertility rate (i.e. the number of children per couple) was reduced from 6.0 in the 1970s to 1.8–1.85 after the 1990s, lower than the population replacement rate. It is predicted that China's population growth will be halted in 20–30 years, once the total population reached 1.5–1.6 billion. Thus, the fuse of the Chinese "population bomb" will be snuffed, providing the fundamental condition for sustainable development in the 21st century.

However, food production will need to be increased by 20% in the next 20–30 years in order to match the Chinese population increase from 1.32 billion in 2007 to 1.5 or 1.6 billion. This will allow for the modest annual consumption of 380 kg of food per capita.

Rice, maize and wheat are the traditional food crops in China, and their yields have been increased to over 300 kg per mu (4.5 ton/ha). This constitutes a real challenge for agricultural technologies under the strain of the continuing decrease of arable land, water shortage in northern China, and adverse weather conditions. The authors of this book thus recommend that the further development of root and tuber crops, such as potatoes and sweet potatoes, should be one of the important strategic measures to counter this problem.

Tudou, the Chinese name for potato (*Solanum tuberosum*), originating from Andes in South America, was first brought to the European continent by Spanish colonists in the 16th century. From Europe, the potato crop was distributed all over the world by various means. In 2007, potatoes were planted in 160 countries around the world; they have become the third-largest food crop, behind only rice and wheat, with total planted area of 20 million hectares and total production of over 300 million tons.

The potato tuber contains many important nutrients, such as glucides, proteins (essential amino acids), minerals, vitamins (primarily vitamin C, which is not found in other grain foods) and fat, and is easier to digest compared to other foods. The potato tuber is a good source of wholesome nutrition, containing high levels of potassium and abundant soft dietary fibers, but low levels of sodium, and has a low fat content.

The potato also has some unique benefits, unfamiliar to most. For example, it is ideal as infant food due to its complete range of nutrients, abundant vitamins, and soft texture. It has been reported that fresh mashed potatoes can be externally applied to heal bone fractures. Freshly extracted potato juice is very helpful in controlling several conditions, such as constipation, gastric ulcers, redundant acidity in the stomach, duodenum ulcers, and nasosinusitis. The potato is beneficial for cancer patients, especially for those undergoing chemotherapy, because of its tender fibers, high potassium, and several special vitamins (namely, vitamins A and B6). It is also regarded as an anti-senescence food because of its high vitamin C, E and B5 content, as well as its anthocyanin component, which can protect cells from attacks by free radicals. Due to the potato's resistant starch content, low caloric value and low fat, it is also popular in the beauty and health industries.

The potato crop began to be widely planted in the coastal and inland regions after its introduction into China during the late Ming Dynasty (1600s). It had become one of the most important foods in the Chinese diet because of the crop's tolerance to drought, ability to adapt to poor fertility, short growing period, good taste, and high yield potential. Though the history of potato planting in China goes back only 400 years, China has become the biggest potato producer in the world since the late 20th century, accounting for one-fourth of the global planting area and one-fifth of global production.

On the one hand, the current average yield of potatoes in China is very low, about one-third to one-half of the yield in developed countries, so there is plenty of room for yield increases. On the other hand, there are over 300 million hectares of winter fallow rice fields, and some of them can be used for potato production without any influence on rice production because of the short growing period of potatoes (less than 3 months for early and medium varieties). Thus there is potential for increase in potato planting area. With the remarkable increase in potato yield by new varieties and technologies and the increase of potato planting area, the potato can play an important role in solving the food security problem and also aid in the relief of future natural disasters in China.

The United Nations has announced 2008 as the International Year of the Potato. This is only the second time an entire year has been dedicated to a crop (after the International Year of Rice in 2003). This indicates how important the two crops are for the world, and China happens to be the biggest producer for both crops in terms of the total planting area and production. Production and consumption is likely to increase due to the potato's abundant and complete nutritional qualities, as well as the healthy and unique Chinese cooking technology. The International Year of the Potato aims to raise the profile of this globally important food crop and commodity, emphasizing its biological and nutritional qualities, and thus promote its production, processing, consumption, marketing and trade.

This book, edited by Dr. Dongyu Qu and Dr. Kaiyun Xie, comprehensively introduces the biological strengths and nutritional value of potatoes, as well as the current situation and future trends of potato production in China. With input from people in the potato industry, over 300 recipes for dishes and staple foods have been collected. They are valuable references, not only for all the provinces in China, but also for people around the world.

J. Song

President Emeritus
Chinese Academy of Engineering
(June 12, 2008)

The Biology of the Potato

The potato is a tuber crop that originated in the Andes of South America. It is known as papa in Spanish, pomme de terre in French, and Solanum tuberosum in Latin. In China, the potato has more than 20 different names. Among them, the following names are most common: tudou in northeast China, shanyao in northern China, and yangyu in both northwest and southwest China. In Chinese, the scientific name for potato is malingshu.

According to its botanical taxonomy, the potato is an annual herbaceous plant with both cultivated and wild species, and belongs to the Tuberosa series, Petota section, Solanum genus, Solanaceae family. Based on its set of chromosomes, potato is a multiploid plant. The basic number of chromosomes in a potato cell is 12 (n=12) and there are diploid (2n=24), triploid (3n=36), tetraploid (4n=48), pentaploid (5n=60), and hexaploid (6n=72).

Potato morphology

As an annual herbaceous plant, the potato plant is comprised of roots, stems, leaves, flowers, fruits and seeds (see Figure 1). Its morphology includes the tuber—a transformed stem, and the most important economic organ—which is different from other plants. The potato's lifecycle doesn't always include the full cycle of planting, emergency, flowering and fruiting; an ideal harvest may be obtained without the two key stages of flowering and fruiting, which are common for most other crops. The most common seeds for potatoes are called seed tubers (or seed potatoes), which are the storage organs of potatoes. This is different from other crops, which usually use seeds as planting material. The real seeds (true potato seeds, or TPS) from the pollinated potato flowers can also be used for multiplication of progenies, but they are mostly used for potato breeding, and not for potato production.

Roots: Potato roots vary according to the planting materials used. A fiber root system will develop if seed tubers are used, and all the roots will be adventitious roots, without differentiation between main and lateral roots. A tap root system will develop if true seeds are used as the planting material, with tap roots and lateral branches. Adventitious roots are produced first from junctures between the seed tuber and the primary buds and more and more adventitious roots will be produced from the knots of underground stems with the growing of buds. Most of the adventitious roots are white, but can be colorful for some varieties. The adventitious roots are distributed within 30 cm of the topsoil.

A tap root system will be formed when the true seeds are used as planting materials. The tap root will be produced from the radicle and extended to the soil. The first lateral roots will be produced when the tap root reaches a length of 3 cm, and additional lateral roots may be produced as the plant continues to grow. These lateral roots are distributed in a netlike structure in the soil.

Stem: There are several types of stems for potato plants, including an upper stem, underground stem, creeping stem (stolon) and tuber (transformed stem). All of the stems originate from the same tissue and organ, but they are quite different in shape and function.

The upper stems are the upper branches developed from the eyes of seed tubers or from the young seedlings of true seeds. They are also called main stems and there may be several main stems in one plant. The knot of the upper stem is round and the stem cross section can have three, four or multiple

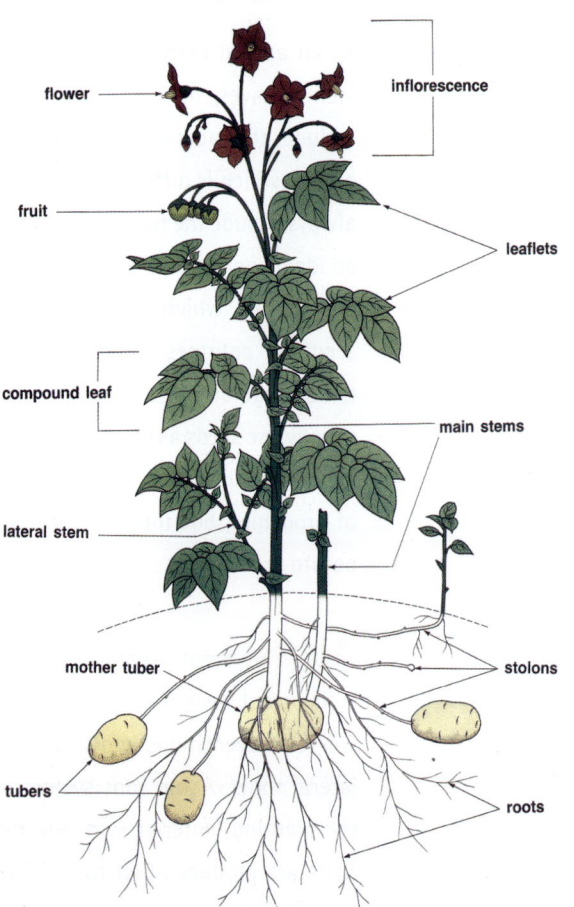

Figure 1: Potato plant (Source: CIP)

ridges. There may also be margin wings with different shapes. The stem color is generally green, but can vary according to different varieties. The stem shape in cross section, the wings' characteristics and the stem color are the key indicators for identifying different varieties.

The underground stems are the parts that produce the tubers, and they vary according to the planting depth and the hilling situation during the growth period. Generally, they are 10 cm long and have eight knots. One to three stolons will be produced from the axil in each knot and the stolons will develop tubers after swelling. The stolons are the organs that produce tubers and are generally white, but may be colorful for some varieties. Normally, one main stem can produce 4–8 stolons and 20–50 stolons can be formed in one plant. Generally, the more stolons there are the more tubers that will be produced. The stolons are geotropic and apheliotropic and most of them are distributed in the soil at a depth of 5 cm to 20 cm. The stolons can develop into new lateral stems, not tubers, if they are not covered well and exposed on the soil surface.

The potato tuber is an economic organ, a propagating organ and also a transformed stem. There are eyebrows, eyes and lenticels in the tubers. The end attached to the stolon is called the basal end, or heel, and the other end is called the apical end, or distal end. Potato tubers vary in shape, skin color and flesh color according to the different varieties. For a particular variety, the tuber shape, skin color and flesh color will not change under normal cultivation conditions and are important indicators for identifying different varieties. Changes in cultivation conditions and planting locations can result in the tuber flesh color ranging from heavy to light for the varieties with colored tuber flesh.

Besides glucides, tubers also contain proteins, vitamins, dietary fibers and minerals. The nutritional value of tubers will be discussed in detail in the second part in this chapter.

Leaf: The well-developed potato leaf is an odd pinnate compound leaf with several leaflets. Most potato varieties will have compound leaves with 7, 9, 11, 13 or 15 leaflets each. The leaflet at the end of the compound leaf is called the terminal leaflet and the other opposite pairs of leaflets are called the lateral leaflets. There can be interjected leaflets or small split leaflets between two pairs of the lateral leaflets. There are some tiny leaflets, called as small leaflets, in the petiolules of the lateral leaflets or in the juncture of the leaflets and the petiole. In the upper area of the juncture of the petiole and the main stem, there is a pair of leaf-shaped structures, called as stipules or leaf ears. For a particular variety, the terminal leaflet, pairs of leaflets, the leaf margin, the surface flatness, occurrence of hairs, and the shape of the stipules are very stable and they are indicators for the identification of different varieties. However, the first leaf of the potato plant is a single leaf regardless of whether tubers or true seeds are used as the planting material.

Flower: Potato flowers are attached to one or several inflorescences, which are called ramificate cymose inflorescences. Normally, there are 2–5 branches in each inflorescence and 4–8 flowers in each branch. Each flower will be connected to the branch or sub-branch from the basal and connected to the basal of the calyx by the flower stalk. There is an absciss layer in the upper part of the flower stalk, also called the knot of the flower stalk, where the flower buds and flowers will fall off.

Each flower comprises four components: calyx, corolla, stamen and pistil. The basal of the calyx is cylindraceous, has five splits at the apical end, and is green in color. The basal of the corolla is funnel-form, has five splits at the apical end, and is pentacle-like. When there are additional petals inside or outside the corolla, they are called inside double petal or outside double petal corollas. The common colors for the corollas are white, light red, purple, amaranthine, and blue.

The stamen comprises five anthers, which are alternately arranged with petals and embrace the pistil in the middle. Different potato varieties can be identified from the calyx, corolla, shape of stamen and pistil, and the fertility of the anthers. The potato is a self-pollinated crop because there is nectar in the flower and the natural hybrid rate is very low.

Fruit: Potato fruits are the berries of the solanaceae family and are similar to the fruits of the berry tomato. Most of the pericarps are green, although they may be brown or purple-green. The fruit is normally divided into two or three locules. Each fruit usually has 100–250 seeds, but can have up to 500 seeds or no seeds. Around 5–7 days of successful pollination, the ovary will start to swell and the fruit will be ripen 30–40 days later. In the meantime, the pericarp will become soft, yellow-white or white, and emit a special fragrance.

Seed: Potato seeds are very small and weigh 0.3–0.6 grams per 1,000 seeds. The seeds are shaped like flat eggs and the end attached to the fruit is a little bit smaller and yellow or dark gray. The dormancy for newly harvested seeds is about six months. A higher sprouting rate can be obtained after storing seeds for one year. Potato seeds can be stored for 20–30 years in low temperature and low moisture conditions. Seeds are used in important gene banks around the world to store the wild potato germplasm.

The potato's nutritional value

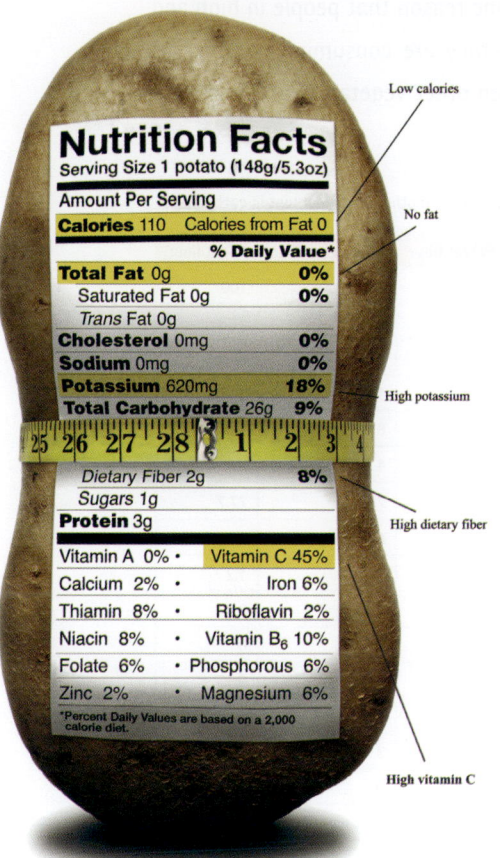

Figure 2: Potato nutrition facts (Source: United States Potato Board)

The potato's nutritional value refers mainly to the nutritional value of tuber when it is used as food. The many differences in potato variety, cultivation conditions and other factors make it difficult to clearly define the nutritional value of a potato. However, the United States Potato Board has developed a Nutrition Facts table based on a 148 g potato (see Figure 2).. So in 2008, the International Year of the Potato, the Journal of Food Composition and Analysis, under the guidance of the United Nations' Food and Agriculture Organization (FAO), is advocating to collect information about the nutritional composition of potato varieties and potato products. It is going to publish a special issue to describe the potato's nutritional value. Before the publication of this special issue, we present here a table comparing the nutritional composition of the potato versus other foods (see Table 1), based on information from the website http://www.swcfcx.cn/.

From Table 1, we can see that the potato contains high level of vitamin C. This explains why Western people do not need to eat other vegetables after they eat potatoes, and it is the same reason that people in high and cold regions in China remain healthy—they are consuming potatoes as their main food in the long winter, when other vegetables and fruits are difficult to obtain.

Table 1: Comparison of the nutritional composition of potatoes and other foods (content in each 100 g)

Nutrition	Fresh tuber	Flake	Rice	Wheat flour	White corn flour	Millet flour
Edible part(g)	94	100	100	100	100	100
Water(g)	79.8	12	13.3	12.7	13.4	11.8
Energy(K cal)	76	337	346	344	340	356
Energy(K J)	318	1410	1448	1439	1423	1490
Protein(g)	2	7.2	7.4	11.2	8	7.2
Fat(g)	0.2	0.5	0.8	1.5	4.5	2.1
Carbohydrates(g)	17.2	77.4	77.9	73.6	73.1	77.7
Dietary fiber(g)	0.7	1.4	0.7	2.1	6.2	0.7
Ash(g)	0.8	2.9	0.6	1	1	1.2
Vitamin A(mg)	5	20	0	0	0	0
Carotene (mg)	30	120	0	0	0	0
Vitamin B1(µg)	0.08	0.08	0.11	0.28	0.34	0.13
Vitamin B2(mg)	0.04	0.06	0.05	0.08	0.06	0.08
Vitamin B5(mg)	1.1	5.1	1.9	2	3	2.5
Vitamin C(mg)	27	0	0	0	0	0
Vitamin E(T)(mg)	0.34	0.28	0.46	1.8	6.89	0
a-E	0.08	0.28	0	1.59	0.94	0
(β-γ)-E	0.1	0	0	0	5.76	0

Nutrition	Fresh tuber	Flake	Rice	Wheat flour	White corn flour	Millet flour
δ-E	0.16	0	0	0.21	0.19	0
Calcium (mg)	8	171	13	31	12	40
Phosphorus (mg)	40	123	110	188	187	159
Potassium (mg)	342	1075	103	190	276	129
Sodium (mg)	2.7	4.7	3.8	3.1	0.5	6.2
Magnesium (mg)	23	27	34	50	111	57
Iron (mg)	0.8	10.7	2.3	3.5	1.3	6.1
Zinc (mg)	0.37	1.22	1.7	1.64	1.22	1.18
Selenium (μg)	0.78	1.58	2.23	5.36	1.58	2.82
Copper (mg)	0.12	1.06	0.3	0.42	0.23	0.32
Manganese (mg)	0.14	0.37	1.29	1.56	0.4	0.55
Iodine (mg)	1.2	0	0	0	0	0

Source: http://www.swcfcx.cn/

Glucides: The glucides in potato tubers can be divided into single glucides (reducing sugars, including sucrose and fructose) and poly-glucides (starch, including amylose and amylopectin). The content of glucides ranges from 13.9% to 21.9%, and 85% of this is starch. The reducing sugars will produce a brown color when a potato is fried in the oil, and their content is one of the important indicators when determining varieties for chipping purposes. The ratio between amylose and amylopectin will affect the dietary quality of potato tubers, and it is one of the important indicators for starch content. A potato tuber contains about 0.6% to 0.8% of coarse fiber, which is also called as dietary fiber, and this content is 2–14 times that of millet, rice and wheat flour.

Protein: Generally, the protein content in potato tubers is 1.6% to 2.1%, but the highest can be over 3%. Potato protein is similar to the protein found in meat; the digestible composition is high and it can be easily absorbed by the human body. The amino acids of potato protein are very abundant, including all of the necessary amino acids.

Minerals: Potato tubers contain high levels of potassium, calcium, phosphorus and iron, and also contain many of the necessary nutrients for humans and animals, such as magnesium, sulfur, chloride, silicon, sodium, boron, manganese, zinc and copper. Because of the alkaline minerals in the potato tuber, it is considered an alkaline food, which means it can neutralize the acidity of acidic food (rice, wheat flour, fish, and animal products) and keep the balance between acidity and alkalinity.

Vitamins: Potato tubers contain more kinds and higher levels of vitamins than most other crops, including vitamins A, B1, B2, B3, B5, B6, C, H, K and M. Of them, the content of vitamin C is the highest, and can reach 20 to 40 mg per 100 g of fresh tubers.

Fat: The fat content in potato tubers is very low, usually about 0.1%. So, the potato is considered to be a typical low-fat food.

Special nutritional and medicinal functions of potatoes

Baby food: One of the best foods for babies is that made from mashed fresh potatoes or dehydrated potatoes. There are three main reasons for this. First, the potato contains a complete range of nutrients, including those necessary for growth and development of human beings, such as proteins, glucides, fat, vitamins and minerals. Some ingredients can't be found in other grain crops.

Second, potatoes contain high levels of vitamins A and C, both of which help in the development of the human body, especially for the infants and young children. The level of vitamin A intake recommended by the FAO and World Health Organization (WHO) is 300~725 μg per day for the children at 1 to 15 years. Vitamin C has about ten functions in the human body; one of the most important being the synthesis of collagen, which is the basic component in gristles, bones, teeth and blood vessel epidermises. However, other grain foods don't contain vitamin C.

Lastly, potato is very tender, which is suitable for the digestive organs of young infants.

Medicinal food: According to the theory of traditional Chinese medicine, the potato is sweet and smooth and is good for the intestines, stomach, spleen and detumescence. The potato is suitable for patients recovering from diseases of the stomach and spleen, as well as indigestion. As a medicinal food, the potato can be used in two main ways: externally and internally.

People in the Andes of South America, where the potato originated, have used potatoes externally to treat bone fractures, headaches, rheumatism, indigestion and others diseases. Fresh potato slices can be plastered on affected areas of the body to reduce bumps created when muscles cannot properly absorb the medicine from an intramuscular injection. Mashed fresh potatoes can also cure skin burnt by fires.

According to the practices of Mr. Wang Shanggong, fresh extracted potato liquid can control and cure many diseases, such as constipation, gastric ulcers, heavy acidity, duodenum ulcers, high blood pressure, diabetes, hepatitis, and the spread of cancer cells. It is also useful for treating nasosinusitis, the exclusion of toxins, and the banting.

Recovery food for cancer patients: Normally chemotherapy is applied for the recovery of early-stage cancer patients whose cancerous tissues will be cut by surgery. In this stage, the vomit reaction is very common for patients. Mashed potatoes from flakes or from boiled fresh potatoes is the best food for patients undergoing chemotherapy treatment. The dietary fibers in potatoes are very tender and do not stimulate the intestines or stomach. Potatoes also contain a high level of potassium, which can cure indigestion. Vitamin B6, which is found in potatoes, can also help to control vomiting, while the complete set of nutrients in potatoes is helpful for the overall recovery of patients.

The liquid from potato tubers is also good for the stomach. The high levels of vitamin A and carotene (which can be converted to vitamin A once ingested) can maintain the integrity of epithelia, control the development of tumors in epidermises, relieve the toxins of carcinogen, and facilitate the recovery of the cancerous cells.

Anti-senescence food: The potato's anti-senescence functions are a result of the high content of several vitamins (C, E and B5), its excellent dietary fibers and its high potassium content. As mentioned before, vitamin C, while found in the potato tuber, is not present in other grain foods. Vitamin C is an effective antioxidant, which can protect the health of cells in the body. It is also good for tooth health, protects the body's immune system, and is the main component for synthesizing collagen, which is a kind of structural protein that exists largely in the skin, bones, muscles and gums.

Vitamin E has a wide range of functions in the body, including improving metabolism. It is also an excellent antioxidant and it can slow down senescence, maintain the integrity of red cells, facilitate the synthesis of cells, protect against pollution, and cure sterility.

Vitamin PP is an important element in the oxidation function of the metabolism of proteins, fats, glucides, and over 40 other biochemical reactions. It also maintains the normal functioning of the nervous system, digestive system and skin. The dietary fibers in potato tubers can reduce the cholesterol content in the blood and the risk of heart disease, maintain peristalsis in the intestines, and reduce the risk of colon cancer. High potassium foods, such as the potato, can also reduce the rate of apoplexy. Consuming 5–6 potatoes every week can significantly decrease the risk of apoplexy.

The latest research shows that some purple flesh potato tubers have very high anthocyanin content. Anthocyanin is thought by some researchers to be the seventh nutriment after water, protein, fat, carbohydrates, vitamins and minerals. Anthocyanin is a strong oxidant and its efficiency is much higher than vitamin C and vitamin E in terms of the elimination of free radicals. Anthocyanin can also increase the elasticity of the blood vessels, improve the cycle system and skin smoothness, control inflammation and hypersensitivity, and improve joint tenacity. Anthocyanin is helpful in controlling the many diseases related to free radicals, such as cancer, heart disease, premature senility and arthritis.

Weight management food: The potato's abundant dietary fibers can increase the feeling of satisfaction in the stomach and reduce the intake of superfluous food. Potato starch has high amylopectin content and can't be digested by normal amylase. Potato starch is sometimes also called a resistant starch. The potato's low- calorie and low-fat qualities are helpful to manage one's weight, and superfluous fat can be burnt if more potatoes have been eaten.

Chinese Potato **Recipes**

China is a nation that places great importance on its cuisine. The potato's place in the national cuisine is now well-established, with many region-specific practices and recipes. Because of the wide territory and diversified food resources and eating customs, the potato recipes here are organized according to four large regions: northeast China, north China, northwest China and southwest China. Among them, northeast China comprises Heilongjiang, Jilin and Liaoning; north China comprises Inner Mongolia, Hebei and Shanxi; northwest China comprises Shaanxi, Ningxia, Gansu and Qinghai; and southwest China comprises Hubei, Chongqing, Sichuan, Yunnan and Guizhou. Western-style recipes and those from other regions are summarized separately.

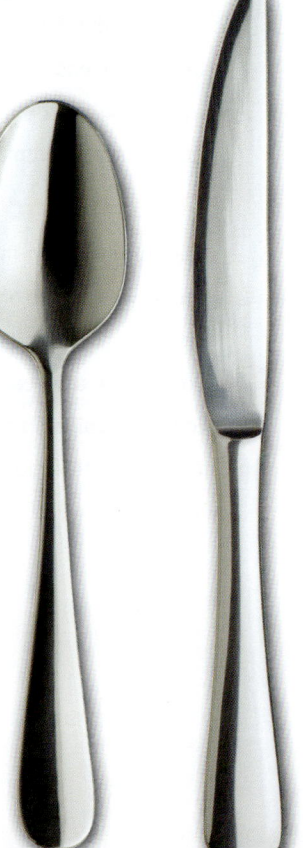

To make it easier for vegetarians and Muslims to enjoy these potato recipes, we have indicated each recipe's suitability for these two groups. Of course, anyone can enjoy any of the dishes if one or several of the ingredients or seasonings are excluded from the recipe. Especially for many dishes in which chicken essence is added, we list them as unsuitable for vegetarians, but they can become vegetarian if you don't include this seasoning.

Readers will notice that a number of seasonings are used in most recipes. This is because traditional Chinese dishes are expected to have good color, be sweet-smelling and taste delicious. However, it is possible to make a delicious potato dish using only some of the seasonings listed in a recipe. It is important to note that although all the amounts for ingredients and seasonings are indicated by weight (grams), it is just an approximate weight because it is unlikely that a cook will have a precise weight scale in the kitchen. This then leads to one of the many fascinating points of Chinese cuisine—that the same dish may taste very different when it is prepared by different cooks.

Potato Recipes from
Northeast China

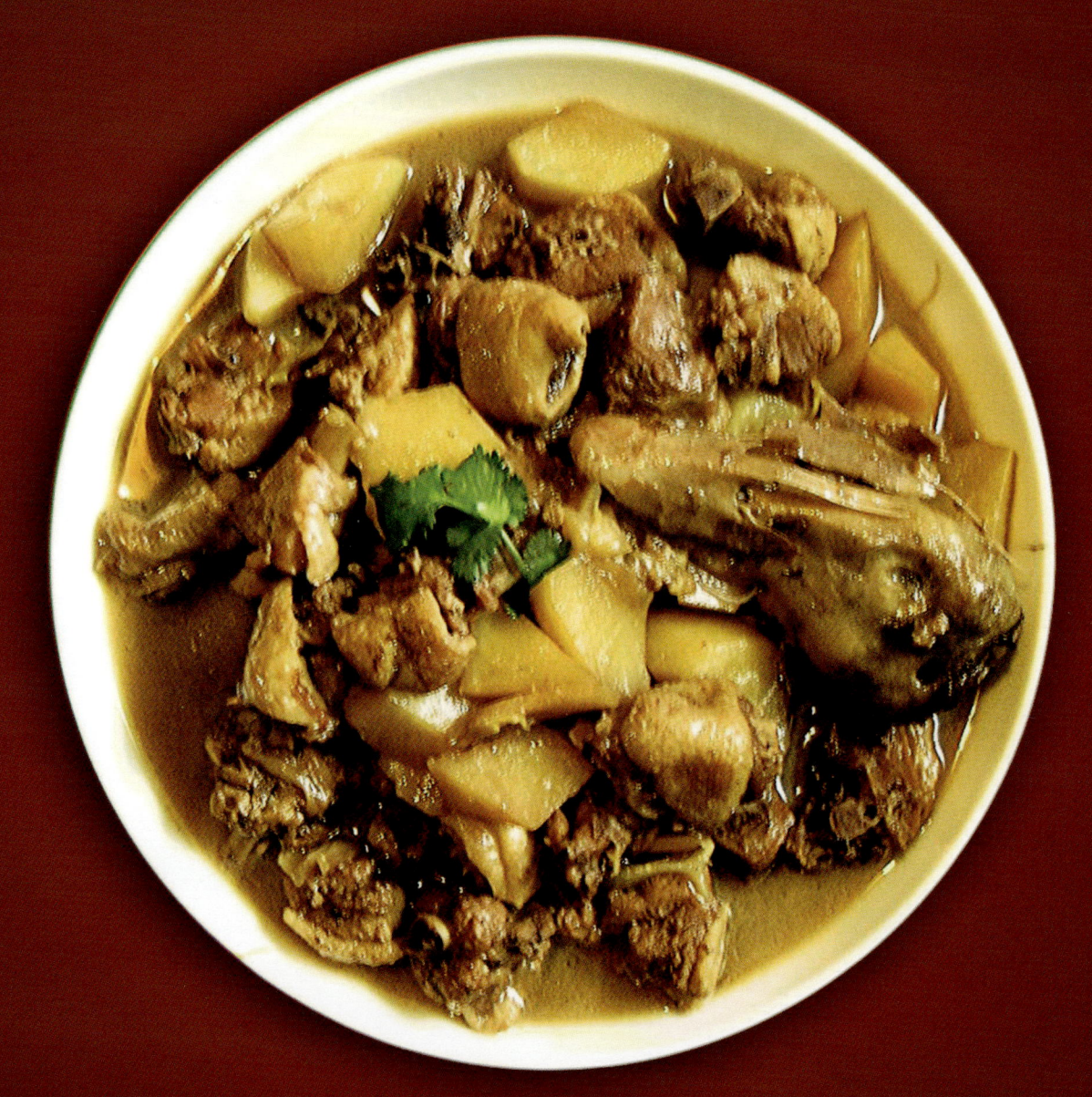

Braised Potato with Goose
Da E Men Tudou

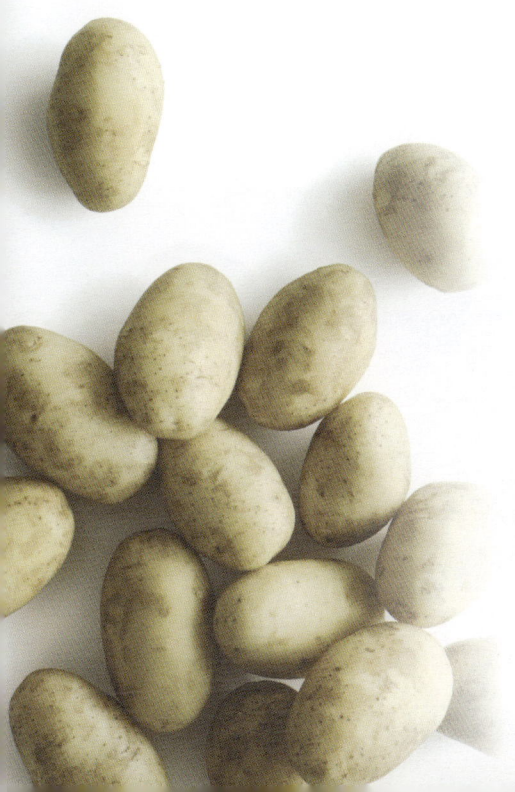

Ingredients:
Potato 300 g, Goose 500 g

Seasonings:
Salt, gourmet powder and wheat flour to taste

Preparation:
1. Dice goose and potatoes into irregular pieces.
2. Braise goose for 9 minutes with soup stock. Put potatoes and stew together, season with salt, gourmet powder and wheat flour to taste, then serve.

Vegetarian: ✗   Muslim: ✓

Cooked potato chips
Peng Tudou Pian

Ingredient:
Potato 500 g

Seasonings:
Vegetable oil 750 g, minced green onion, salt, chicken essence, Chinese prickly ash, aniseed

Preparation:
1. Peel potatoes and cut them into thick slices of 3-5 mm.
2. Heat the oil in the wok untill the oil temperature is about 140°c, then fry the sliced potatoes until they turn brown. Remove the fried slices from the oil and drain. Set aside for about 10 minutes.
3. Heat wok and put in vegetable oil. When the oil is bubbling, add the dried potato pieces. Remove as soon as they start to bulge.
4. Keep a little oil in wok, heat it, add the seasonings and stir-fry the potato chips.

Vegetarian: ✗   Muslim: ✓

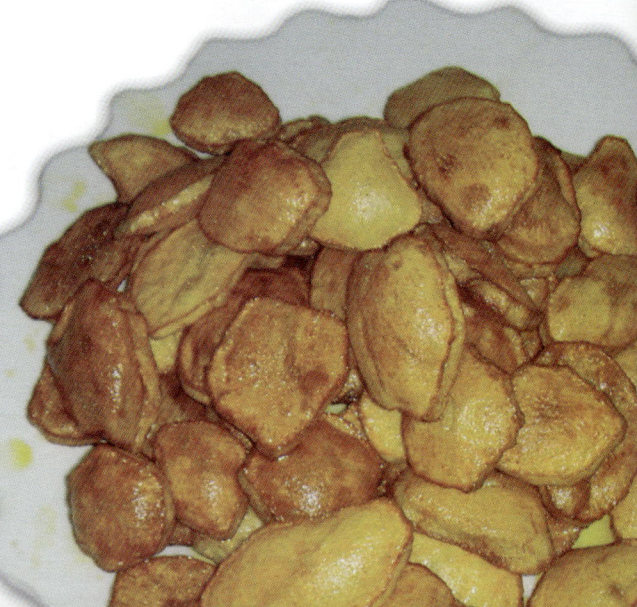

Flavored Mashed Potatoes
Fengwei Tudou Ni

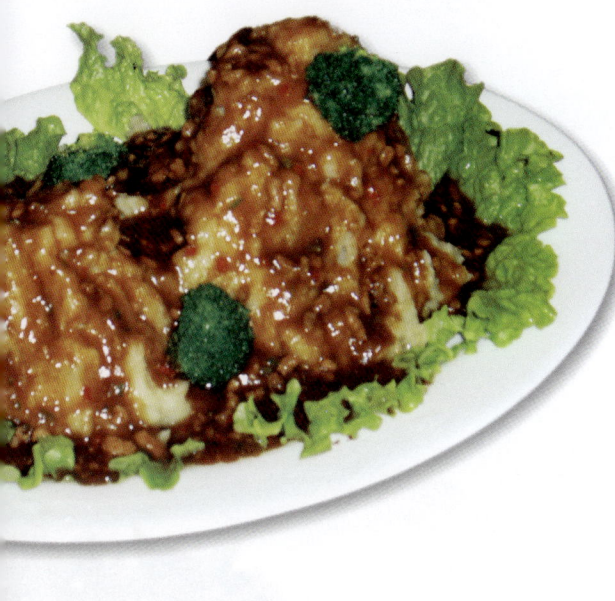

Ingredients:
Potato 500 g, minced meat 50 g.

Seasonings:
Minced green onion

Preparation:
1. Peel potatoes and steam them well in a steamer tray, then mash them.
2. Heat oil in wok, add minced meat and stir-fry. Add fresh-tasting soup, using wet starch to thicken soup. Put the soup on the mashed potatoes, sprinkle minced green onion.

Vegetarian: ✗   Muslim: ✗

Fried lichen and potato chips
Dipi Tudou Pian

Ingredients:
Potato 300 g, lichen 100 g

Seasonings:
Salt and gourmet powder to taste

Preparation:
1. Peel potatoes and cut into diamond-shape pieces; fry to golden yellow.
2. Put oil in wok, add lichen and stir-fry with potato pieces. Season to taste.

Vegetarian: ✓   Muslim: ✓

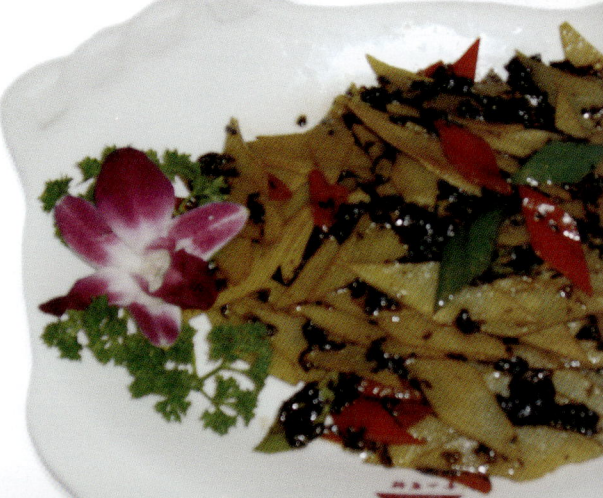

Fried Potato Cake I
Jian Tudou Bing

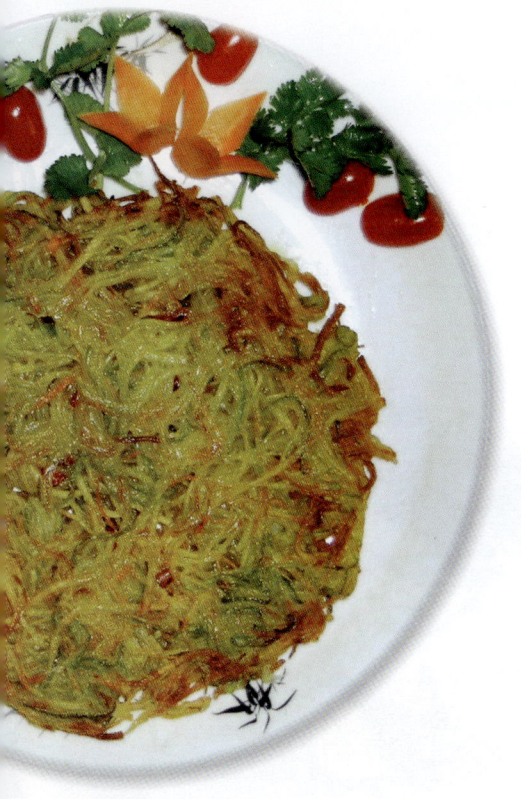

Ingredients:
Potato 300 g, carrot 50 g, green pepper 50 g

Seasonings:
Green onion 20 g, starch, salt and gourmet powder to taste

Preparation:
1. Peel and shred potato and carrot, shred green pepper to strings, add starch, salt and gourmet powder and mix evenly to form a paste.
2. Put a little oil in pan, put the paste in the pan to make a cake, fry both sides of the cake to golden brown.

Vegetarian: ✓   Muslim: ✓

Fried potato chips with green pepper
Chao Tudou Pian Qingjiao

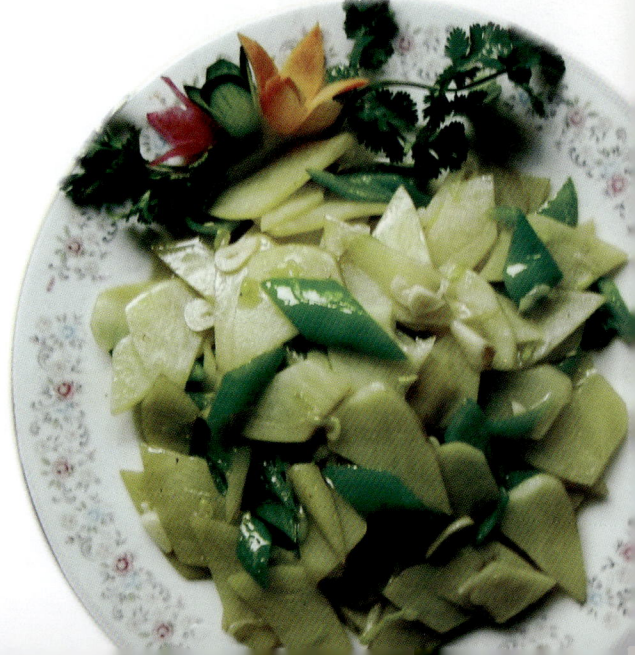

Ingredients:
Potato 400 g, pork 75 g, green pepper 150 g

Seasonings:
Onion, ginger, garlic and coriander to taste

Preparation:
1. Slice potatoes, pork and green pepper. Heat oil in a pan and fry green onion and garlic until they give off aroma. Add pork and stir-fry, then add a little soy sauce.
2. Fry potato slices in a wok until medium done, then add green pepper and fry together until cooked. Remove and serve.

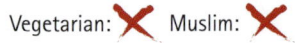

Fried potato chips with spicy cabbage
La Baicai Chao Tudou Pian

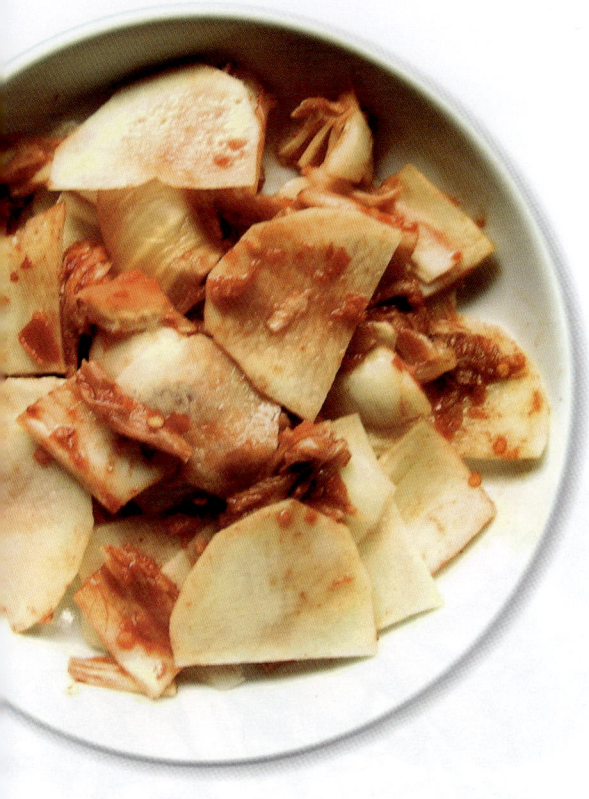

Ingredients:
Potato 200 g, spicy cabbage 200 g (can be adjusted according to individual taste)

Seasonings:
Vegetable oil 50 g

Preparation:
1. Slice potatoes.

2. Put a little oil in wok and heat. Add potato chips to stir-fry until medium done, then add the spicy cabbage and continue to stir-fry. When potatoes are well-cooked, remove and serve.

Vegetarian: ✓   Muslim: ✓

Fried potato strips with garlic bolt
Zha Tudou Tiao Chao Suantai

Ingredients:
Potato 300 g, garlic bolt 250 g

Seasonings:
Green onion, ginger, garlic to taste

Preparation:
1. Cut potatoes into thick strips, fry to golden brown. Cut garlic into sections and quick-boil.
2. Put a little oil in wok and fry green onion, ginger and garlic to give off aroma. Add a little cooking liquor, salt, gourmet powder and soy sauce, then add potato strips and garlic bolt and fry together until almost done. Mix with starch to thicken soup, then serve.

Vegetarian: ✓   Muslim: ✓

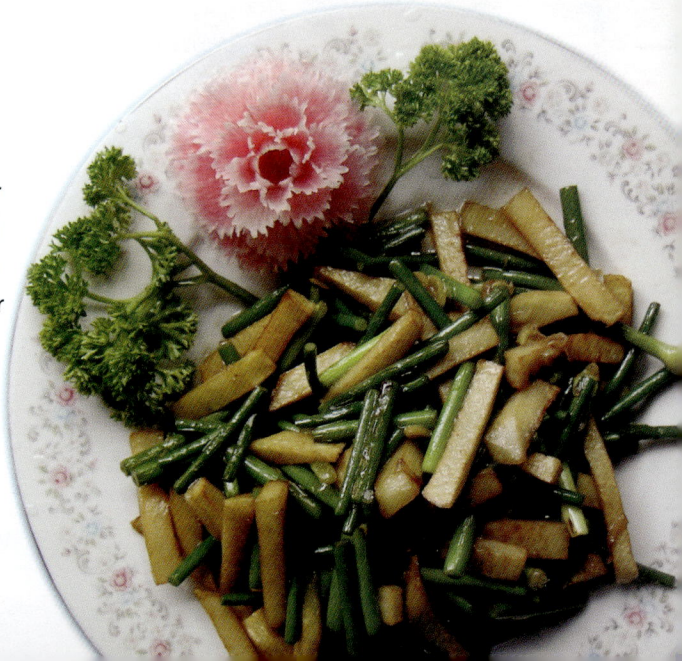

Fried shredded potato
Suchao Tudou Si

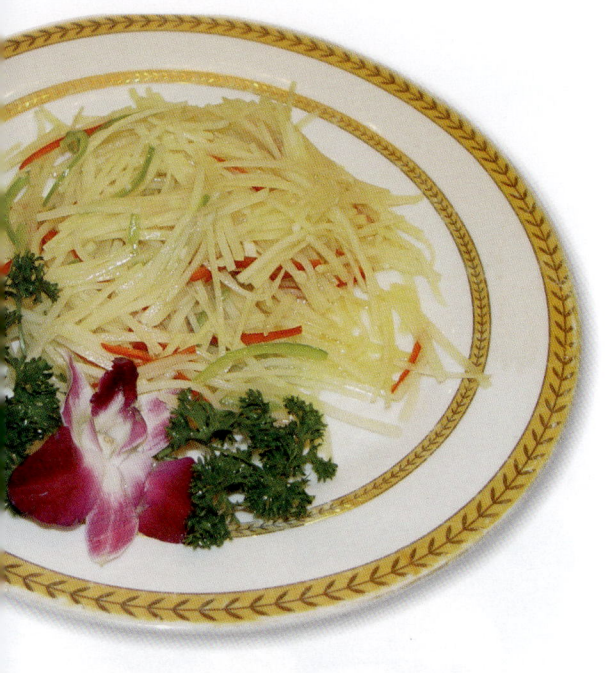

Ingredients:
Potato 400 g, small amount of green pepper and red pepper

Seasonings:
Salad oil 50 g, vinegar 5 g, green onion 3 g, ginger 3 g, salt 1 g

Preparation:
1. Peel and shred potatoes into strings. Boil water and add potato strings in to boil for half mature. Remove and set aside.
2. Heat salad oil in another wok. Fry green onion and ginger until it gives off aroma.
3. Add the potato strings, green pepper and red pepper and quick-fry. Add seasonings to taste, and add a little vinegar before removing from heat.

Vegetarian: ✓   Muslim: ✓

Golden fried potato balls
Zha Huangjin Tudou Qiu

Ingredients:
Potato 500 g, sweet round dumpling stuffing 300 g, bread crumbs 300 g

Seasoning:
Vegetable oil 250 g

Preparation:
1. Steam potatoes, then peel and mash them.
2. Wrap sweet round dumpling stuffing to make several ping pong-size balls. Coat the balls with bread crumbs, and then deep-fry in a wok until they turn golden brown.

Note: Crisp outside and tender inside, pleasant to the taste buds.

Vegetarian: ✓   Muslim: ✓

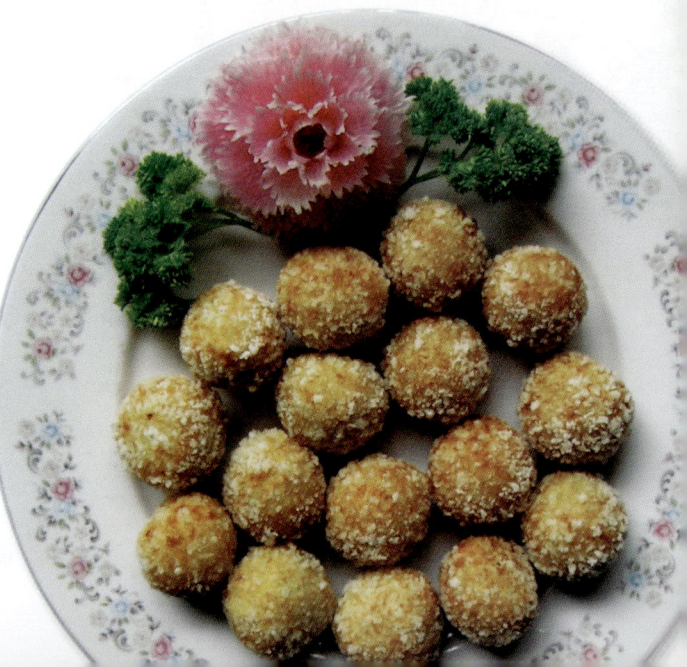

Mashed potatoes with sauce
Jiaozhi Tudou Ni

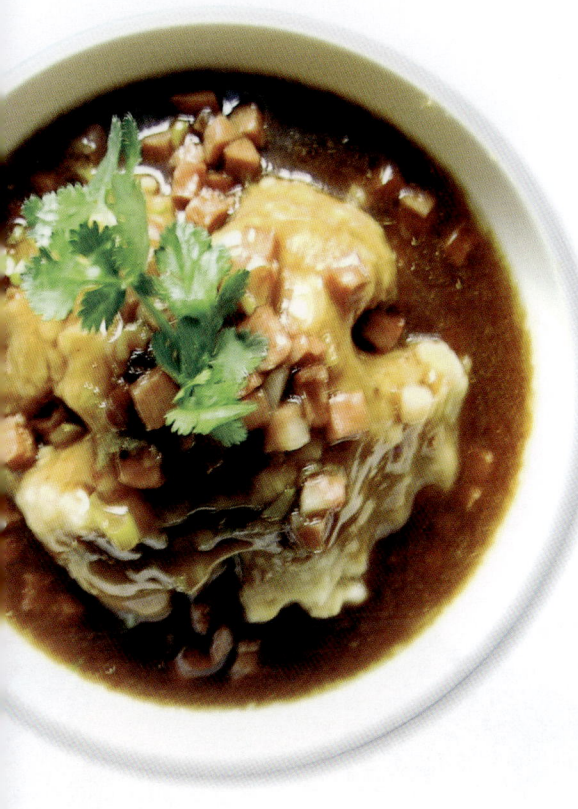

Ingredients:
Potato 600 g, ham 100 g

Seasonings:
Green onion 30 g, salt, gourmet powder and soy sauce, starch solution, to taste

Preparation:
1. Peel and mash potatoes, then mix evenly with seasonings.
2. Put a little oil in a wok and fry minced green onion to give off aroma. Add diced ham and fry, add soup stock to taste, a little salt, gourmet powder and soy sauce. Thicken the soup with starch solution and then sprinkle it on the mashed potatoes.

Vegetarian: ✗   Muslim: ✗

Mixed shredded potatoes
Ban Tudou Song

Ingredients:

Potato 400 g, salad oil 1 kg

Seasonings:

Salt and coriander to taste

Preparation:

1. Peel potatoes and shred into small strings. Heat salad oil in a pan, add potato strings and fry to golden yellow.//
2. Add coriander strips, mix evenly and season to taste.

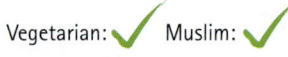

Vegetarian: ✓   Muslim: ✓

Potato and cabbage soup
Hongcai Tang

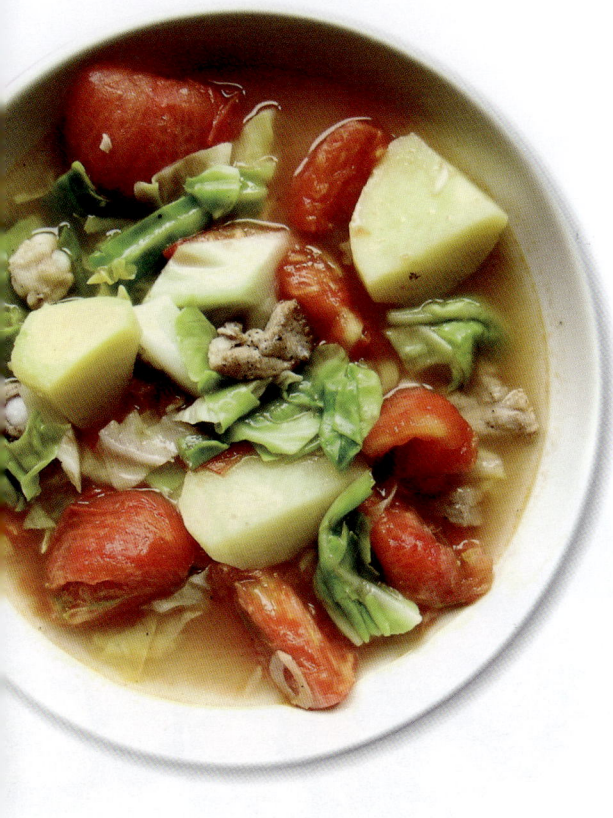

Ingredients:
Cooked beef 250 g, carrot 100 g, potato 500 g, cabbage 200 g

Seasonings:
Tomato, onion, garlic, pepper, bay leaves, cream, gourmet powder and butter to taste

Preparation:
1. Slice cooked beef, dice potatoes, cut cabbage and tomato into pieces, shred carrot and onion, mince garlic.

2. Stir-fry carrot and onion with butter, add tomato pieces, bay leaves, pepper, white sugar, white vinegar and salt, then simmer for 15 minutes.

3. Add cabbage, beef, tomato and minced garlic to stew until done. Add gourmet powder and cream, then serve.

Vegetarian: ✗   Muslim: ✓

Potato balls
Tudou Li Wanzi

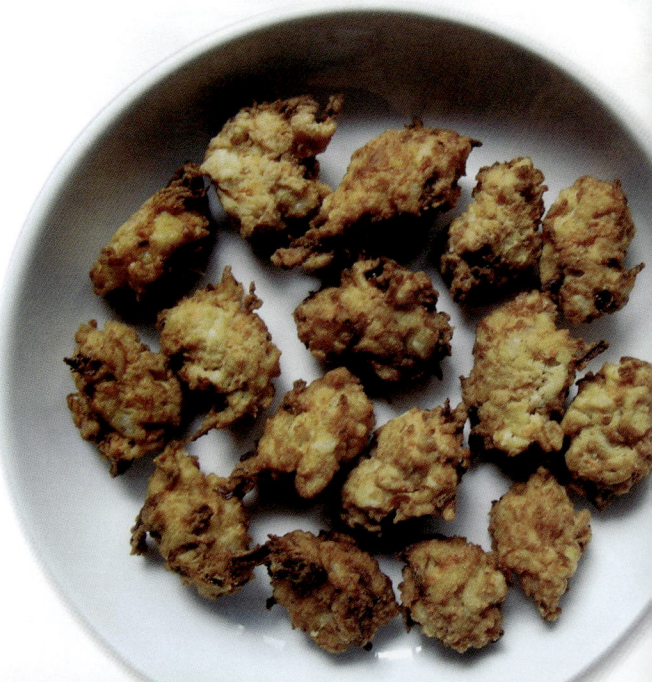

Ingredients:
Potato 200 g, carrot 100 g

Seasonings:
Refined salt 5 g, soy sauce 2 g, Shao liquor 2 g, flour 75 g, green onion and ginger 5 g, cooked lard 500 g (consumed 100 g), salt with Chinese prickly ash 2 g, gourmet powder 2 g

Preparation:
1. Shred and dice potatoes, or mash potato into pieces (not paste).
2. Add flour, salt and gourmet powder. Adjust the amount of flour you use; too much flour will make the meatball hard, too little will make it soft. Keep oil medium-hot when frying.

Vegetarian: ✗   Muslim: ✗

Potato Cake I
Tudou Bing I

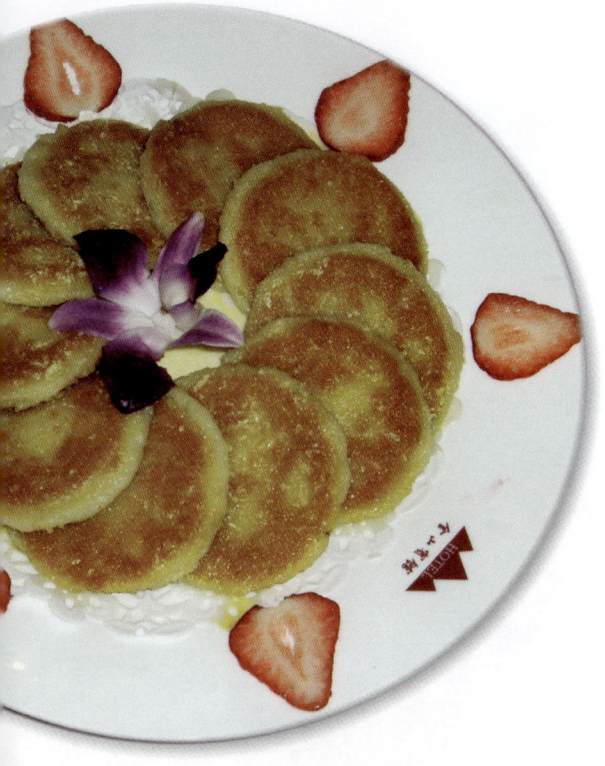

Ingredients:
Potato 400 g, glutinous rice flour 80 g

Seasonings:
Bread crumbs and egg to taste

Preparation:
1. Peel potatoes and put on steamer tray to steam well.

2. Mash potatoes and mix well with glutinous rice flour to make a cake, coat with egg and bread crumbs and fry.

Vegetarian: ✗   Muslim: ✓

Potato salad with green vegetables
Qingcai Tudou Shala

Ingredients:
Potato 100 g, tomato 25 g, lettuce 10 g, cauliflower 25 g, carrot 25 g, cucumber 50 g, peas 10 g, egg 2

Seasonings:
Salad dressing, tri-flavored juice, white sugar, salt, gourmet powder and cream

Preparation:
1. Peel cooked potatoes and carrots and slice into small, thick pieces. Stew cauliflower and peas well and slice them into small pieces. Slice cooked eggs into large piece; slice lettuce, tomato and cucumber into small pieces.
2. Add seasonings, mix evenly and serve.

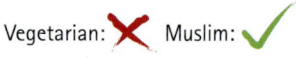

Vegetarian: ✗   Muslim: ✓

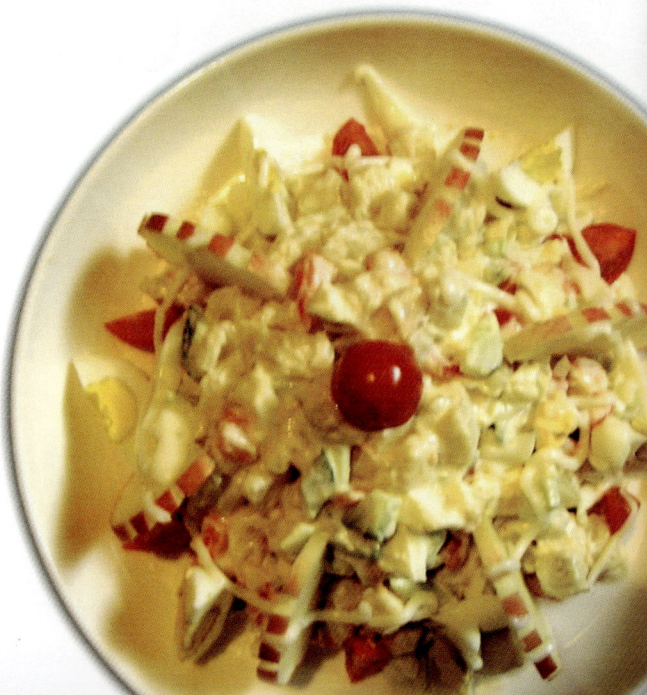

Seasoned potato strings and noodles
Qiang Tudou Si, Fensi

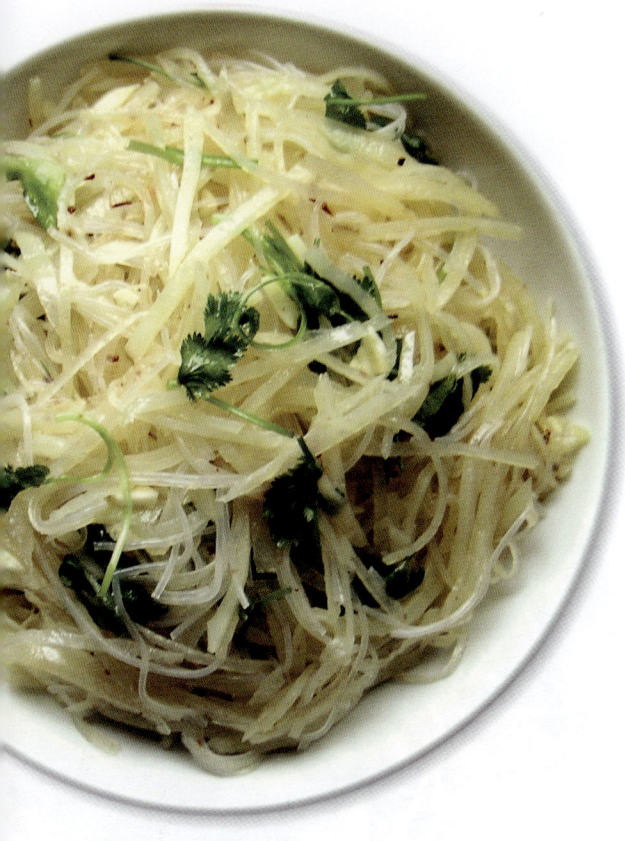

Ingredients:
Potato 300 g, potato noodles 100 g

Seasonings:
Onion, ginger, garlic, coriander, to taste

Preparation:
1. Cut potatoes into strings; quick-boil potato noodles, potato strings. Shred green onion, ginger and garlic, and place all in a dish.
2. Add Chinese prickly ash oil, chili oil, sesame oil, salt, gourmet powder, mix evenly and serve.

Vegetarian: ✓   Muslim: ✓

Shredded potato and bean salad
San Si Bao Dou

Ingredients:
Potato 350 g, green onion 100 g, coriander 50 g, fried peanut 100 g

Seasonings:
Salt and gourmet powder to taste

Preparation:
1. Peel and shred potatoes, then fry well. Shred green onion and cut coriander into sections. Put them together with the fried peanut in a dish.
2. Add salt and gourmet powder, mix them evenly.

Vegetarian: ✓   Muslim: ✓

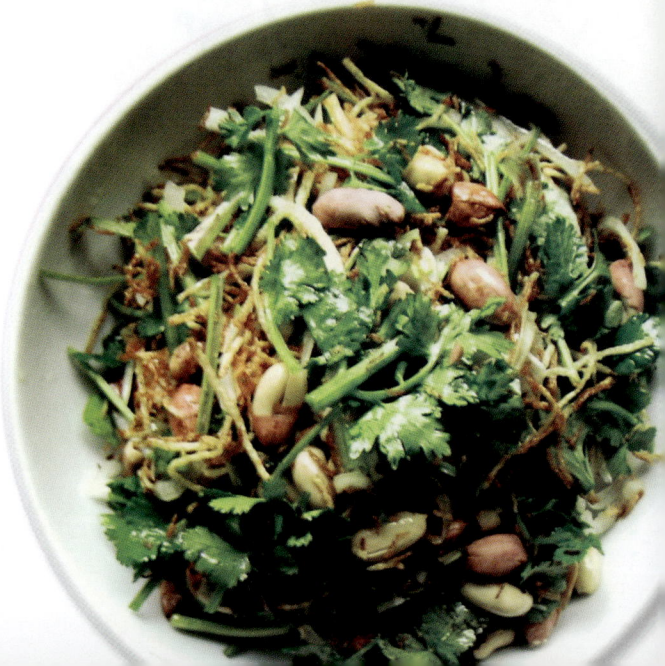

Steamed potato and eggplant served with soy sauce
Nongjia Dajiang Zheng Tudou Qiezi

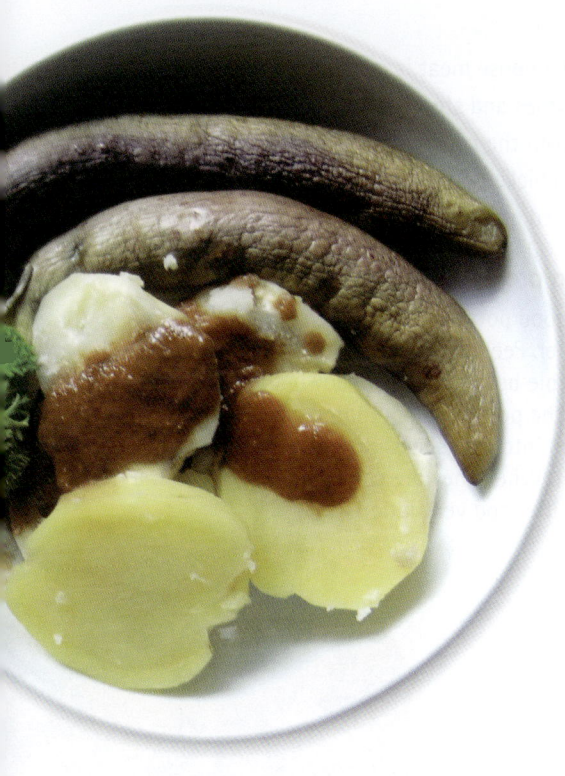

Ingredients:
Potato 400 g, eggplant 300 g, soy sauce 50 g

Preparation:
1. Peel potatoes, cut into cubes and steam.
2. Steam eggplant.
3. Use soy sauce for dipping when served.

Vegetarian: ✓   Muslim: ✓

Stewed potato chips with goose
Tudou Gan Dun Da E

Ingredients:
Goose 500 g, dried potatoes

Seasonings:
Garlic, salt, onion, chicken essence, soup stock, cooking oil, Chinese prickly ash, aniseed, soy sauce

Preparation:
1. Slice garlic, clean the dried potatoes, clean goose and chop it into pieces (can be large or small pieces, as preferred).

2. Put the cleaned goose pieces into boiling water and quick-boil. Take out and set aside.

3. Heat oil in wok and fry ginger, Chinese prickly ash and onion until they give off aroma, then add goose pieces and fry. Add yellow wine, soy sauce and sugar in turn (more sugar is better). Boil first, then turn to medium heat to stew for 30 minutes. Ensure there is sufficient cooking liquor in the wok; do not let it dry out.

4. When goose meat is medium-cooked, add potatoes and stew for 10–20 more minutes. Thicken the cooking liquor on high heat, add salt and chicken essence to taste, and sprinkle with minced green onion.

How to prepare dried potato chips:
Select good potatoes, clean them, then steam in a steamer. Peel cooked potatoes by hand as soon as possible before they cool down, then set aside, letting the potatoes cool thoroughly. Slice cooled potatoes into thin slices; dry the potato slices in sunlight. When they are completely dry, store in a place with good ventilation.

Vegetarian: ✗   Muslim: ✗

Stewed potatoes with cowpeas
Tudou dun Doujiao

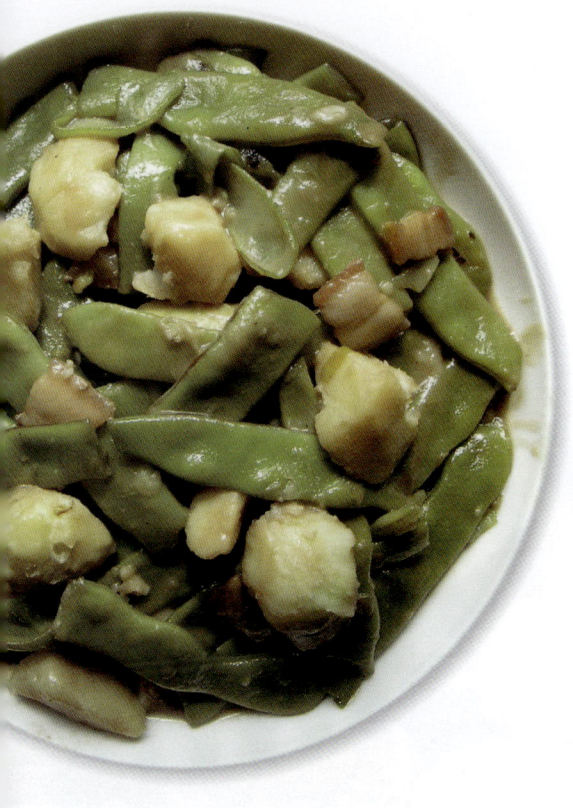

Ingredients:
Potato 300 g, cowpeas 200 g, pork 25 g

Seasonings:
Green onion 20 g, salt to taste, a little soy sauce

Preparation:
1. Peel potatoes and dice into irregular pieces. Clean cowpeas and cut them into sections.

2. Heat oil in wok, fry pork and minced green onion together until it gives off aroma. Add cowpeas and stir-fry until their color changes to dark green.

3. Add potatoes and continue to stir-fry, add a little light soy sauce, fry to give off aroma. Add some water and cover the pot to simmer until the potatoes and cowpeas are well cooked. Wait until the cooking liquor is almost dry, put in salt and gourmet powder, then serve.

Vegetarian: ✗ Muslim: ✗

Stewed potatoes with curry chicken
Tudou Dun Gali Ji Kuai

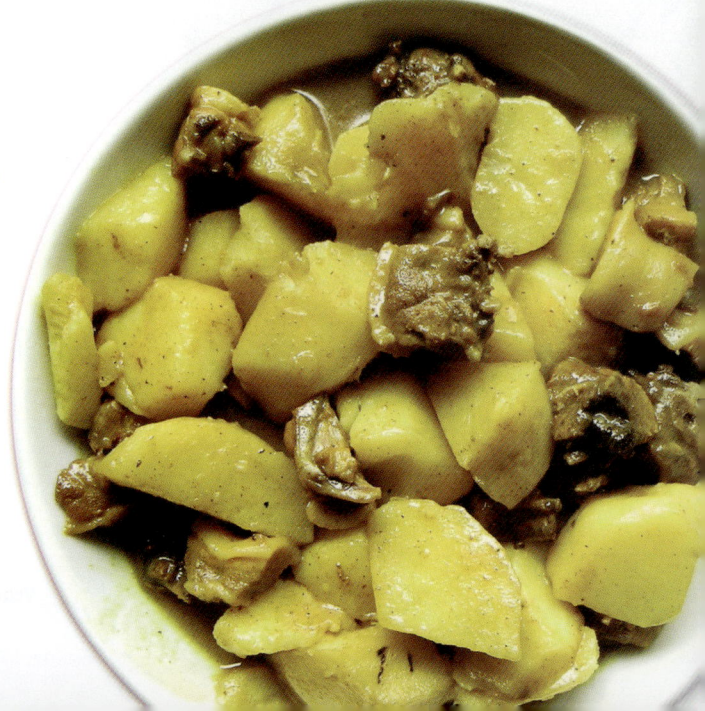

Ingredients:

Chicken 300 g, potato 400 g

Seasoning:

Curry to taste

Preparation:

1. Dice chicken and stew with curry until almost cooked.
2. Add diced potatoes and stew together, add seasonings, then remove.

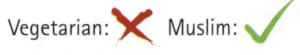

Stewed potatoes with eggplant in thick sauce
Tudou Jiang Dun Qiezi

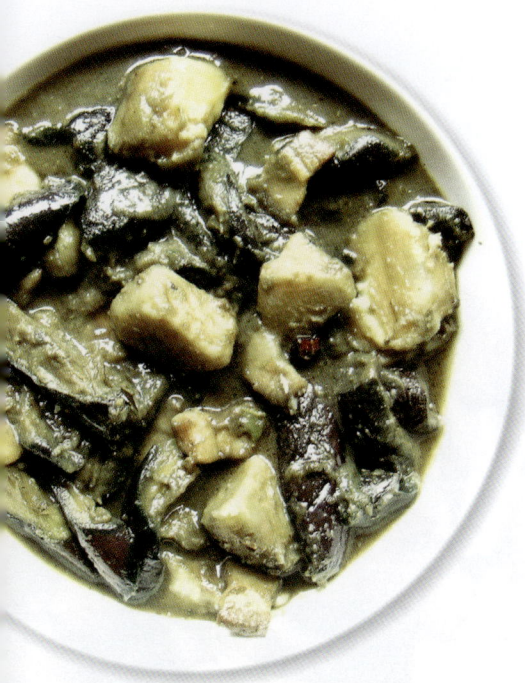

Seasonings:

Thick sauce, ginger, garlic piece, aniseed, soy sauce, salt and chicken essence, to taste

Preparation:

1. Peel potatoes and scoop into suitable pieces with a teaspoon; rinse and set aside. Clean eggplant and break into pieces by hand (it tastes better than when it's cut with a knife).

2. Heat oil in wok, and then fry ginger, garlic and aniseed to give off aroma. Add potatoes and stir-fry, then add thick sauce (special sauce in northeast China) to fry for a moment. Add one teaspoon of soy sauce and soup ingredients, then cook on high heat until it boils. Change to medium heat to stew slowly until medium-done, add salt to taste, change to low heat, and stew until potatoes can be easily poked with chopsticks. Add chicken essence and stir-fry for a few seconds, then remove.

Vegetarian: ✘   Muslim: ✓

Ingredients:

Potato 500 g, eggplant 250 g

Stewed potatoes with yellow sturgeon
Xunhuangyu Men Tudou

Ingredients:
Yellow sturgeon 400 g (Shi's yellow sturgeon, a fish variety in Heilongjiang and the Wusuli River), potato 300 g

Seasonings:
Green onion, ginger, garlic, cooking wine, soy sauce, gourmet powder and salt to taste

Preparation:
1. Chop yellow sturgeon into sections, roll potatoes when dicing.
2. Put a little oil in a wok and fry green onion, ginger and garlic until they give off aroma, then add yellow sturgeon and stir-fry. Then fry with cooking wine and soy sauce before adding soup stock, potatoes and salt to stew well. Add gourmet powder before serving.

Vegetarian: ✗   Muslim: ✗

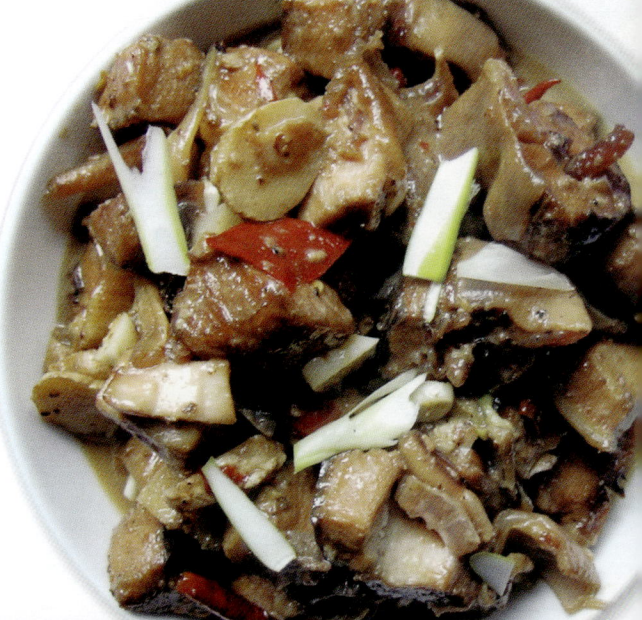

Stewed small potatoes I
Youmen Xiao Tudou I

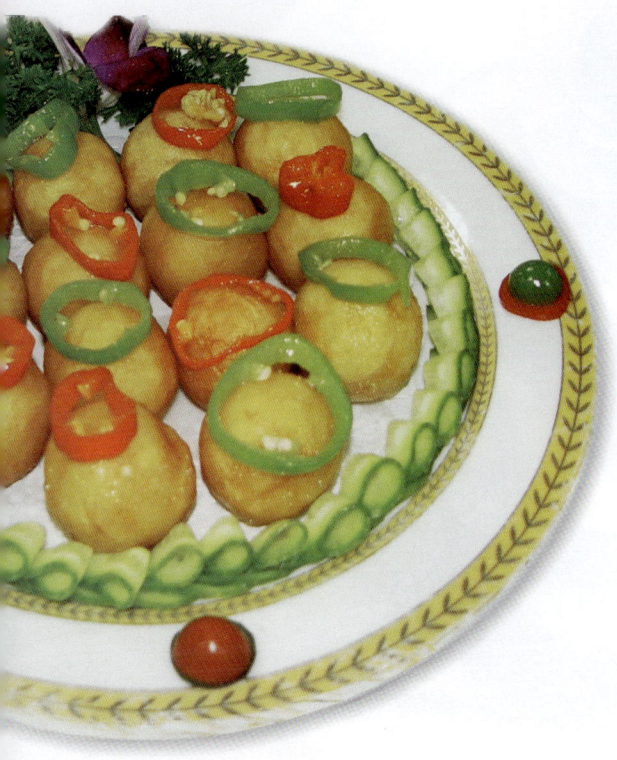

Ingredients:
Potato 1,000 g, a little green pepper, red pepper and green onion

Seasonings:
Soup stock, green onion 5 g, salt 1 g

Preparation:
1. Peel potatoes. Put soup stock in the pressure cooker and simmer potatoes in it for 7 minutes, remove.

2. And then Fry the potatoes in a wok.

Vegetarian: ✘   Muslim: ✘

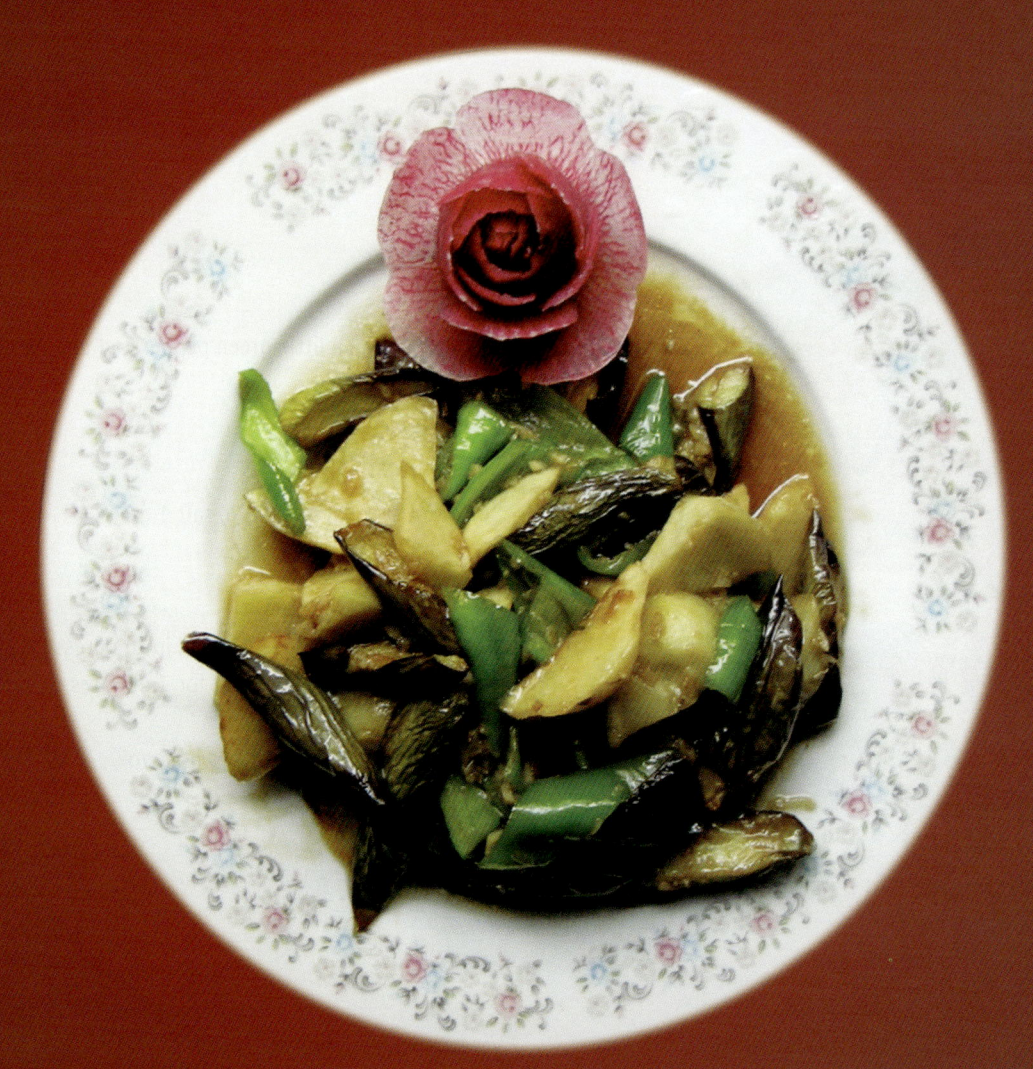

Stir-fried potato, green pepper and eggplant
Di Sanxian

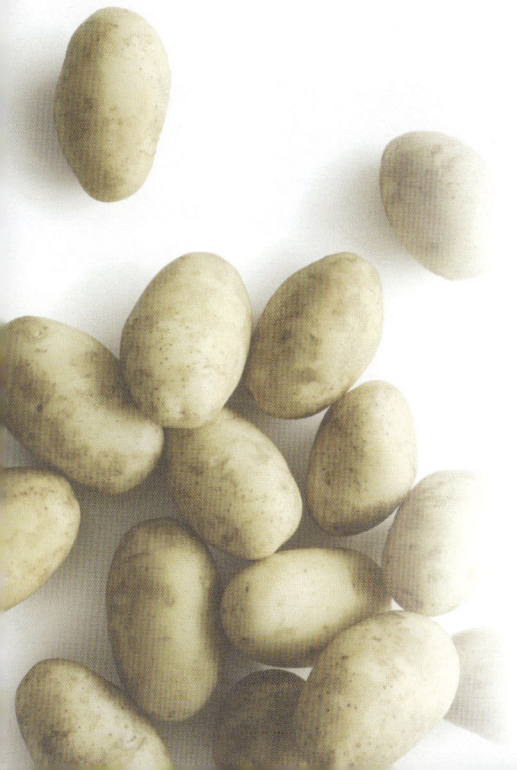

Ingredients:
Potato 300 g, eggplant 300 g, green bell pepper 100 g

Seasonings:
Green onion, ginger, garlic to taste

Preparation:
1. Dice potatoes and the peeled eggplants into irregular pieces and deep-fry. Slice the green bell pepper.

2. Heat the oil, fry the green onion, ginger and garlic until they give off aroma. Add some water to taste, then put salt, gourmet powder, soy sauce, and a little white sugar.

3. Fry the deep-fried potatoes and eggplants together with the green peppers, adding starch to thicken soup, and put a little Chinese prickly ash oil.

Vegetarian: ✓   Muslim: ✓

Potato Recipes from North China

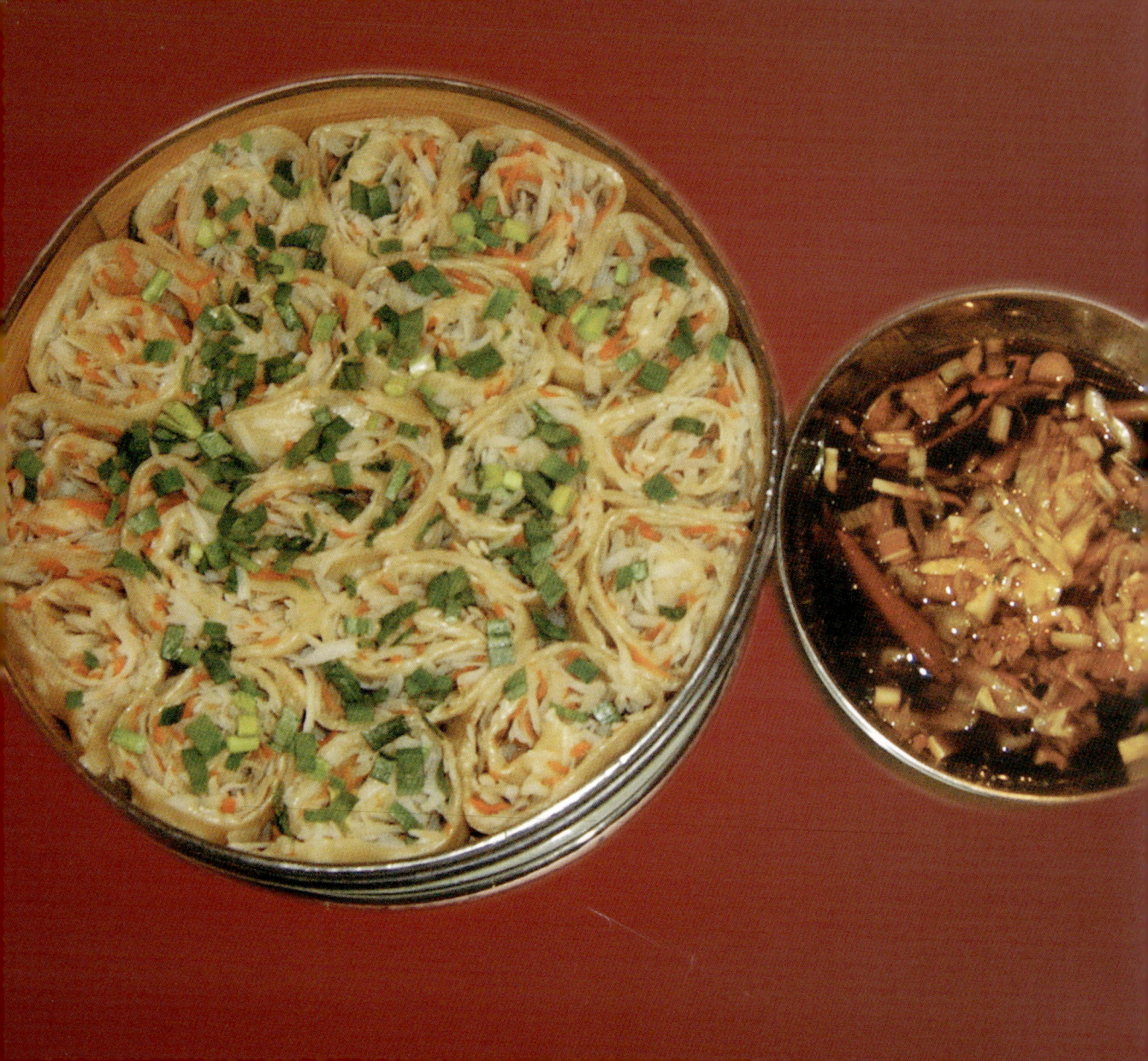

Bag-shaped oat potato pie
Malingshu Tuntun

Ingredients:
Potato 500 g, oat flour 300 g

Seasonings:
Refined salt 3 g, minced green onion 10 g, minced garlic 10 g, pickled vegetable 50 g, mung bean sprouts 10 g, spinach 20 g, carrot 10 g, soy sauce 5 g, vinegar 5 g, gourmet powder 1 g, sesame oil 10 g

Preparation:
1. Shred carrot, put the spinach sections and mung bean sprouts into boiling water to stew for a moment, then remove. Mix with refined salt, minced green onion, minced garlic, sliced pickled vegetables, sliced carrot, soy sauce, vinegar, gourmet powder, sesame oil and some water to make thick sauce.

2. Knead the oat flour dough and roll with a rolling pin until 0.5 cm thick. Sprinkle the dough with sliced potatoes, roll up and cut into sections, steam in a steamer, then served with thick sauce.

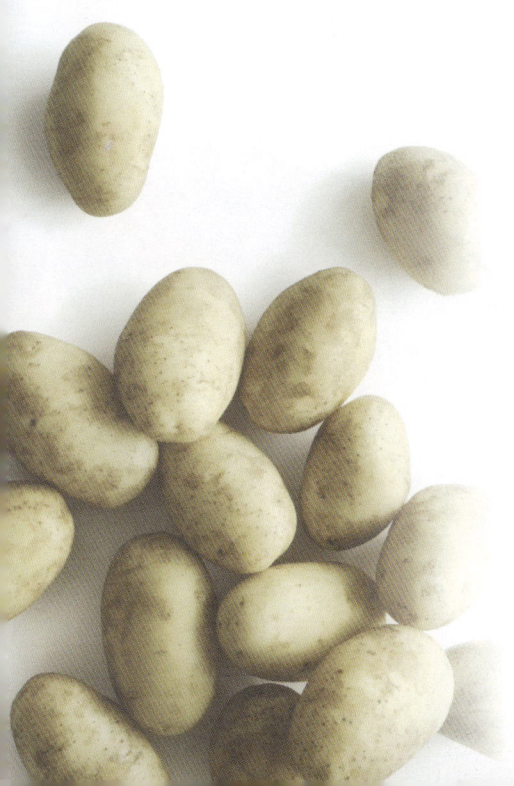

Vegetarian: ✓   Muslim: ✓

Baked potato cake
Lao Malinghshu Yangzi

Ingredients:
Potato 400 g, oat flour 250 g, linseed oil 50 g

Seasonings:
Refined salt 3 g, Chinese prickly ash 3 g, green onion 10 g, gourmet powder 1 g

Preparation:
1. Peel and mash cooked potatoes and put in a basin.
2. Add refined salt, Chinese prickly ash, minced green onion and gourmet powder to make potato dough. Roll to make several cake-like circles.
3. Heat a frying pan, add linseed oil, and fry both sides of the potato cake until golden brown.

Vegetarian: ✓   Muslim: ✓

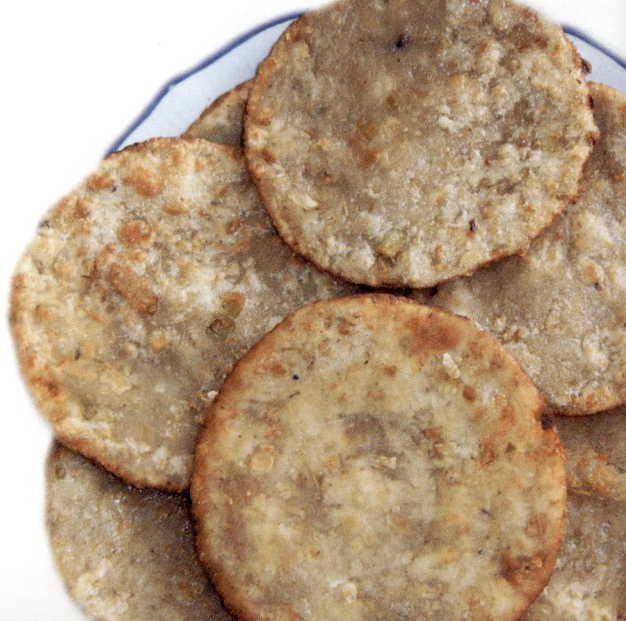

Black soy sauce potatoes
Jiangyou Malingshu Tiao

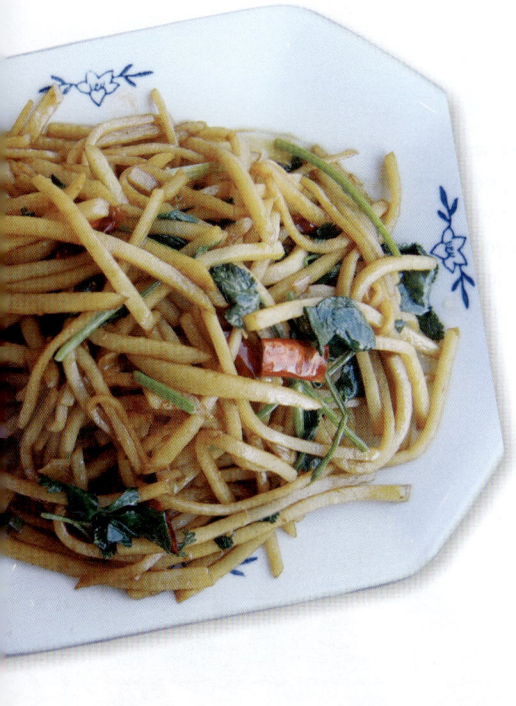

Ingredient:
Potato 300 g

Seasonings:
Celery leaf 20 g, a little red pepper 5 g, black soy sauce 5 g, table salt 5 g, chicken essence 3 g, Chinese prickly ash 3 g, green onion 5 g, garlic 5 g, fresh ginger 5 g, vegetable 20 g

Preparation:
1. Clean the potatoes and cut them into strips. Heat the oil in frying pan over high heat, add the Chinese prickly ash and fry it until it smokes, then discard it. Add red pepper, green onion, garlic and ginger and stir-fry.
2. Add the potato strips and black soy sauce, add some water and stir-fry them until cooked. Add the celery leaf and stir-fry a little bit, then add some chicken essence and table salt before serving.

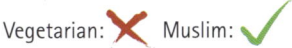

Vegetarian: ✗   Muslim: ✓

Braised beef with potato
Malingshu Shao Niurou

Ingredients:
Beef 300 g, potato 300 g

Seasonings:
Linseed oil 200 g, scallion 10 g, ginger 15 g, garlic 10 g, light soy sauce 10 g, white sugar 5 g, Chinese prickly ash 3 g, star anise 5 g, salt 10 g, chicken essence 5 g, cooking wine 5 g

Preparation:
1. Peel potatoes and chop them into pieces, then put into a wok and fry to golden brown; remove and drain off. Dice the beef and scald in boiling water. Remove and drain well. Slice the ginger and garlic; cut scallion into sections.
2. Heat oil in a wok and fry the scallion, ginger and garlic. Stir-fry the beef thoroughly with soy sauce, sugar and cooking wine.
3. Add some water and put the gauze-wrapped Chinese prickly ash and star anise into the wok. After 1 hour of soft spirit stewing, add the fried potatoes, salt and gourmet powder and continue stewing until cooking liquor dries up. Remove to a dish, sprinkle with sliced scallion, and serve.

Vegetarian: ✗   Muslim: ✗

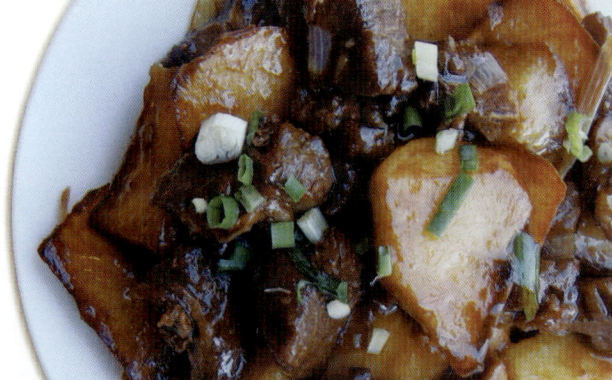

Braised Potato Pieces
Hongshao Shukuai

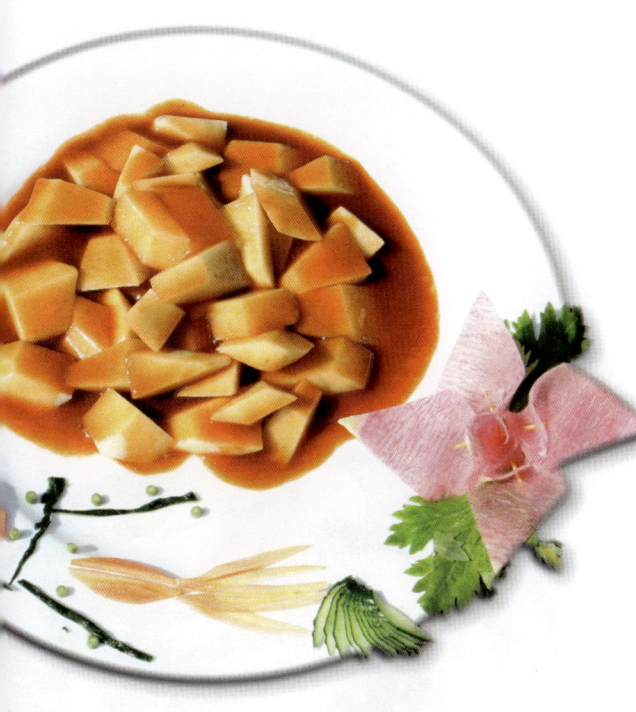

Ingredient:
Potato 500g

Seasonings:
Cooking wine, salt, gourmet powder, a little sugar

Preparation:
Cut potato into pieces and heat oil in a wok. Fry the potato pieces well and remove. Put them into the wok again to braise with the seasonings.

Vegetarian: ✓   Muslim: ✗

Braised potato, cabbage and tofu
Malingshu Baicai Tofu

Ingredients:
Potato 300 g, pakchoi 100 g, tofu 300 g, tomato 150 g, soup stock 200 g

Seasonings:
Gourmet powder 5 g, sesame oil 5 g, salt 5 g

Preparation:
1. Peel potatoes and cut them into strips. Clean the pakchoi and cut into pieces. Cut tofu into strips and dice the tomatoes.
2. Mix the potato strips, pakchoi, tofu and tomato into soup stock over low heat.
3. About 10 minutes later, add gourmet powder, sesame oil and salt, then serve.

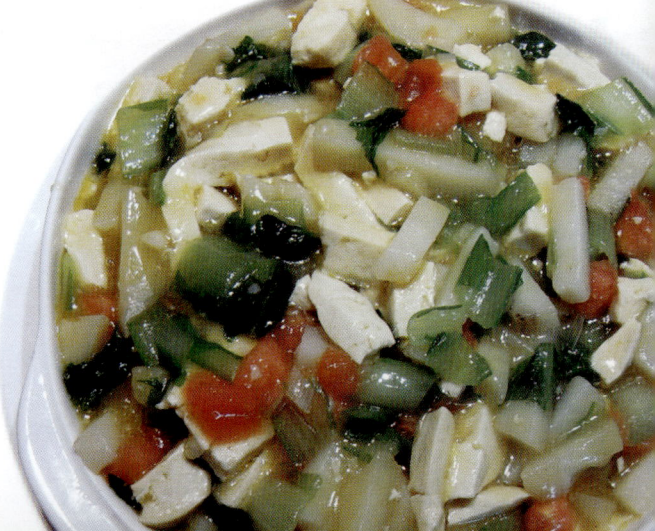

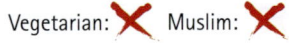

Vegetarian: ✗   Muslim: ✗

Braised potatoes
Malingshu Dahuicai

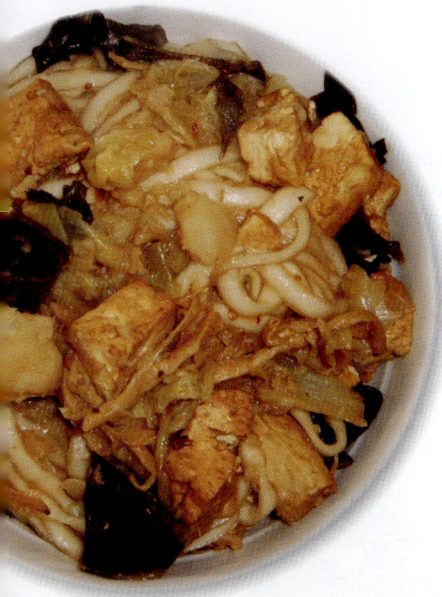

Preparation:

1. Clean the potatoes and peel and dice them. Put pieces into water to remove starch, then drain.

2. Dice the tofu and heat the oil in a frying pan. Deep-fry the tofu pieces to a golden brown, then remove. Put the day lily and kelp into warm water, then remove and cut into pieces. Cut the cabbage into small pieces.

3. Put oil in frying pan and heat, then add potato pieces and stir-fry. Add pork broth to frying pan, and add noodles, kelp, tofu, day lily, cabbage and fungus. Then add some water into frying pan, along with green onion, ginger and garlic. Mix broad bean paste and table salt, and boil for five minutes, then remove and season with chicken essence.

Ingredients:

Potato 200 g, cabbage 150 g, kelp 150 g, raised edible fungus 50 g, fresh potato noodles 100 g, tofu 100 g, day lily 50 g, vegetable oil 200 g

Seasonings:

Green onion 10 g, ginger 5 g, garlic 5 g, salt 5 g, chicken essence 3 g, broad bean paste, pork broth

Vegetarian: ✗   Muslim: ✗

Braised potatoes and cabbage
Malingshu Baicai Hui Fenkuai

Ingredients:
Potato 300 g, pakchoi 150 g, potato starch 500 g, alum 3 g, water 1500 g

Seasonings:
Red pepper 5 g, cooking wine 10 g, salt 5 g, gourmet powder 3 g, soy sauce 10 g, Chinese prickly ash 3 g, green onion 10 g, ginger 5 g, lard 50 g

Preparation:
1. Make some bean jelly with potato starch.
2. Clean and peel potatoes and cut them into chips. Put the chips into water in order to remove starch. Clean the pakchoi and cut into pieces. Heat the oil in a frying pan over high heat and add the Chinese prickly ash. Fry until it smokes, then discard the fried prickly ash.
3. Lightly fry the red pepper, green onion, ginger and garlic. Mix the cooking wine and soy sauce, add the pakchoi and potato chips and stir-fry. Add some water and bring to a boil. While the water is boiling, add bean jelly. Boil the soup for about 3 minutes. Mix table salt and gourmet powder, then serve.

Vegetarian: ✘   Muslim: ✘

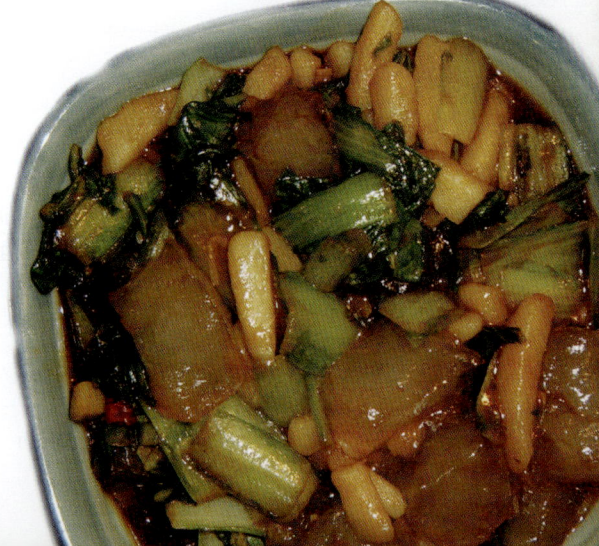

Braised potatoes and tofu with spareribs
Malingshu tofu Dun Paigu

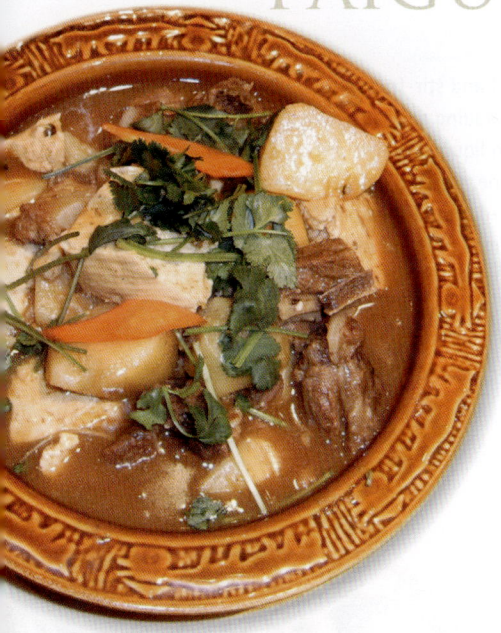

Seasonings:
Cilantro 5 g, carrot 5 g, scallion 20 g, ginger 15 g, garlic 10 g, Chinese prickly ash 3 g, star anise 5 g, salt 10 g, gourmet powder 2 g, cooking wine 5 g

Preparation:
1. Chop spareribs into 5 cm sections; peel potatoes and chop them into pieces; chop tofu into pieces; cut ginger, garlic, carrots and scallion into small pieces.

2. Put water into wok. After it boils, drop in spareribs to clean. Empty the wok and add oil. Fry the scallion, ginger, garlic for flavor, then stir-fry with the spareribs.

3. Add the cooking liquor, Chinese prickly ash, star anise, cooking wine, salt and gourmet powder and braise the spareribs. When cooked to medium-done, add the potatoes and tofu and cook 10 minutes. Remove into a soup wok, dressing it with carrot pieces and cilantro and serve.

Ingredients:
Potato 200 g, tofu 200 g, pig spareribs 200 g, lard (refined) 30 g

Vegetarian: ✗   Muslim: ✗

Braised potatoes with cowpeas and spareribs
Malingshu Doujiao Dun Paigu

Ingredients:
Potato 300 g, cowpea 150 g, spareribs 300 g

Seasonings:
lard (refined) 30 g, scallion 20 g, ginger 15 g, garlic 10 g, soy sauce 10 g, vinegar 5 g, Chinese prickly ash 3 g, star anise 5 g, salt 10 g, chicken essence 5 g, cooking wine 5 g

Preparation:
1. Chop the spareribs into 5 cm-long sections; peel potatoes and chop them into pieces; cut cowpeas into 5 cm-long sections; slice ginger and garlic; and cut scallion into sections.

2. Boil water in a wok, then add the spareribs. Remove the spareribs and rinse the froth from the wok.

3. Heat the oil and stir-fry the spareribs. Fry a little bit more after adding soy sauce and vinegar. Then add the cooking liquor, Chinese prickly ash, star anise, cooking wine, salt and chicken essence. Once cooked to medium-done, add the potatoes and cowpeas. Cook with medium heat until ready.

Vegetarian: ✗ Muslim: ✗

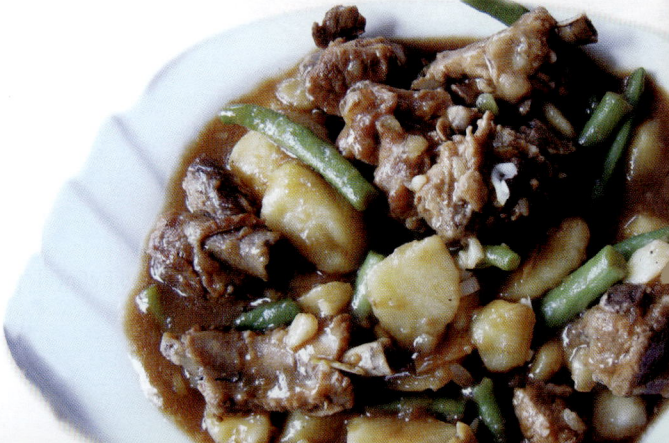

Braised potatoes with fish-shaped oat noodles
Malingshu Hui Youmian Yu

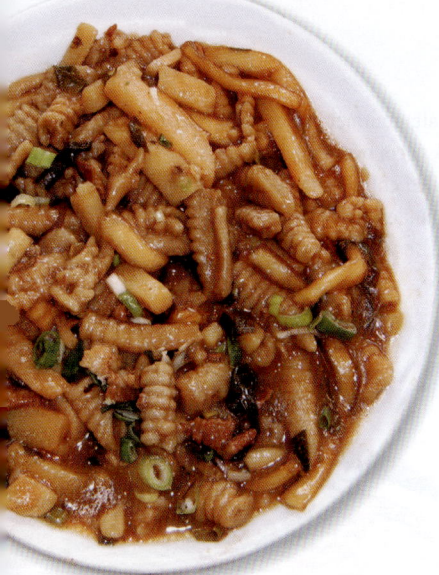

Preparation:

1. Mix oat flour with warm water to make dough, and cut into fish-shaped pieces using a special knife. Steam the pieces for 10 minutes and set aside. Peel and dice potatoes and slice the cleaned side pork (with skin) into thin pieces.

2. Mince the green onion and ginger and slice the garlic. Heat oil in wok and add Chinese prickly ash to fry until it gives off smoke, then remove. Stir-fry the side pork, adding green onion, ginger and garlic until they give off aroma. Then add soy sauce, vinegar and cooking wine to stir-fry for a moment. Add the potato pieces, Chinese toon leaf and water, and boil over high heat. Change to low heat to stew well, adding fish-shaped oat noodles, with salt and gourmet powder, to stir-fry evenly. Remove and sprinkle with minced green onion, then serve.

Ingredients:

Potato 300 g, side pork (with skin) 150 g, oat flour 300 g, lard (refined) 30 g

Seasonings:

Chinese toon leaf 10 g, green onion 10 g, ginger 5 g, garlic 5 g, Chinese prickly ash 3 g, salt 5 g, gourmet powder 2 g, soy sauce 5 g, vinegar 5 g, cooking wine 5 g

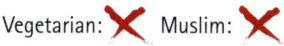

Braised Sheep Entrails with Noodles
Guozai Fentiao Yangza

Ingredients:
Potato starch 500 g, alum 3 g, cooked lamb tripe 150 g, cooked sheep lung 150 g, cooked sheep liver 100 g, cooked sheep face 100 g, cooked sheep intestines 100 g

Seasonings:
Salt 3 g, gourmet powder 5 g, chicken essence 5 g, chaffy dish flavoring 50 g, vegetable oil 50 g, dry paprika 5 g, fermented black beans 20 g, green onion 5 g, ginger 5 g, soup stock from sheep bones 500 g

Preparation:
1. Make potato starch into some fresh noodles.
2. Cut sheep tripe, lung, liver, face and intestines into pieces about 0.3 cm thick. Put some oil into a pot and heat, then add dry paprika, green onion, ginger, fermented soybeans, and chaffy dish flavoring and stir-fry them over high heat. While the aroma is coming out, add the sheep tripe, lung, liver, face and intestines and stir-fry for two more minutes.
3. Mix soup stock, salt, gourmet powder and chicken essence, and cook them over high heat, bringing to a boil. Place the boiled entrails into a wok and served the dish with fire under the wok, adding the fresh noodles when it is served.

Vegetarian: ✗   Muslim: ✓

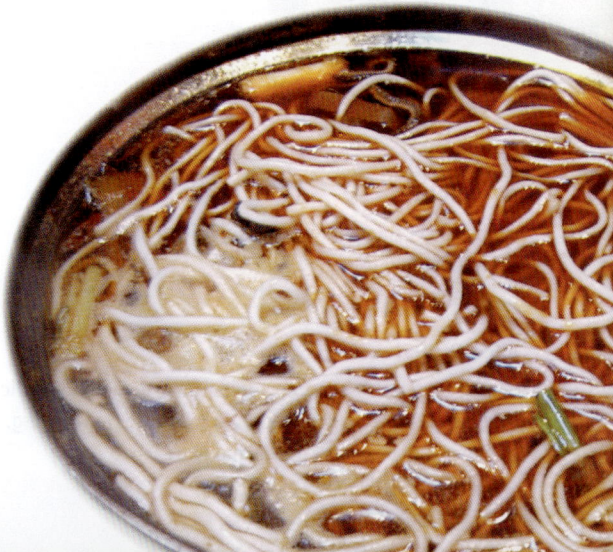

Braised side pork and rape with potatoes

Wuhuarou Youcai Hui Malingshu

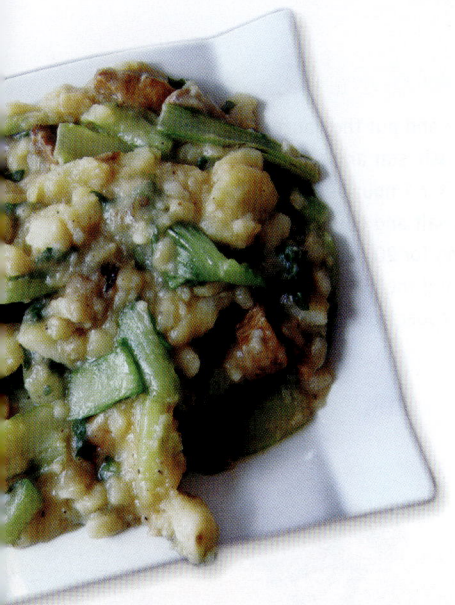

Seasonings:

Onion 10 g, ginger 5 g, garlic 5 g, Chinese prickly ash 3 g, salt 5 g, gourmet powder 2 g, soy sauce 5 g, vinegar 5 g, cooking wine 5 g

Preparation:

1. Peel potatoes and cut them into pieces; clean the side pork and slice; cut the cleaned rape into sections; mince onion, ginger and garlic.

2. Heat oil and fry Chinese prickly ash until it smokes, then discard. Stir-fry side pork, then add onion, ginger and garlic and stir-fry until they give off aroma. Add soy sauce, vinegar and cooking wine and fry for a moment, then add potato pieces, rape and water and stew over high heat until it boils. Reduce to low heat and stew well, adding salt and gourmet powder.

Ingredients:

Potato 300 g, side pork 150 g, rape 150 g, lard (refined) 30 g

Vegetarian: ✗   Muslim: ✗

Braised sirloin with potatoes
Malingshu Dun Niunan

Ingredients:
Sirloin 300 g, potato 300 g, green pepper 25 g, red pepper 25 g

Seasonings:
Scallion 10 g, ginger 10 g, garlic 10 g, Chinese prickly ash 3 g, soy sauce 5 g, white sugar 5 g, star anise 5 g, dried orange peel 5 g, salt 10 g, gourmet powder 2 g, cooking wine 5 g

Preparation:
1. Dice sirloin and put into boiling water to scald; peel potato and chop into pieces.
2. Heat oil in a wok and fry the scallion, ginger and garlic for flavor, then add sauce and sugar to stir-fry with spareribs.
3. Add some water and put the gauze- wrapped Chinese prickly ash, star anise and dried orange peel into the wok. After 1 hour of soft spirit stewing, add the potato, salt and gourmet powder and continue stewing for 20 minutes. Braise until cooking liquor dries up and the meat is cooked. Then add green and red pepper, cook for a while, and serve.

Vegetarian: ✗   Muslim: ✗

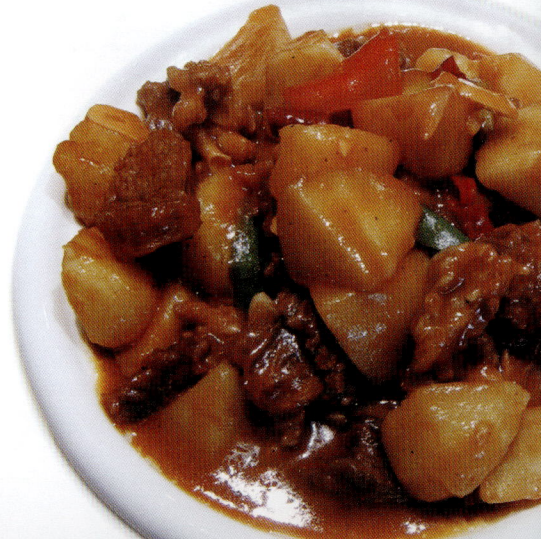

Braised small potato balls with oxtail
Xiao Tudou Shao Niuwei

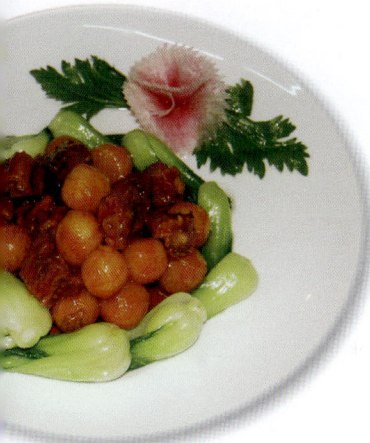

Ingredients:
Potato 500 g, oxtail

Seasonings:
Salad oil 1,100 g, oyster oil 15 g, green onion 30 g, fresh ginger piece 15 g, garlic cloves 10 g, cooking wines, light soy sauce 30 g, dark soy sauce 30 g, salt 30 g, a little chicken essence, a little white sugar

Preparation:
1. Clean oxtail, chop into 3 cm sections and blanch. Put the oxtail and potatoes in water with a little salt and bring to a boil; remove and put them on a plate.
2. Heat salad oil in a wok over low heat, then add 5 cm green onion sections, fresh ginger piece and garlic cloves and stir-fry. Add the oxtail to stir-fry for two minutes, then add cooking wine, light soy sauce and dark soy sauce.
3. Add 500 g water in the wok, wait for it to boil, and then add salt. Stew over low heat for 30 minutes until almost cooked, then add a little chicken essence and white sugar. Remove the oxtail and set aside. Remove all the seasonings, keeping only the soup.
4. Peel potatoes and make potatoes into small balls with a 2 cm diameter, then quick-boil in water.
5. Heat 1,000 g of salad oil over medium heat, and deep-fry the potato balls until golden yellow, then remove and set aside.
6. Heat 25 g of salad oil in wok and add a little minced green onion and oyster oil to fry, then add the oxtail soup, cooked oxtail and fried small potatoes. After it boils, stew for 2 more minutes and thicken soup with starch.
7. Heat 5 g of salad oil and add salt and chicken essence. Then add quick-boiled rape, stir-fry, thicken soup, and remove.
8. Serve cooked small potatoes and oxtail on a plate with fried oilseed rape.

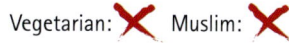

Vegetarian: ✗   Muslim: ✗

Camel palm encircled with shredded potato
Tuozhang Tudou Si

Ingredients:
Potato 100 g, camel palm 300 g

Seasonings:
White sugar 100 g

Preparation:
1. Cook camel palm well.
2. Cut potatoes into strips and deep-fry. Then add the fried white sugar. Place potato on a plate, encircling the cooked camel palm and serve.

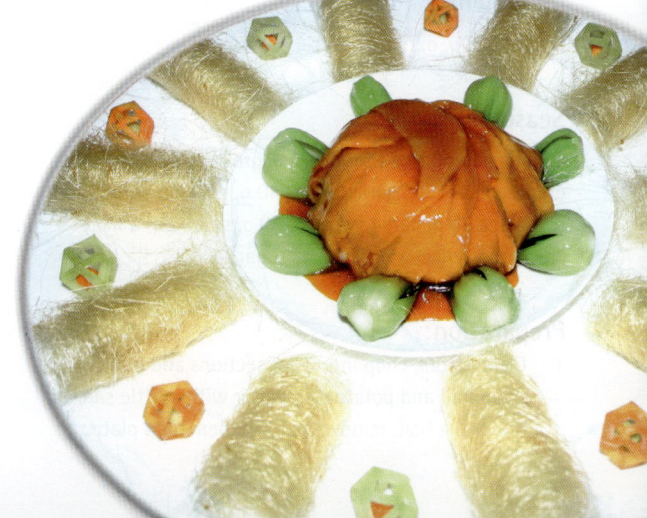

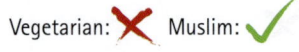

Chinese chess fun
QI QU

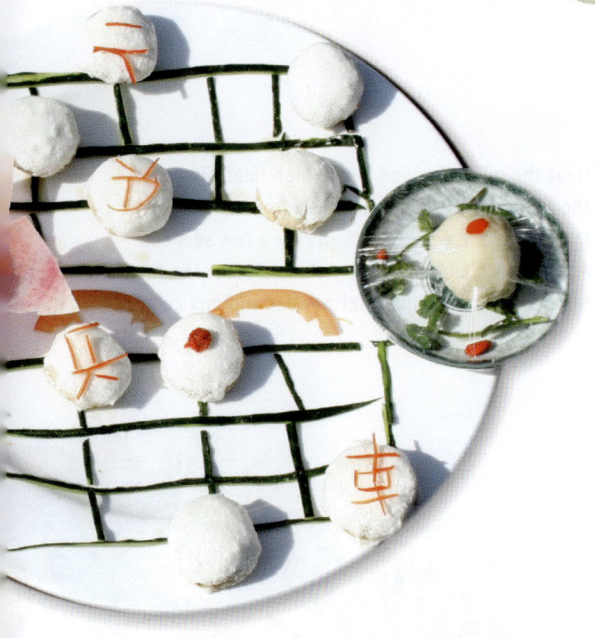

Ingredient:
Mashed potatoes 400 g

Seasonings:
Whisked egg, salt, minced meat, minced green onion and ginger, gourmet powder to taste

Preparation:
Season the mashed potatoes, then add wheat flour and form into the shape of chess pieces. Smear pieces with whisked egg, steam for 2 minutes, remove and place on the "chess board" in a dish. Use carrot strings to make the Chinese chess characters on the chess men.

Vegetarian: ✗   Muslim: ✗

Cold potato strings in oil, vinegar and spices
Liangban Malingshu Si

Ingredients:
Potato 300 g, cucumber 50 g, mung bean sprouts 50 g, soybean sprout 50 g

Seasonings:
Leek 30 g, Chinese prickly ash 3 g, vegetable oil 20 g, sesame oil 5 g, table salt 5 g, vinegar 10 g, gourmet powder 3 g

Preparation:
1. Peel potatoes and chop them into strings, then put the potato strings in clean water to wash off the starch. Blanch the potato strings, soybean sprouts and mung bean sprouts in boiling water, cool them down after removing from water.
2. Slice the cleaned cucumber and leek. Lay out potato strings, soybean sprouts, mung bean sprout and cucumber on plate.
3. Heat the oil in the wok over a high heat. Then fry the Chinese prickly ash and discard when black. Put the leek in the wok and stir-fry for a few seconds. Add the leek and oil to the dish, add some sesame oil, table salt, vinegar, gourmet powder and mix evenly.

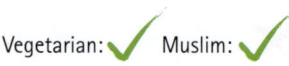
Vegetarian: ✓   Muslim: ✓

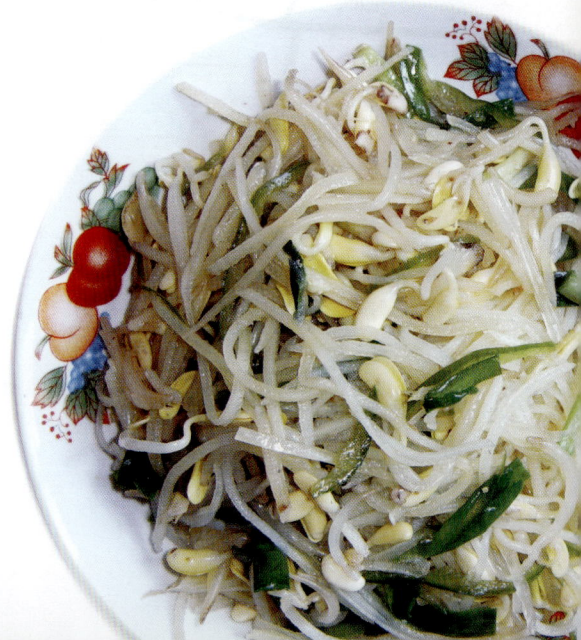

Countryside Tricolor Potatoes
Nongjia Tianyuan Sanse

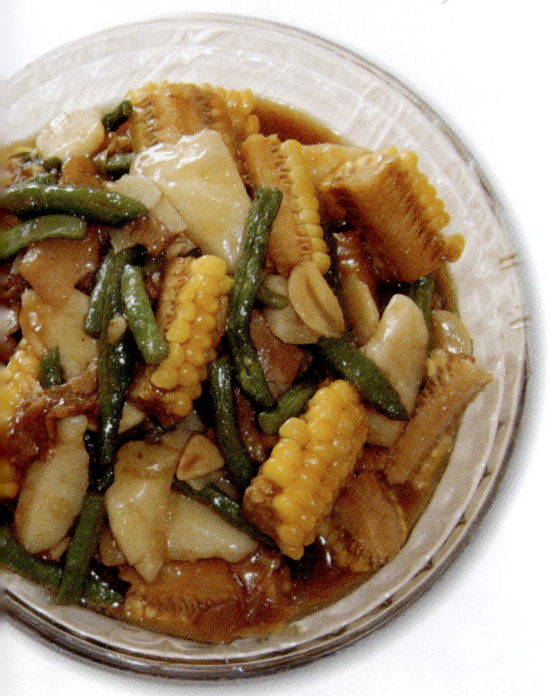

Seasonings:

Lard (refined) 30 g, onion 5 g, ginger 5 g, garlic 5 g, Chinese prickly ash 3 g, salt 5 g, gourmet powder 2 g, soy sauce 5 g, vinegar 5 g, cooking wine 5 g, wet starch 10 g

Preparation:

1. Peel potatoes and cut them into strips; quick-boil the cowpeas for 1 minute.

2. Slice cleaned side pork, boil corn cob well and cut into four portions, then cut them into 4 cm long sections, mince green onion and ginger, slice garlic.

3. Heat oil in wok and fry Chinese prickly ash until it gives off smoke, the discard. Stir-fry side pork, then add green onion, ginger, garlic and stir-fry until they give off aroma. Add soy sauce, vinegar and cooking wine to stir-fry for a moment, then add potato pieces, cowpeas, corn and water. Boil on high heat and then change to low heat to stew, adding salt and gourmet powder. Then use wet starch to thicken soup, remove and serve.

Vegetarian: ✗   Muslim: ✗

Ingredients:

Potato 300 g, corn cob 200 g, cowpea 100 g, streaky pork 150 g

Deep-fried potato doughnuts
Youzha Malingshu Guozi

Ingredients:
Potato 400 g, flour 150 g, potato starch 100 g

Seasonings:
Linseed oil 300 g, white sugar 50 g, alum 2 g

Preparation:
1. Peel cooked potatoes and mash them with a grater in a basin.
2. Add flour, potato starch, white sugar and alum to make dough. Cut into 16 cm² diamond. Heat oil to 180°C and fry to golden brown.

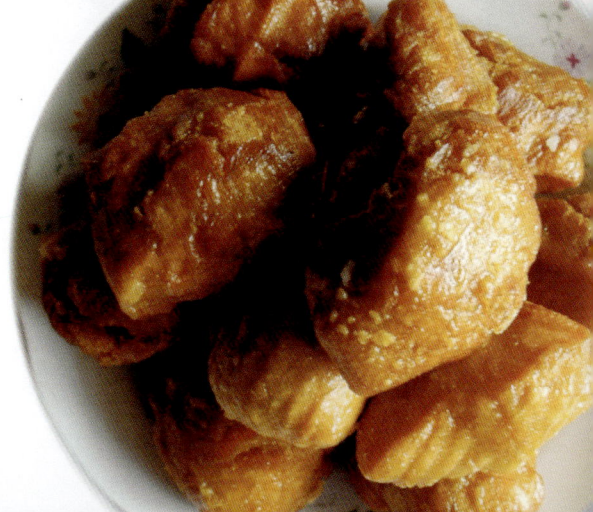

Vegetarian: ✓   Muslim: ✓

Deep-fried potato strips with tomato sauce
Mizhi Shasi Tudou Tiao

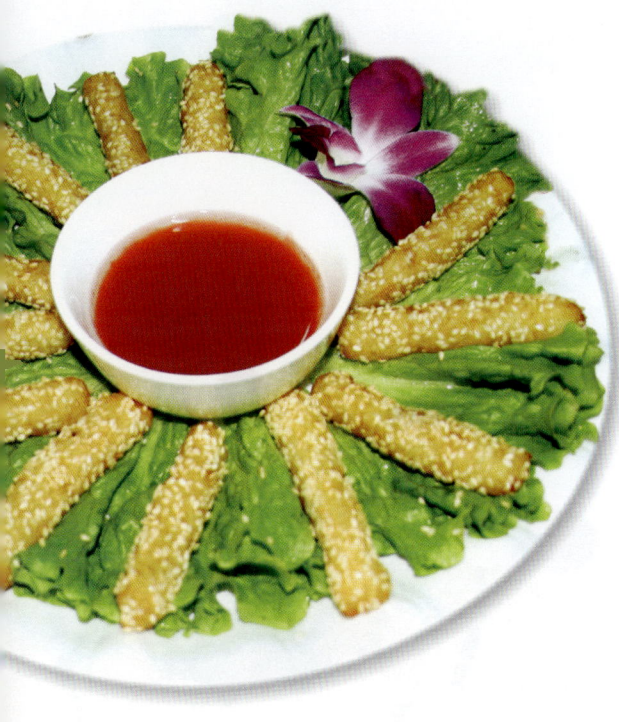

Ingredients:
Potato 300 g, sesame seed 50 g

Seasonings:
Tomato sauce 50 g, sesame seeds

Preparation:
1. Peel potatoes and cook well.
2. Mash cooked potatoes into paste and knead into figure-shaped strips.
3. Coat potato strips with sesame seeds.
4. Heat the oil over medium heat and deep-fry potato strips until they turn golden brown.
5. Serve with tomato sauce.

Vegetarian: ✓   Muslim: ✓

Drunk potato
Zuijiu Malingshu

Ingredients:
Fresh potato 500 g

Seasonings:
Beer 150 g, wheat starch 50 g, white sugar 50 g

Preparation:
1. Peel potatoes and steam them well, then mash into potato paste. Mix potatoes with wheat starch, white sugar and beer to make dough.
2. Form the potato dough into gourd shapes, coat with bread crumbs and deep-fry them in the oil, then serve.

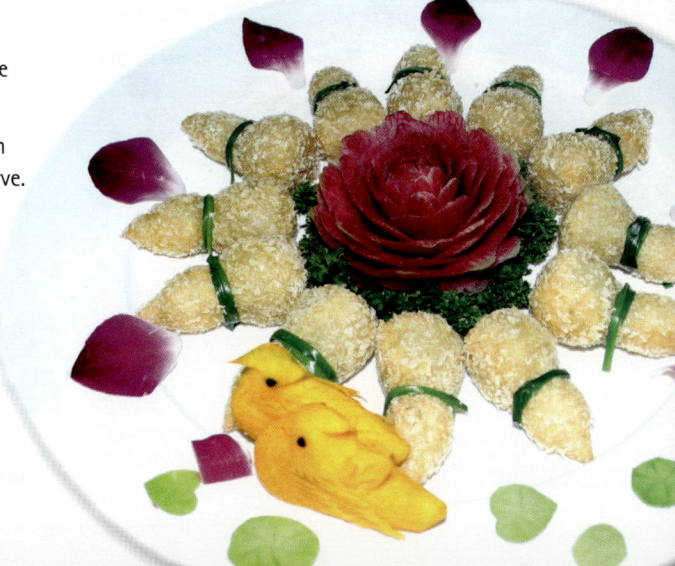

Vegetarian: ✓ Muslim: ✗

Egg, shredded bottle gourd and potato cake
Jidan Hulusi Malingshu Bing

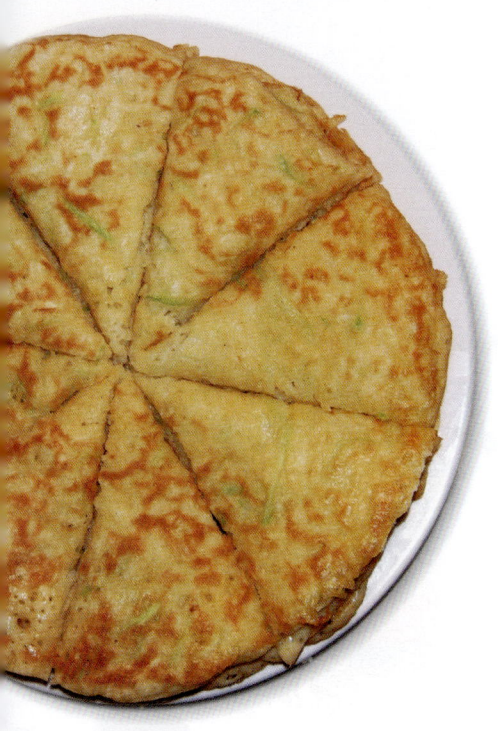

Ingredients:
Potato 400 g, wheat flour 150 g, potato starch 100 g, cucurbit 100 g

Seasonings:
Linseed oil 50 g, refined salt 3 g, minced green onion 10 g

Preparation:
1. Shred pumpkin into thin strings, whisk eggs in a large bowl and add salt. Add pumpkin strings and minced green onion into bowl and stir evenly.
2. Peel cleaned potatoes, mince them with a potato grater. Put minced potato in a bowl together with wheat flour, starch and egg mixture and roll.
3. Heat the pan, add linseed oil and fry the cake until both sides turn golden brown.

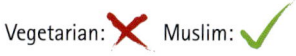

Elegant taste
Ya Qu

Ingredient:
Mashed potatoes 1,000 g

Seasonings:
Eggs, sesame seeds and garlic bolt, sweet spicy chicken sauce to taste, a little wheat flour, 1 or 2 live goldfish

Preparation:
1. Wrap garlic bolt in the mashed potatoes, sprinkle with wheat flour and coat with whisked egg and sesame seeds.
2. Heat the oil and fry to golden yellow, place in the sweet spicy chicken sauce cup and garnish with goldfish.

Note: Crisp outside, tender inside, with a distinctive sour and sweet flavor.

Vegetarian: ✗   Muslim: ✗

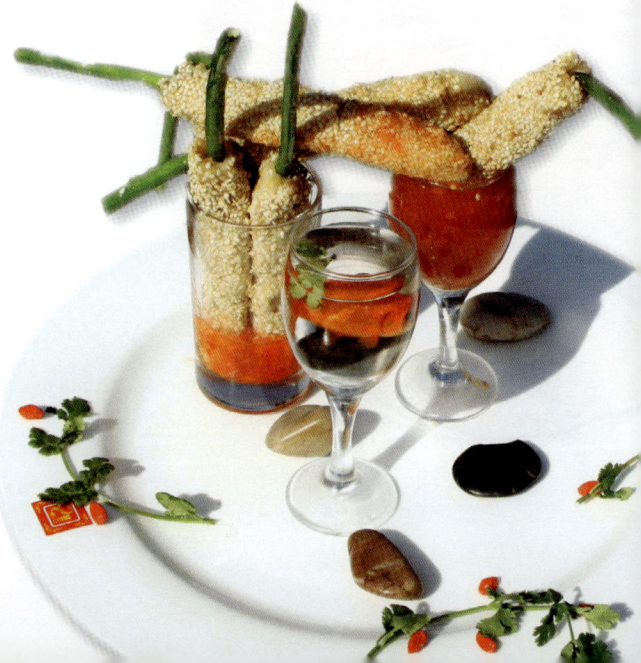

Fish-Shaped Potato
Malingshu Yu

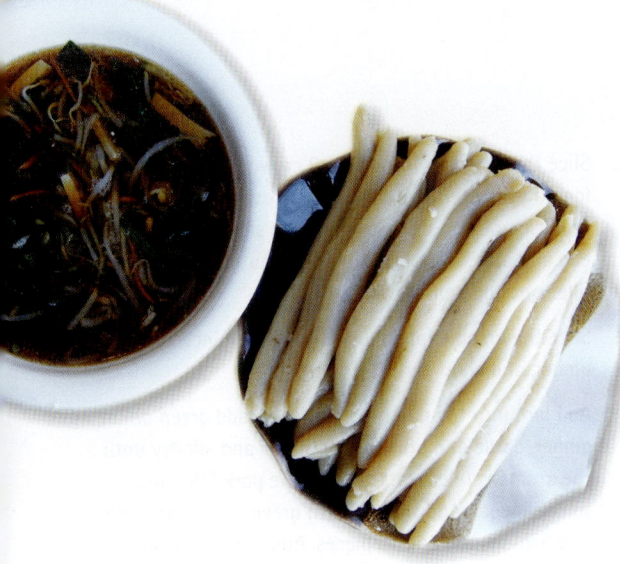

Ingredients:
Potato 500 g, flour 125 g, starch 125 g

Seasonings:
Spinach 50 g, dried tofu 50 g, soybean sprout and mung bean sprout 50 g each, red radish 50 g, cucumber 100 g, soybean sauce 10 g, vinegar 10 g, sesame oil 5 g, table salt 5 g, chili oil 5 g, vegetable oil 20 g, Chinese prickly ash 3 g, gourmet powder 3 g, green onion 10 g, ginger 5 g, garlic 5 g

Preparation:
1. Steam potatoes, then peel and mash into potato paste. Add starch and flour, mix together, and knead into dough. Divide the dough into small sections and make fish-shaped strips. Steam the strips for about 10 minutes over high heat.

2. Blanch spinach, soybean sprouts and mung bean sprouts in boiling water. Drain and cool. Chop cucumber and radish into strings and dried tofu into strips. Put all into a bowl.

3. Heat oil in the wok over high heat. Fry the Chinese prickly ash until it smokes, then discard. Put minced green onion, ginger and garlic in and stir-fry for a few seconds. Put the oil into the bowl, add a little bit of sesame oil, chili oil, table salt, soybean sauce, vinegar, gourmet powder, and 300 g of cool boiled water, then serve with the fish-shaped potato strips.

Vegetarian: ✓   Muslim: ✓

Fish-shaped potato with fried pork fillet
Guoyourou Malingshu Yu

Ingredients:
Potato 500 g, flour 125 g, starch 125 g, pork loin 200 g, lard 500 g

Seasonings:
Green vegetable 50 g, red pepper 25 g, chili 5 g, garlic 5 g, vinegar 20 g, Chinese prickly ash, water 5 g, green onion stalk 20 g, soybean sauce 15 g, fresh ginger 15 g, table salt 5 g, cooking wine 5 g, starch 50 g, gourmet powder 5 g, 1 egg

Preparation:
1. Steam the potatoes, then peel and mash them into potato paste. Add starch and flour; mix them together and knead into dough. Divide the dough and make small fish-shaped strips, then steam them for about 10 minutes over high heat.
2. Slice the pork loin into fillets 2 cm wide and 2 cm long. Put them into a bowl and mix with some Chinese prickly ash, water, soybean sauce, table salt, egg and starch. Marinate for 60 minutes. Deep-fry the fillet until golden brown.
3. Slice the green pepper and chili, finely minced the ginger, and chop garlic into fine slices.
4. Add lard into the pan over high heat, add green onion, ginger, garlic and green vegetable in and stir-fry until the aroma is released, then add the pork fillet and some vinegar. Add the chopped green pepper and chili and fish-shaped potato pieces. Add some cooking wine, gourmet powder and soybean sauce and stir-fry a little bit, then serve.

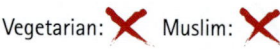

Vegetarian: ✗   Muslim: ✗

Fish-shaped potato-oat flour noodles
Tudou Yuzi

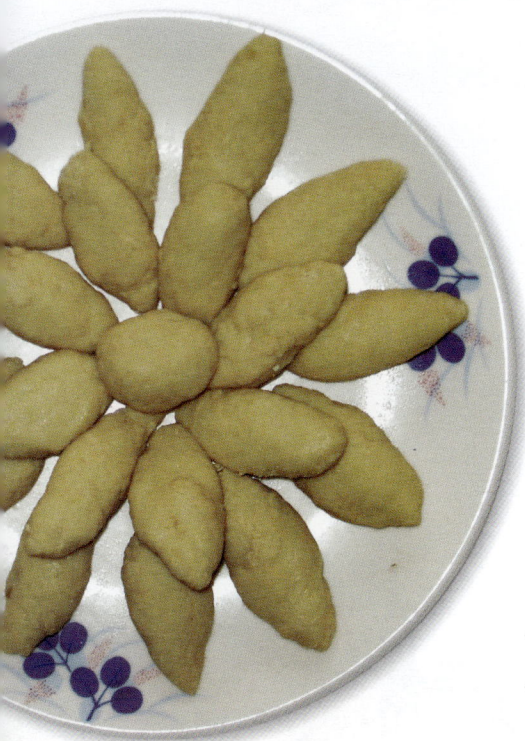

Seasonings:
Refined salt 10 g, cooking oil, Chinese prickly ash, soy sauce, starch, chicken essence, rice wine

Preparation:
1. Boil cleaned potatoes, then peel while hot and mince with a grater. Use a pestle to finely mash.
2. Evenly mix 200 g of oat flour with the mashed potatoes, then knead repeatedly in an iron saucepan to ensure toughness of the dough. Add 50 g of oat flour into the dough and knead evenly, divide into several 30 g pieces. Knead the pieces into an ellipse shape, put on a steamer tray and let stand.
3. Put 500 ml of water in steamer and bring to a boil over high heat, then put steamer tray in and steam for about 6 minutes.
4. Add oil into the wok, mix the soup stock, soy sauce, salt, chicken essence and rice wine.

Ingredients:
Potato 500 g, oat flour 250 g

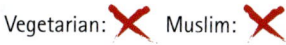

Vegetarian: ✗ Muslim: ✗

Flavored potato balls
Fengwei Tudou Qiu

Ingredients:
Potato 500 g, Chinese chives 200 g, steamed bread 100 g, bean or sweet potato starch noodles 50 g

Seasonings:
Salad oil 250 g, dried steamed bread crumbs

Preparation:
1. Select fresh potatoes with enough starch, peel them and steam well. Mash the cooked potatoes, and knead into 20 identical-sized balls; mince steamed bread.
2. Coat potato balls with minced steamed bread, then deep-fry over high heat until golden brown.
3. Serve the fried potato balls on sweet potato (bean) starch noodles.

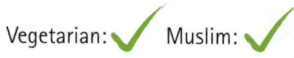

Vegetarian: ✓   Muslim: ✓

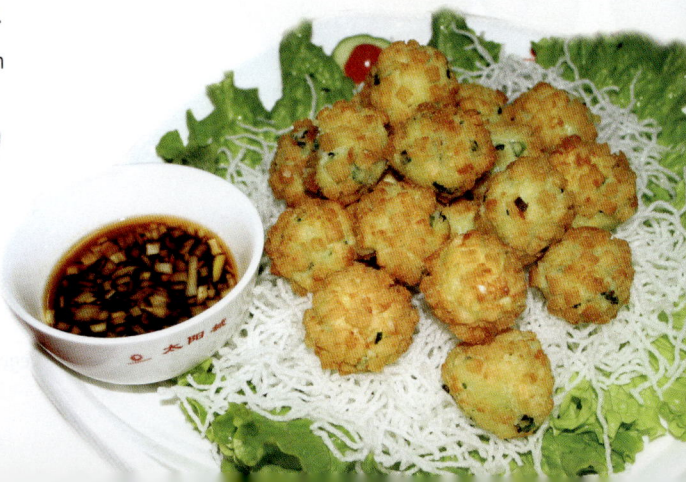

Fried Chicken-Flavored Potato
Youzha Malingshu Su Jitui

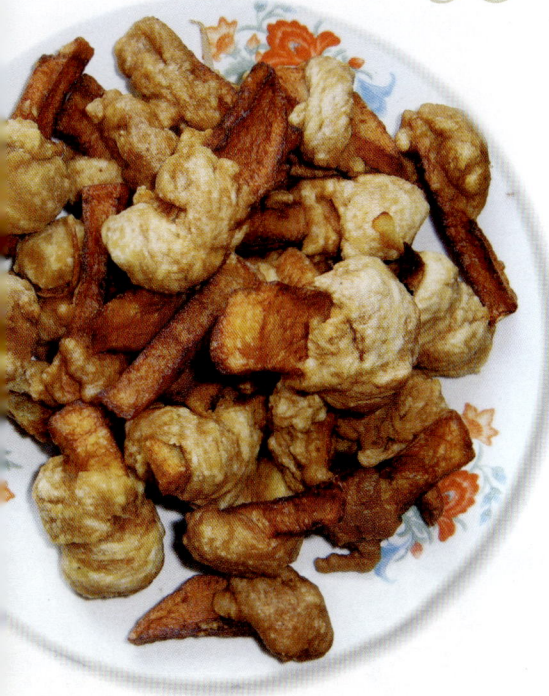

Seasonings:

Oil 300 g, Chinese prickly ash powder 3 g, refined salt 3 g, fermented dough 30 g, fluffy soda 2 g

Preparation:

1. Peel potatoes, cut them into strips, and wash in clear water to remove excessive starch. Remove from water and drain.

2. Put 150 ml of warm water and fermented dough into a bowl. Add fluffy soda, and dissolve the fermented dough, then add wheat flour, Chinese prickly ash and refined salt to make dough. Let the dough stand for fermenting.

3. Put the fermented dough on a smooth surface (smear a little oil on it to prevent sticking). Roll the dough into 1 cm thick, 2 cm wide, and 10 cm long pieces, and roll each piece together with a potato strip. Deep-fry the pieces until the potato strips become deep yellow and the surface of dough turns to golden brown, then serve.

Ingredients:

Potato 300 g, wheat flour 300 g

Vegetarian: ✓   Muslim: ✓

Fried Chinese sauerkraut and noodles
Suancai Chao Fentiao

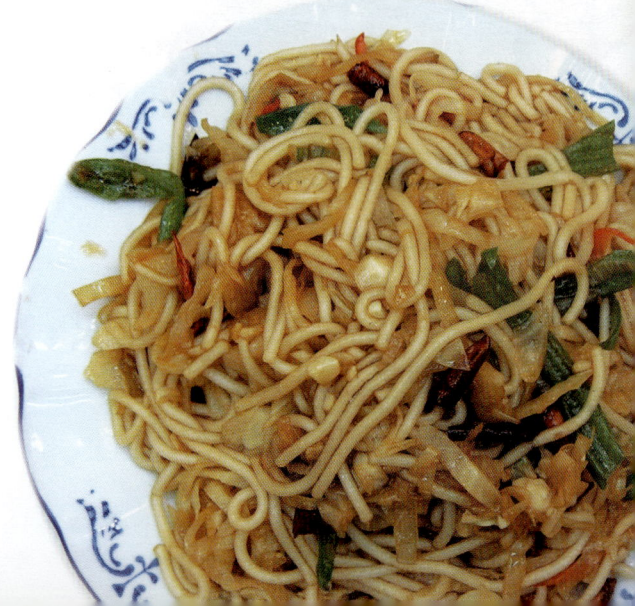

Ingredients:
Potato starch 500 g, alum 3 g, Chinese sauerkraut 200 g

Seasonings:
Red pepper 5 g, green and red paprika 10 g each, table salt 5 g, chicken essence 3 g, Chinese prickly ash 3 g, green onion 10 g, garlic 5 g, fresh ginger 5 g, vegetable oil 20 g

Preparation:
1. Make some fresh noodles with potato starch.
2. Cut the Chinese sauerkraut into strips. Heat the oil in frying pan over a high heat. Fry the Chinese prickly ash until it smokes, then remove and discard. Add a little red pepper, green onion, garlic, ginger and stir-fry. Add potato noodles and green and red paprika strings and stir-fry. Mix with some chicken essence and salt, then serve.

Vegetarian: ✗   Muslim: ✓

Fried Chinese sauerkraut and potato chips
Suancai Malingshu Tiao

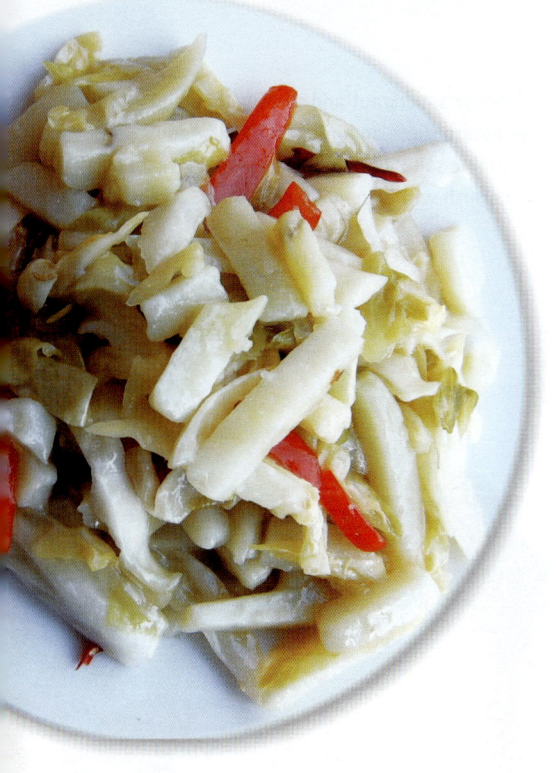

Ingredients:
Potato 300 g, Chinese sauerkraut 200 g

Seasonings:
Red pepper 5 g, green and red paprika 20 g, table salt 5 g, chicken essence 3 g, Chinese prickly ash 3 g, green onion 10 g, garlic 5 g, fresh ginger 5 g, vegetable 20 g

Preparation:
1. Peel potatoes and cut them into chips. Put the chips into water to remove starch, then blanch them. Cut the Chinese sauerkraut into pieces.

2. Heat oil over high heat, and fry the Chinese prickly ash until it smokes, then discard. Add a little red pepper, green and red paprika, green onion, ginger and garlic lightly quick-fry. Add the Chinese sauerkraut pieces and potato chips and stir-fry. Season with table salt and gourmet powder, then serve.

Vegetarian: ✗   Muslim: ✓

Fried Chinese sauerkraut and potato slices
Suancai Malinghsu Ni

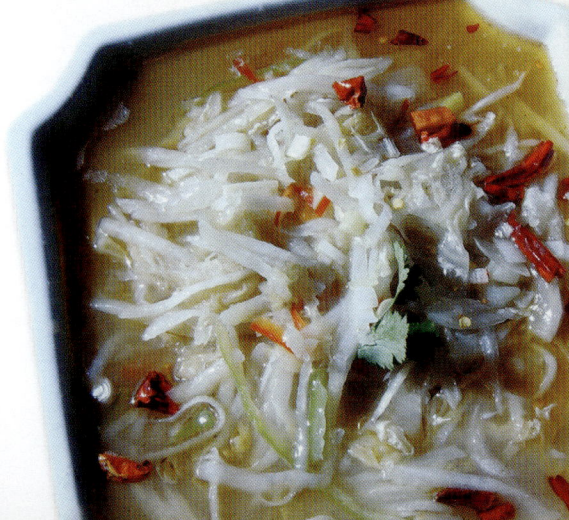

Ingredients:
Potato 300 g, Chinese sauerkraut 200 g

Seasonings:
Green paprika 10 g, red paprika 10 g, coriander 5 g, chicken essence 3 g, Chinese prickly ash 3 g, green onion 10 g, garlic 5 g, fresh ginger 5 g, sesame oil 5 g, vegetable oil 20 g

Preparation:
1. Clean and peel the potatoes, then cut them into strings. Wash strings in clean water to remove starch. Cut the Chinese sauerkraut to pieces.

2. Heat oil in frying pan over a high heat and fry the Chinese prickly ash until it smokes, then discard. Add a little red pepper, green and red paprika, green onion, ginger and garlic and lightly quick-fry.

3. Add the Chinese sauerkraut and stir-fry, then add water and potato slices and bring to a boil. Add sesame oil, table salt and gourmet powder. Place on a plate and garnish with coriander, then serve.

Vegetarian: ✗   Muslim: ✓

Fried mashed potatoes, carrots and mushrooms
Jinsha Fengguang

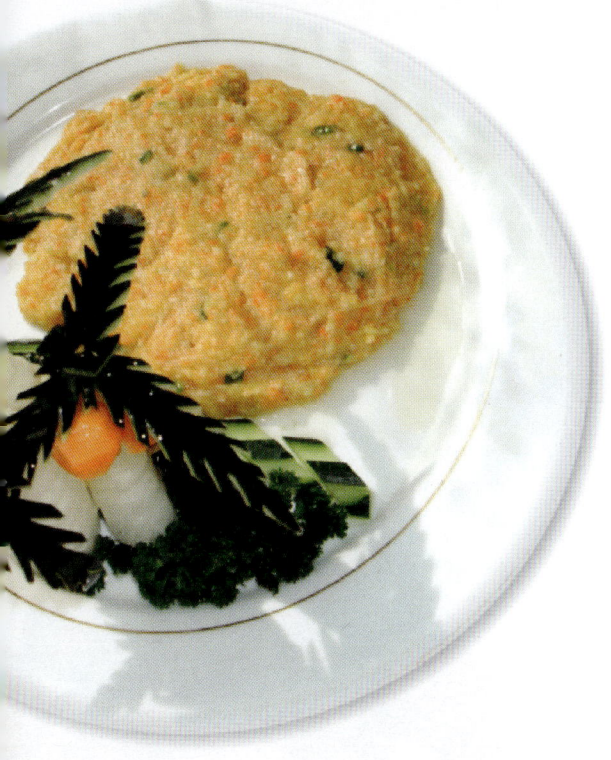

Ingredients:
Potato 1,000 g, carrot 500 g, dried mushrooms 100 g

Seasonings:
Salad oil 20 g, salt 9 g, gourmet powder 3 g, chicken essence 5 g, chili pepper 1 g

Preparation:
1. Make potato and carrot pastes and mix them evenly.
2. Mince the dried mushrooms.
3. Put the minced mushrooms into the potato and carrot paste, add salt, gourmet powder, chicken essence, chili pepper and then stir evenly.
4. Heat the oil to medium-hot, add the mixture paste mixture and fry for 1 minute until it turns golden yellow and breaks into small pieces. Garnish with minced green onion and serve.

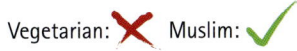

Vegetarian: ✗   Muslim: ✓

Fried potato balls
Youzha Malingshu Wanzi

Ingredients:
Potato 500 g, starch 150 g, linseed oil 300 g

Seasonings:
Refined salt 3 g, Chinese prickly ash powder 3 g, green onion 10 g, granulated sugar 5 g, gourmet powder 1 g

Preparation:
1. Boil and peel potatoes, then mince with a potato grater. Put potatoes in a bowl and add flour, refined salt, Chinese prickly ash powder, green onion, granulated sugar and gourmet powder, and then knead into dough.

2. Heat linseed oil, knead the dough into small balls of identical size and fry in the oil until golden brown. Remove, drain and serve.

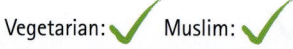
Vegetarian: ✓   Muslim: ✓

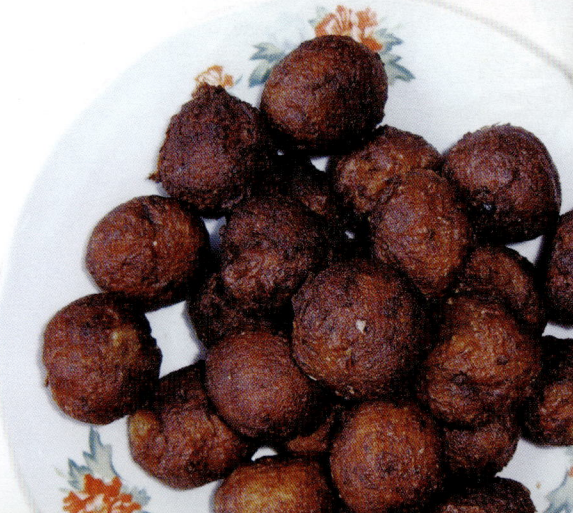

Fried Potato Cake II
Xiangjian Tudou Bing I

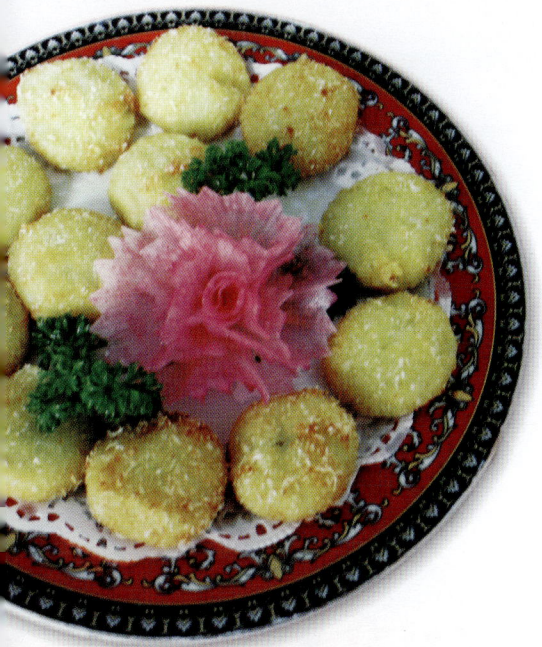

Preparation:

1. Peel and dice fresh potatoes, then steam for 10 minutes.

2. Mash the steamed potatoes; mix well with concentrated milk, sticky rice and white sugar. Knead into dumplings (knead for 3 to 5 minutes), making 12 dumplings of identical size.

3. Stuff the potato balls with meat fillings such as pork, beef or mutton, or sweet red bean paste.

4. Whisk two eggs. Dip the potato balls in the eggs and then coat them with coconut granules (for sweet taste) or bread crumbs (for salty taste).

5. Knead the potato balls into pancakes and put them on a baking tray, sprinkle with salad oil and bake for about 5 minutes over low heat. Serve while hot.

Ingredient:

Potato 500 g

Seasonings:

Concentrated milk 25 g, sticky rice 60 g, white sugar 20 g, coconut granules (bread crumbs) 50 g, meat filling to taste

Vegetarian: ✘   Muslim: ✘

Fried Potato Slices I
Youzha Malingshu Pian

Ingredients:
Potato 400 g, blending oil 300 g

Seasonings:
Refined salt 3 g, minced dried green onion 1 g, Chinese prickly ash powder 2 g, gourmet powder 1 g

Preparation:
1. Peel and slice potatoes, then wash in water to remove starch and drain.
2. Deep-fry the potato slices in a wok until golden brown. Remove slices and drain oil; sprinkle with salt, minced dried green onion, Chinese prickly ash powder and gourmet powder, then serve.

Vegetarian: ✓   Muslim: ✓

Fried potato strings
YOUZHA MALINGSHU SI

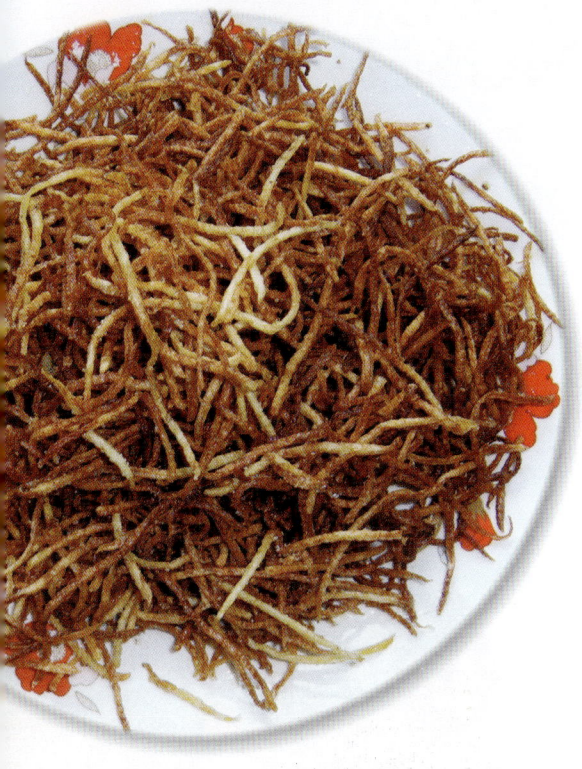

Ingredients:
Potato 400 g, blending oil 300 g

Seasonings:
Refined salt 3 g, Chinese prickly ash powder 2 g, gourmet powder 1 g

Preparation:
1. Peel potatoes and cut them into strings, then wash in water to remove starch and drain.
2. Fry potato strings in cooking oil until golden brown. Remove strings and drain oil; sprinkle with salt, Chinese prickly ash powder and gourmet powder, then serve.

Vegetarian: ✓   Muslim: ✓

Fried potato strings with pickled celery cabbage and mutton fat
Yangyou Suancai Malingshu Si

Ingredients:
Potato 300 g, pickled celery cabbage 200 g

Seasonings:
Mutton fat 50 g, small red pepper 3 g, onion 10 g, ginger 5 g, garlic 5 g, Chinese prickly ash 3 g, salt 5 g, gourmet powder 2 g, soy sauce 5 g, vinegar 5 g, cooking wine 5 g

Preparation:
1. Peel potatoes and cut them into strings, then wash in water to remove starch. Shred pickled cabbage.
2. Fry Chinese prickly ash in wok until it smokes, then discard. Quick-fry small red pepper, minced green onion and ginger, and garlic, then add shredded pickled cabbage, soy sauce, vinegar and cooking wine and stir-fry. Add water and potato strings and boil. Once it boils mix in refined salt and gourmet powder, remove to a dish and sprinkle with minced green onion.

Vegetarian: ✗ Muslim: ✗

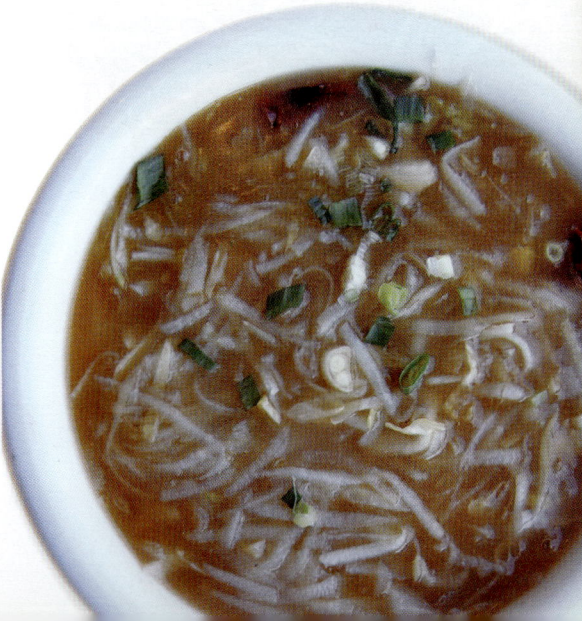

Fried potato strips coated with sugar
Liuli Shutiao

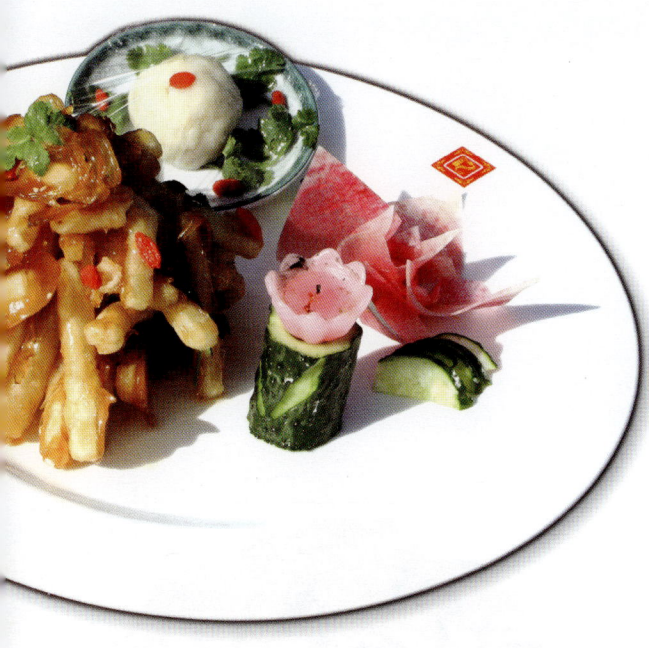

Ingredient:
Potato 500 g

Seasoning:
White sugar 50 g

Preparation:
Cut potatoes into strips, coat them with starch and deep-fry in oil. Combine oil, water and sugar, and fry until it thickens. Then stir-fry potato strips in the mixture, cool and serve.

Vegetarian: ✓   Muslim: ✓

Fried potato strips with chili
Ganbian Tudou Tiao

Ingredients:
Fresh potato 500 g, hot pepper 50 g, pork

Seasonings:
Salt, gourmet powder, garlic, ginger and green onion to taste

Preparation:
1. Cut potatoes into strips.
2. Heat oil and fry potato strips twice with a short interval in between.
3. Add minced pork, dry chili and other seasonings and stir-fry with potato strips for 3 minutes.

Vegetarian: 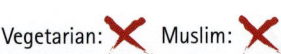 Muslim:

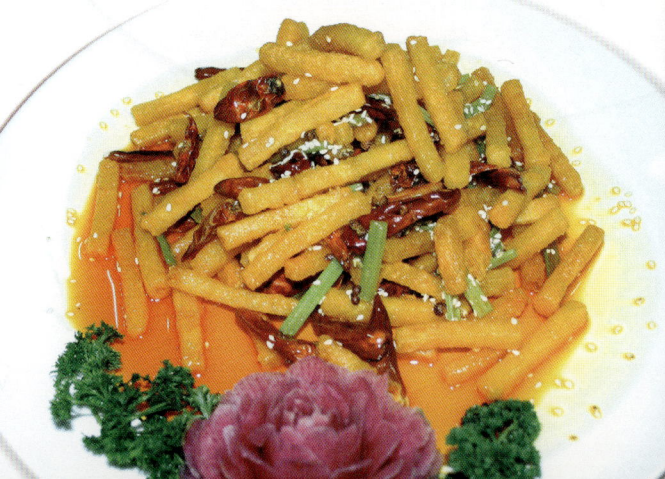

Fried potato strips with pork
Youbailuo Chao Malingshu Tiao

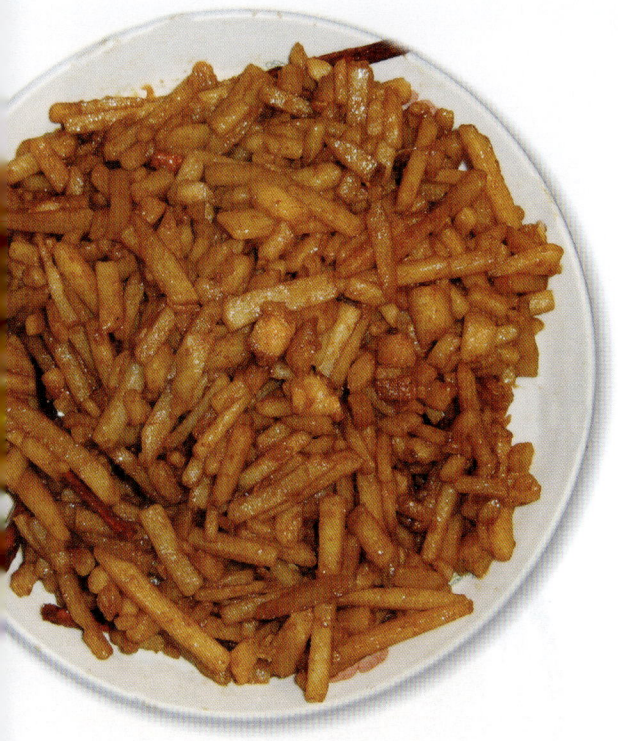

Ingredients:
Potato 400 g, fat pork 150 g

Seasonings:
Small red pepper 3 g, onion 10 g, ginger 5 g, garlic 5 g, Chinese prickly ash 3 g, salt 5 g, gourmet powder 2 g, soy sauce 15 g, white sugar 5 g, vinegar 5 g, cooking wine 5 g

Preparation:
1. Peel potatoes and cut them into strips, then wash to remove starch. Dice fat pork.
2. Deep-fry diced pork over high heat until golden brown, then remove and set aside. Heat oil, and fry Chinese prickly ash until it smokes, then discard. Quick-fry small red pepper, minced green onion and ginger, and garlic, then add fried pork, potato strips, soy sauce, white sugar, vinegar and cooking wine and stir-fry. Add appropriate amount of water and, when boiling, mix in refined salt and gourmet powder, then serve.

Vegetarian: ✗ Muslim: ✗

Fried potatoes with egg
Tudou Jian Dan

Ingredients:
Potato 100 g, 2 eggs

Seasonings:
Pepper and salt

118>

Preparation:
1. Peel and dice potatoes. Whisk the eggs and mix in the ground pepper and salt.
2. Heat oil in wok and fry potatoes.
3. Put the egg fluid in the wok and fry slowly over low heat.
4. Fry both sides until golden yellow, then serve.

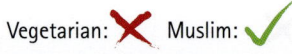

Vegetarian: ✗   Muslim: ✓

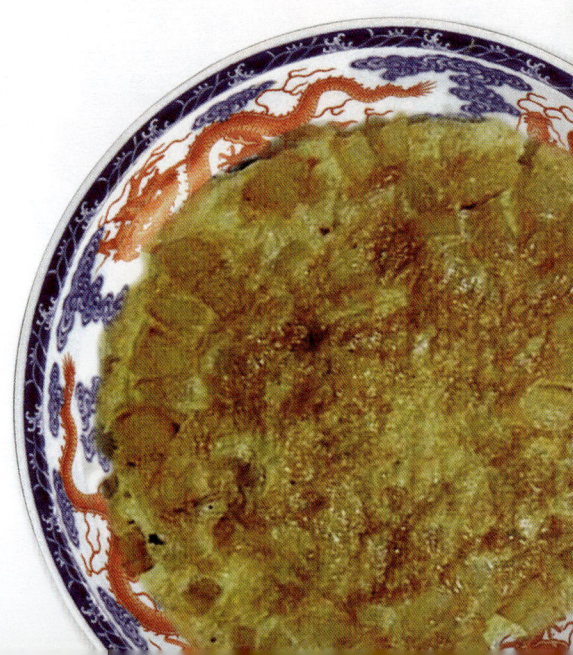

Fried potatoes with soybean sprouts
Tudou Chao Huangdou Ya

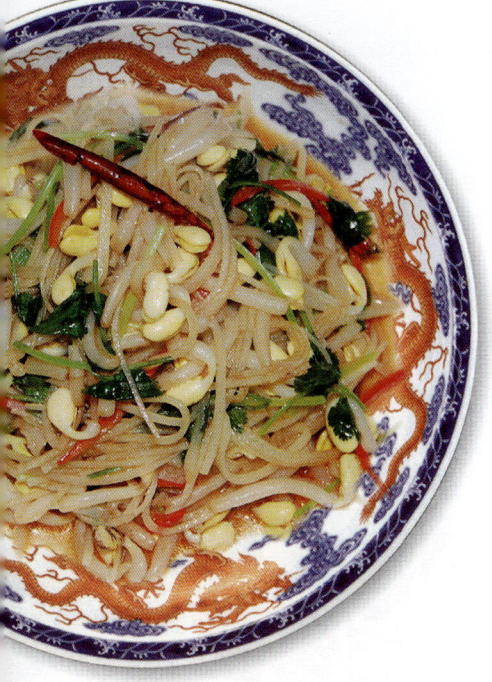

Seasonings:
Salad oil 25 g, dried hot pepper 2 g, chili oil (red) 2 g, salt 3 g, gourmet powder 3 g, black soy sauce

Preparation:
1. Peel potatoes and shred them into strings at 6–7 cm long.
2. Place shredded potato in water to remove starch. then quick-boil the soybean sprouts and potato with a little salt. Put the soybean sprouts in cold water first, when boil, put the potato strings.
3. Put salad oil in wok with dried hot pepper and stir-fry. Add a little shredded onion and ginger, then add the potato strings and soybean sprouts and stir-fry for 30 seconds to 1 minute. Then add a little soy sauce, salt and gourmet powder and stir-fry.
4. Add coriander and stir-fry, then add chili oil (red oil) and serve.

Ingredients:
Potato 250 g, soybean sprout 250 g

Vegetarian: ✓   Muslim: ✓

Fried Shredded Potato Cake I
Xiang Jian Tudou Pai

Ingredient:
Potato 500 g

Seasonings:
Kaka marvelous sauce and white sugar

Preparation:
1. Shred potatoes into medium-thick strings, coat with wet starch and place on a plate to form a cake shape. Heat the oil and deep-fry the potatoes until crisp.
2. Remove to a dish, decorate the dish with some Kaka marvelous sauce and sprinkle with white sugar.

Vegetarian: ✓   Muslim: ✓

Fried shredded potato with Chinese chives and egg (served with cake)
Malingshu Si Jiucai Jidan Dai Bing

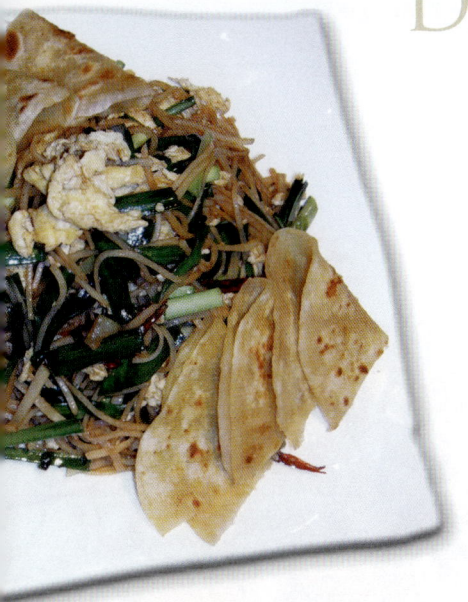

Preparation:

1. Add 75 ml boiling water to wheat flour, knead well and allow to cool. Roll the dough into an oblong shape, then apply linseed oil, roll it up, slice it into small dumplings, roll them into cakes and set aside.

2. Heat pan, put oil on the cake and put in the pan to roast over low heat until both sides of the cake turn golden brown.

3. Peel and shred potatoes and wash in clear water to remove starch, then drain. Whisk egg in a bowl and add salt. Cut Chinese chives into sections.

4. Heat oil in a wok and fry the egg.

5. Heat oil over strong heat, add small red pepper, garlic, soy sauce and potato and stir-fry well. Add the fried egg and Chinese chives and fry slightly. Season with salt and gourmet powder. Blend flavors and remove to a dish, cut the wheat pancake in half and place on dish.

Ingredients:

Potato 150 g, egg 150 g, Chinese chives 100 g, wheat flour 150 g, linseed oil 50 g

Seasonings:

Small red pepper 5 g, soy sauce 10 g, refined salt 5 g, chicken essence 3 g, garlic 5 g

Vegetarian: ✗   Muslim: ✓

Fried side pork with potato
Wuhuarou Jian Malingshu

Ingredients:
Potato 300 g, side pork 200 g, lard 30 g

Seasonings:
Onion 15 g, green onion 10 g, ginger 5 g, garlic 5 g, Chinese prickly ash 3 g, salt 5 g, gourmet powder 2 g, soy sauce 5 g, vinegar 5 g, cooking wine 5 g

Preparation:
1. Boil potatoes and cool slightly, then peel and mash. Clean and slice side pork.
2. Shred onion and mince green onion, ginger and garlic.
3. Heat oil and fry Chinese prickly ash until it smokes, then discard. Stir-fry side pork, then add onion, minced green onion, ginger and garlic to stir-fry until they give off aroma. Add soy sauce, vinegar and cooking wine and fry for a moment. Add potatoes and fry. Add salt and gourmet powder, mix well, then serve.

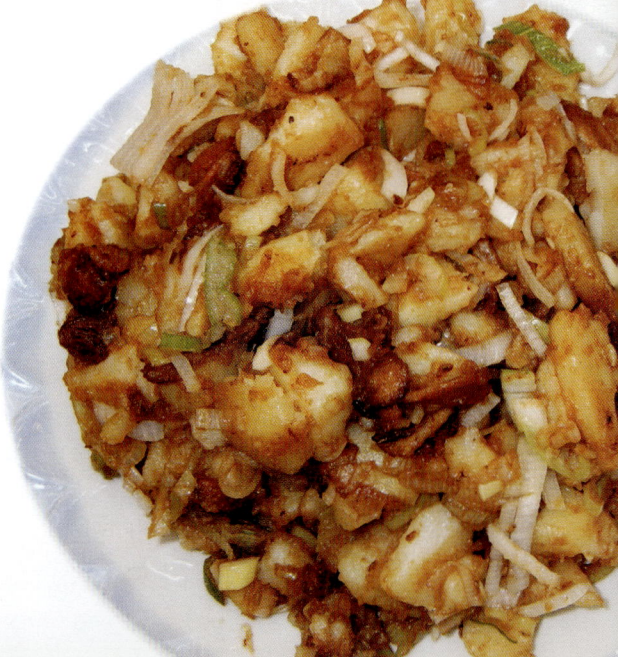

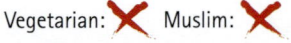

Handmade noodles with potatoes in an earthen pot

Shaguo Malingshu Shouganmian

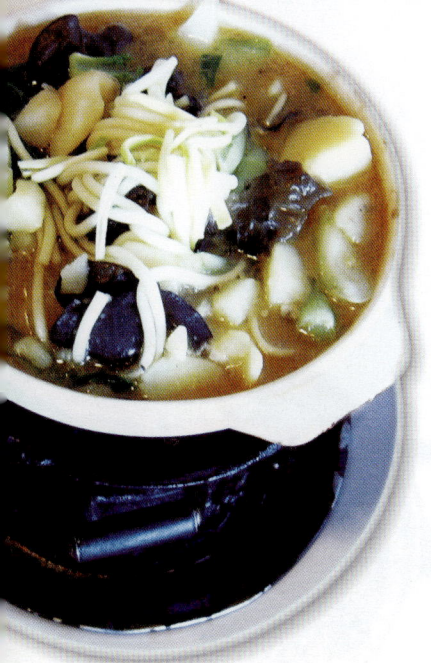

Seasonings:

Table salt 5 g, soy sauce 10 g, chicken essence 3 g, green onion 10 g, garlic 5 g, fresh ginger 5 g, chicken broth 500 g, sesame oil 5 g

Preparation:

1. Clean the rape and chop it into pieces. Clean the potatoes and peel and dice them, then blanch in boiling water.
2. Put the chicken broth into wok and add the diced potato, rape and raised edible fungus into the broth. Mix with table salt, soy sauce, garlic and fresh ginger. Boil the broth for about 5 minutes and then add handmade noodles. When the noodles are done, add green onion, chicken essence and sesame oil, then serve.

Ingredients:

Potato 300 g, handmade noodles 150 g, rape 100 g, raised edible fungus 50 g

Vegetarian: ✘   Muslim: ✔

Hotpot Potato Pieces
Malingshu Huoguo Pian

Ingredient:
Potato 200 g

Seasonings:
Sesame sauce 150 g, fragrant-flowered garlic 10 g, fermented tofu 10 g, chili oil 2 g, cilantro 10 g

Preparation:
1. Peel and slice potatoes.
2. Mix fragrant-flowered garlic, fermented bean curd, chili oil and cilantro in sesame sauce in a bowl to make the hotpot sauce. Put potato pieces into the hot pot to boil. Dip pieces in the hotpot sauce when eating.

Vegetarian: ✓ Muslim: ✓

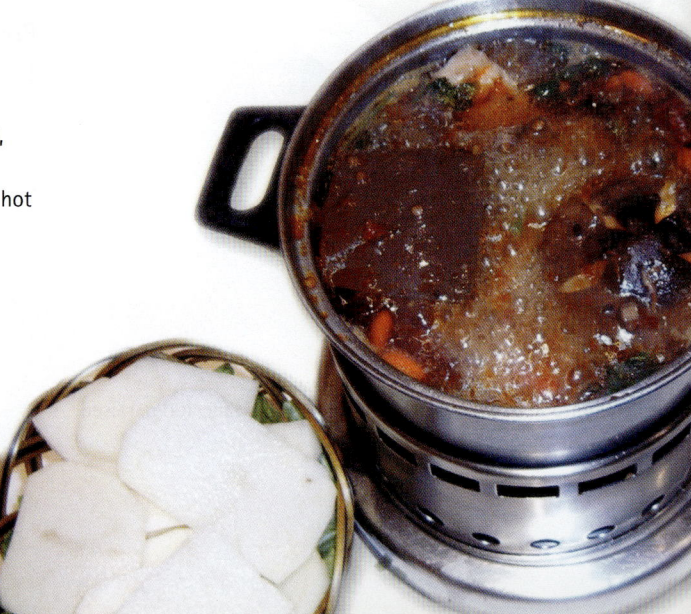

Hunyuan cold potato jelly
HUNYUAN LIANGFEN

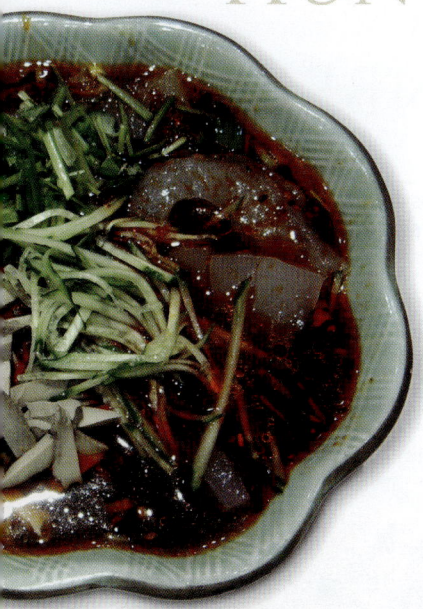

Preparation:

1. Put starch into a big bowl, add water and mix.
2. Boil water in wok, add the starch from bowl and stir until it becomes a paste.
3. Add the alum solution and stir. When the color of the paste changes, stop stirring. It will now turn into potato jelly.
4. Put the jelly in a big bowl, cool and then slice.
5. Heat oil and stir-fry the minced onion for a few seconds, then pour the hot oil over the jelly.
6. Season with some table salt, gourmet powder, sesame oil, vinegar, fried chili oil, dried tofu slices, shredded cucumber, cilantro, and deep-fried broad bean.

Ingredients:
Potato starch 500 g, water 1,500 g

Seasonings:
Alum 3 g, dried tofu 50 g, cucumber 50 g, lotus flower (deep-fry broad bean) 50 g, cilantro 10 g, linseed oil 30 g, green onion 10 g, garlic 5 g, table salt 5 g, green onion 10 g, sesame oil 5 g, table salt 5 g, vinegar 10 g, gourmet powder 3 g, fried chili oil 20 g

Vegetarian: ✓ Muslim: ✓

Mashed Garlic Scallop with Potato Noodles
Suanrong Fensi Zheng Shanbei

Ingredients:
Big scallops 5, potato noodles 30 g

Seasonings:
Salt 2 g, garlic 10 g, green onion 5 g, paprika powder 2 g, cooking wine 15 g, light soy sauce 15 g, vegetable oil 10 g

Preparation:
1. Clean the scallops and put them into the steamer.
2. Put the potato noodles in cold water for about 20 minutes. Lay out the noodles round the scallops in the steamer.
3. Mix the light soy sauce, cooking wine, salt and paprika powder together to make a juice. Fry the garlic in hot oil until it turns yellow. Pour the juice, garlic powder and oil onto the scallops.
4. Steam the scallops over a high heat for about 5 to 8 minutes. Remove from steamer, sprinkle with green onion and serve.

Vegetarian: ✗   Muslim: ✗

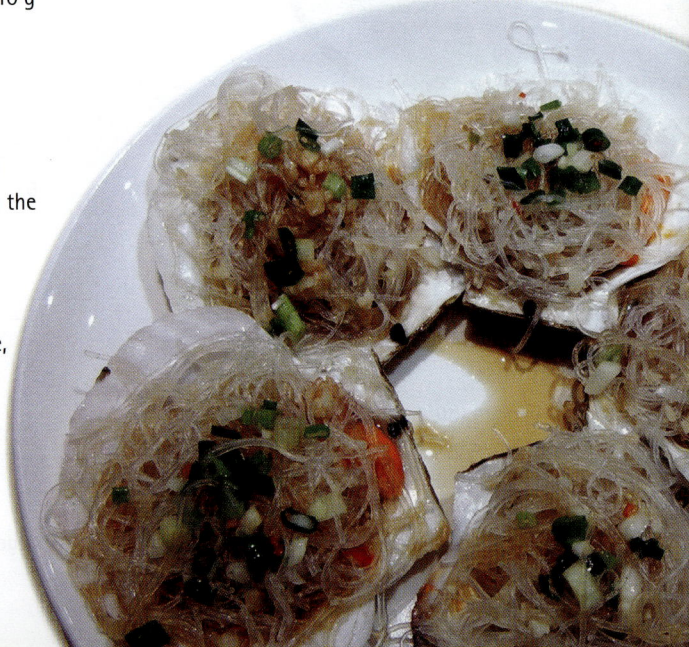

Min Bagu

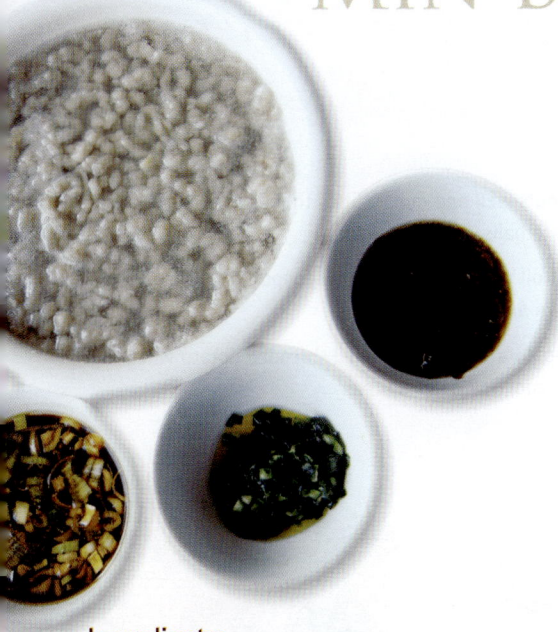

Preparation:

1. Chinese chives thick sauce: Minced Chinese chives, heat oil in wok and stir-fry chives, then remove to a bowl and mix evenly with salt and chicken essence.

2. Fried bean sauce: Stir-fry the minced meat in oil, then add fermented soy paste and fry well.

3. Minced green onion thick sauce: Put minced green onion, soy sauce, vinegar, salt, chicken essence and sesame oil in a small bowl. Add boiled and cool water and mix well.

4. Min bagu: Boil and peel potatoes, then mince with a potato grater. Put the potato paste in a bowl and add oat flour to make dough. Place the dough on Min mian chuang (special tool for make Min mian, a board with many small holes, like a strainer). Make dough into Min bagu and leak into boiling water. Quick-boil to well-done. Serve with minced green onion thick sauce, fried bean sauce or Chinese chives thick sauce.

Ingredients:
Potato 500 g, oat flour 250 g

Seasonings:
Chinese chives 20 g, onion 10 g, soy sauce 5 g, vinegar 5 g, salt 15 g, chicken essence, sesame oil 5 g, minced meat 20 g, fermented soy paste 20 g, vegetable oil 10 g

Vegetarian: ✗   Muslim: ✗

Mini embroidered potato balls
Mini Xiuqiu Wan

Ingredients:
Potato 1,500 g, wheat flour 75 g, salad oil 1,500 g

Seasonings:
Salt 6 g, gourmet powder 3 g, chicken essence 6 g, chili pepper 3 g, Chinese prickly ash 2 g, nuts 20 g

Preparation:

1. Make 500 g of potato paste. Shred 1,000 g of potatoes and put the strings in cold water to remove starch.
2. Steam wheat flour in a steamer.
3. Mix salt, gourmet powder, chicken essence, chili pepper, Chinese prickly ash and well-steamed wheat flour with mashed potatoes, then knead it into balls with a diameter of 3 cm. Put the balls on a plate and set aside.
4. Fry nuts well and mince. Stuff the nuts inside the potato balls.
5. Heat oil to medium hot. Deep-fry potato until golden brown and crisp.
6. Wrap potato balls with fried shredded potato when they cool down, then serve.

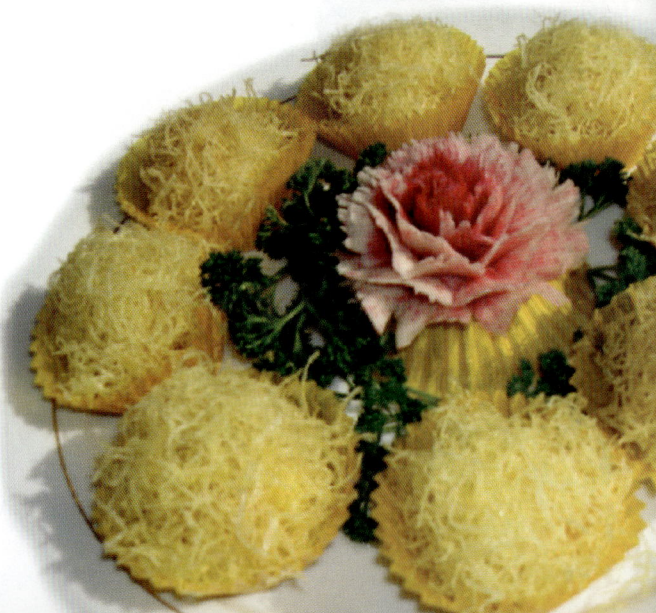

Vegetarian: ✗   Muslim: ✓

Noodles with Potato and Spinach
Malingshu Bocai Gangsimian

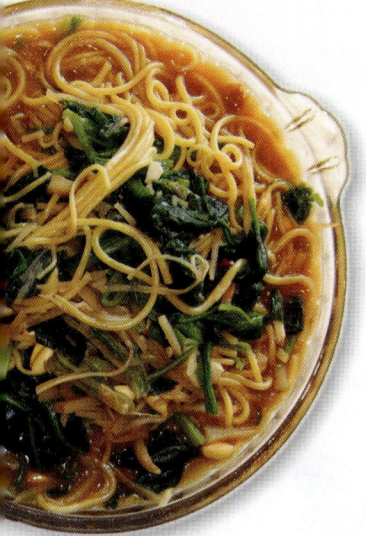

Preparation:

1. Making noodles: Quick-blanch corn flour, then make corn noodles using a special kitchen tool.

2. Clean and peel potatoes and cut them into chips. Put the chips in water to remove starch. Clean the spinach and cut into pieces. Slice the pork.

3. Heat oil in frying pan over high heat. Fry Chinese prickly ash until it smokes, then remove and discard. Stir-fry the pork, then add green onion, ginger and garlic and quick-fry. Add the cooking wine and broad bean paste, then add the potato chips and soybean sprouts and stir-fry.

4. Add some water into the frying pan and bring to a boil, then add the noodles and spinach and cook for about 5 minutes. Season with table salt and serve.

Ingredients:

Potato 200 g, spinach 200 g, noodles 250 g, side pork 50 g, soybean sprout 100 g

Seasonings:

Cooking wine 5 g, salt 5 g, broad bean paste 5 g, Chinese prickly ash 3 g, green onion 5 g, ginger 5 g, garlic 5 g, lard (refined) 50 g

Vegetarian: ✗   Muslim: ✗

Oat dumplings with potato filling
Malingshu Youmian Jiaozi

Ingredients:
Potato 800 g, oat flour 300 g, Chinese chives 150 g

Seasonings:
Refined salt 5 g, Chinese prickly ash powder 3 g, gourmet powder 3 g, chicken essence 3 g, soy sauce 5 g, sesame oil 5 g, vegetable oil 20 g.

Preparation:
1. Clean 300 g of potato, then peel and shred it. Mince Chinese chives and put both in a bowl. Add refined salt, Chinese prickly ash powder, gourmet powder, chicken essence, soy sauce, sesame oil and vegetable oil and mix well. This is now the dumpling filling. Set it aside.

2. Clean remaining potatoes, then boil and peel them and mince with a potato grater. Put the minced potatoes in a bowl, add oat flour and knead into a dough. Divide dough into small pieces to make dumplings. Roll each piece into a small thin cake, then knead the edge of the cake to make it thinner, with a thicker center. Fill the wrapper with dumpling illing; fold the wrapper and pinch the edge tightly from left to right.

3. Put some water in a pot, put the dumplings on a steamer tray and steam for about 15 minutes. Remove and serve.

Vegetarian: ✗   Muslim: ✓

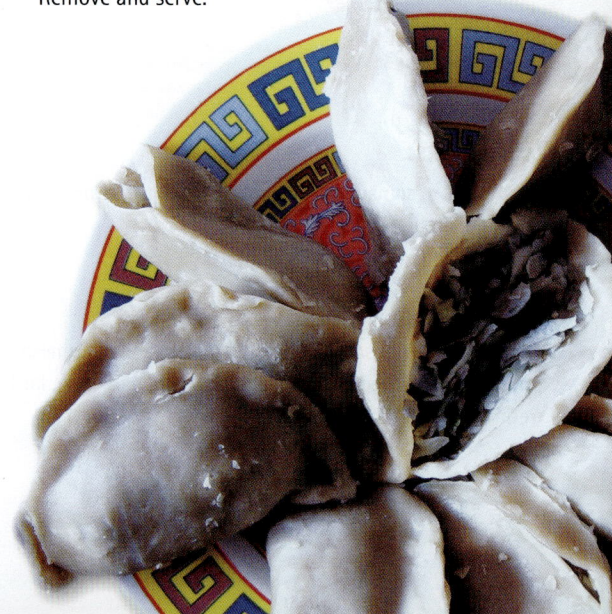

Oat flour-wrapped shredded potato
Youmian Tuntun

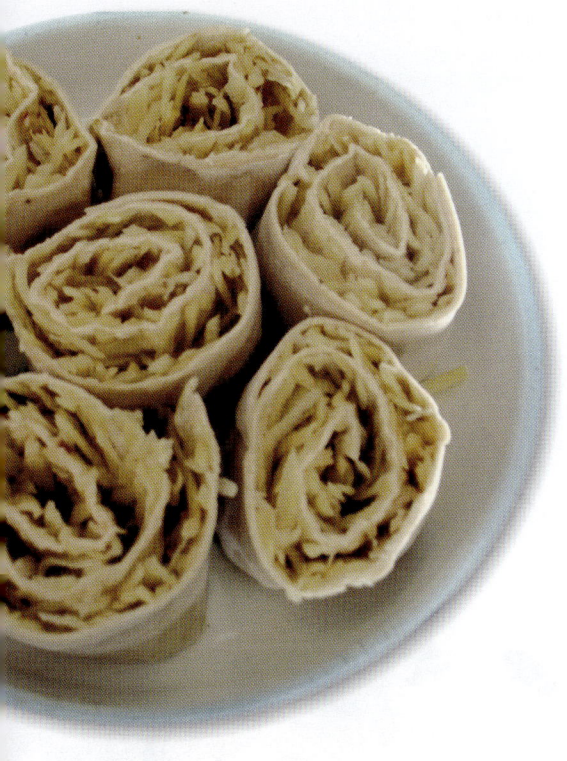

Ingredients:
Potato 150 g, oat flour 100 g

Seasonings:
Different sauces according to individual taste

Preparation:
1. Add boiling water to oat flour and knead well. Peel and shred potatoes, then put in cool water for 5 minutes and remove.

2. Put the oat dough on the rolling board and roll it into a 1 mm-thick big piece. Put the potato strings on the dough piece and then roll it up. Cut the roll into 5 cm sections, put them in a steamer tray, and steam for 10 minutes. Serve with different sauces to taste.

Vegetarian: ✓   Muslim: ✓

Pepper oil-flavored shredded potato
Jiaoyou Tudou Si

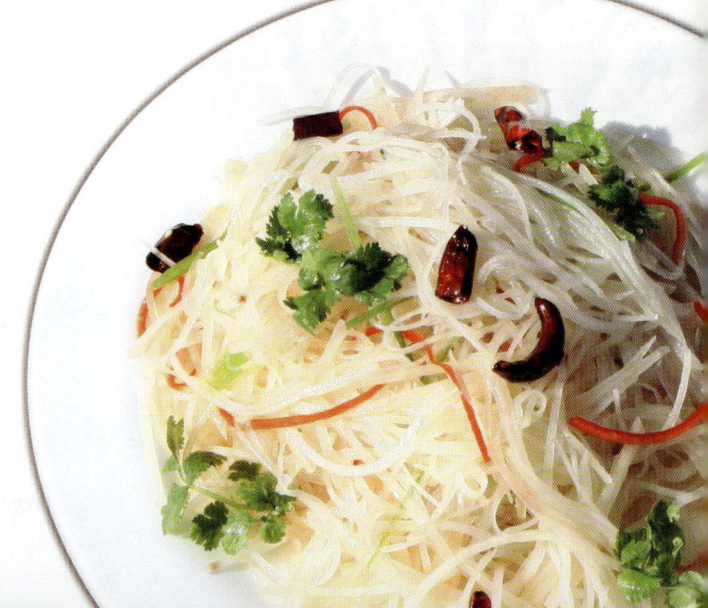

Ingredient:

Potato 500 g

Seasonings:

A little salt, gourmet powder, Chinese prickly ash oil and white vinegar

Preparation:

Finely shred potatoes, then add oil and salt in water to quick-boil the potato strings. When they cool down, add seasonings and mix well.

Vegetarian: ✓   Muslim: ✓

Pickled Chinese cabbage with mashed potatoes
Suancai Tudou Ni

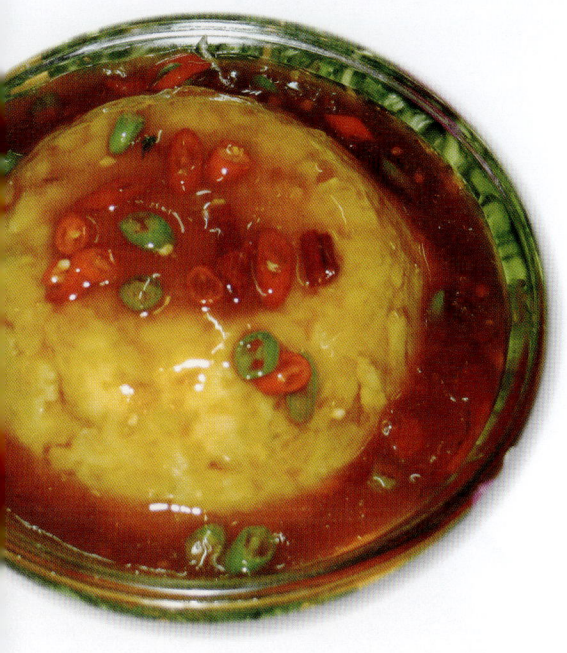

Ingredients:
Pickled Chinese cabbage 250 g, potato 300 g, blade meat (or side pork) 100 g, red and green) bell pepper 50 g

Seasonings:
Green onion, ginger, garlic, a little salt and soy sauce

Preparation:
1. Mince pickled Chinese cabbage, make potato paste, quick-boil and deep-fry the sliced pork.
2. Put meat, green onion, ginger and garlic into wok and fry until it give off aroma, then add minced pickled Chinese cabbage and mashed potatoes with a little salt and soy sauce and stir-fry over medium heat until the mashed potatoes mix evenly with the pickled Chinese cabbage.

Vegetarian: ✗   Muslim: ✗

Potato and millet porridge
Qiangguo Malingshu Xifan

Ingredients:
Potato 300 g, millet 150 g

Seasonings:
Coriander 20 g, green onion 10 g, refined salt 3 g, vegetable oil 20 g

Preparation:
1. Peel potatoes and cut them into pieces.
2. Wash millet then add water. The proportion of millet to water is 1:6. Boil over high heat, add potato pieces, then reduce to low heat and stew for 20 minutes. Remove to a soup dish.
3. Heat oil in the wok, put coriander and minced green onion and fry until it gives off aroma. Then put in the soup dish, mix with salt, and serve.

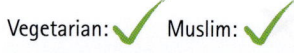
Vegetarian: ✓   Muslim: ✓

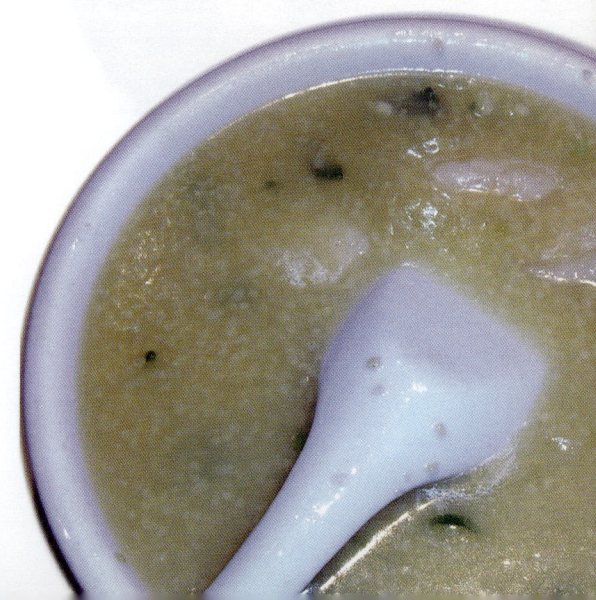

Potato and oat pancake
Tudou Bing II

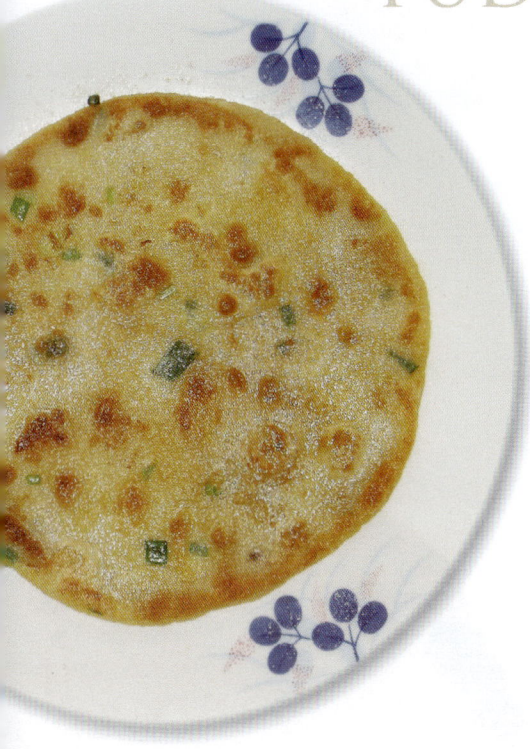

Seasonings:
Minced green onion 40 g, cooking oil 50 g, refined salt 10 g

Preparation:
1. Boil cleaned potatoes, then remove and peel while hot. Mince peeled potatoes with a grater, then use pestle to finely mash them.
2. Put 200 g of oat flour, salt and minced green onion into the mashed potatoes, mix evenly, then knead in the pan repeatedly to make dough.
3. Add 50 g of oat flour into the dough and knead well. Divide into dumpling dough pieces of about 70 g each and roll into cakes.
4. Put 5 g of oil in a flat-bottomed pan and heat. Add the cakes and fry over medium heat. After the cakes become golden yellow, brush oil on both sides, remove and serve while hot.

Ingredients:
Potato 500 g, oat flour 250 g

Vegetarian: ✓   Muslim: ✓

Potato cake II
Malingshu Bing

Ingredients:
Potato 400 g, wheat flour 150 g, potato starch 100 g, linseed oil 50 g

Seasoning:
Refined salt 3 g

Preparation:
1. Boil the cleaned potatoes then mash them into paste with a potato grater.
2. Heat linseed oil in a pan, then fry potato cakes until both sides turn golden brown.

Vegetarian: ✓ Muslim: ✓

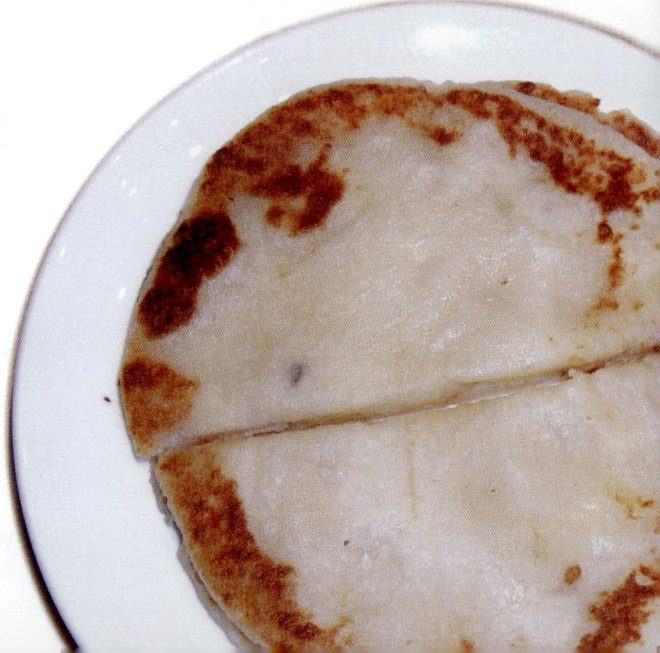

Potato chips with fried pork fillet
Guoyourou Malingshu Pian

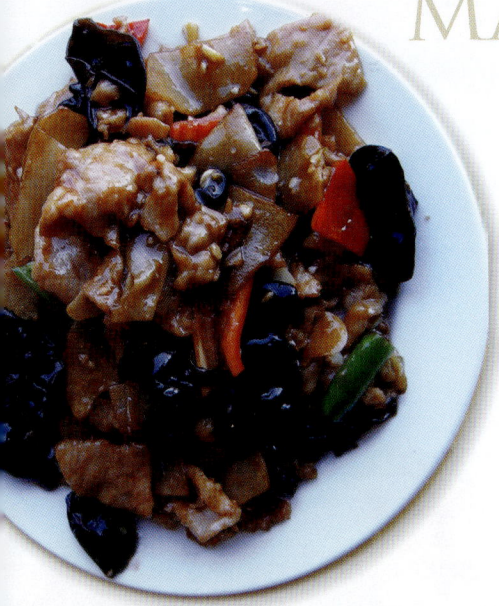

Preparation:

1. Slice the pork loin into fillets 2cm wide and 2cm long. Put it into a bowl and mix with some Chinese prickly ash water, soybean sauce, table salt, egg and starch. Marinate for 60 minutes. Deep-fry the fillet until it turns golden brown, then remove.

2. Clean the potato and cut into chips about the same size as the pork fillets. Fry the potato chips until golden brown.

3. Slice green and red pepper, black agaric, green onion and garlic. Finely mince the ginger.

4. Put lard into the frying pan, heat it and stir-fry the green onion, minced ginger and garlic. Add the pork fillets in, add some vinegar and cook for a little bit, then add the potato chips. Then add black agaric, green and red pepper, some cooking wine, gourmet powder, soybean sauce and wet starch sauce. Stir-fry a little bit and serve.

Ingredients:

Pork loin 200 g, potato 300 g, lard 500 g

Seasonings:

Black agric 15 g, green pepper 25 g, red pepper 25 g, garlic 5 g, vinegar 20 g, Chinese prickly ash water 5 g, green onion stalk 20 g, soybean sauce 15 g, fresh ginger 15 g, table salt 5 g, cooking wine 5 g, wet starch 80 g, gourmet powder 5 g

Vegetarian: ✗   Muslim: ✗

Potato egg cake with sesame seeds
Malingshu Jidan Zhima Bing

Ingredients:
Potato 400 g, egg 120 g, wheat flour 150 g, potato starch 100 g, sesame seed 2 g, linseed oil 50 g

Seasonings:
Minced green onion 10 g, refined salt 3 g

Preparation:
1. Boil cleaned potatoes, then mash with a potato grater.
2. Put mashed potatoes in a bowl, add egg, wheat flour, starch, green onion and refined salt and knead into dough. Roll the dough into a raw cake and sprinkle with sesame seeds.
3. Heat sesame oil and fry the cake until both sides turn golden brown.

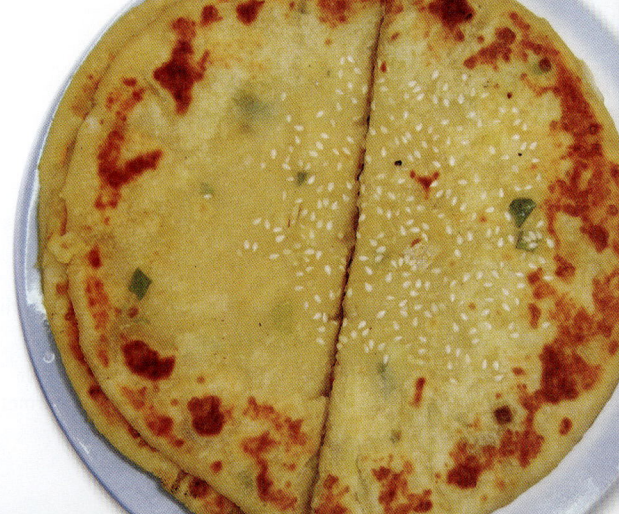

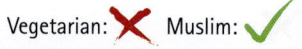

Potato Kuilei
Tudou Kuilei

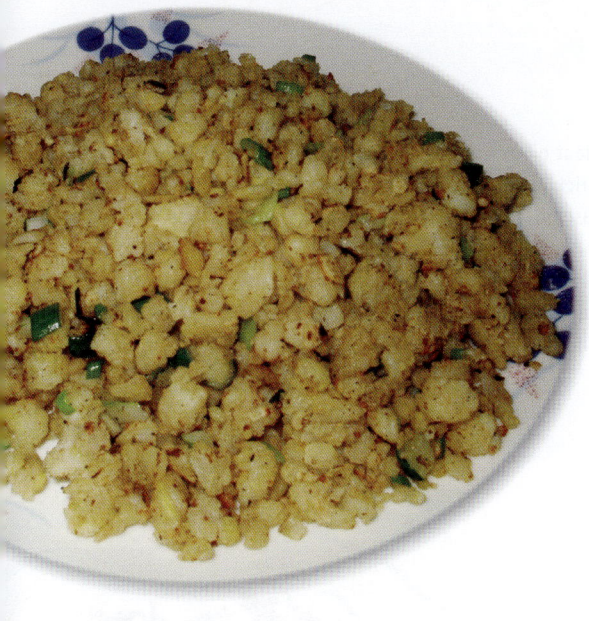

Ingredients:
Potato 500 g, oat flour 200 g

Seasonings:
Cooking oil 5 g, minced green onion 10 g, refined salt 5 g, gourmet powder, Chinese prickly ash 1 g

Preparation:
1. Boil potatoes, then peel while hot and mince with a grater.
2. Mix well with oat flour, refined salt, minced green onion, gourmet powder and Chinese prickly ash.
3. Add oil into wok and heat over high heat, then reduce to medium heat and stir-fry the potatoes until golden yellow. Remove and serve while hot.

Vegetarian: ✓ Muslim: ✓

Potato lambsquarter goosefoot salad in vinegar sauce
Malingshu Ban Huicai

Ingredients:
Potato 200 g, lambsquarter goosefoot 300 g, linseed oil 20 g

Seasonings:
Onion 5 g, ginger 5 g, garlic 5 g, Chinese prickly ash 3 g, salt 5 g, gourmet powder 2 g, vinegar 5 g, sesame oil 5 g

Preparation:
1. Peel potatoes, then boil and dice them.
2. Clean lambsquarter goosefeet, cut into sections, then quick-boil. Remove from boiling water and cool, then mix evenly with the potato pieces.
3. Heat oil in a wok over high heat, then fry Chinese prickly ash until it smokes. Remove the ash and discard. Stir-fry the minced green onion, minced ginger and garlic until it gives off aroma, then put a dish with diced potato and lambsquarter goosefoot, add refined salt, gourmet powder, vinegar and sesame oil and mix evenly.

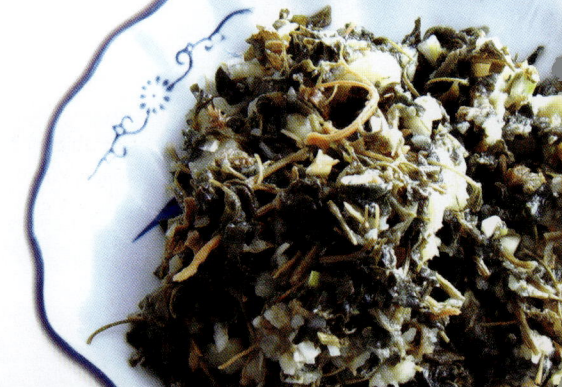

Vegetarian: ✓   Muslim: ✓

Potato noodles mixed with sauce
Jiachang Ban Fen

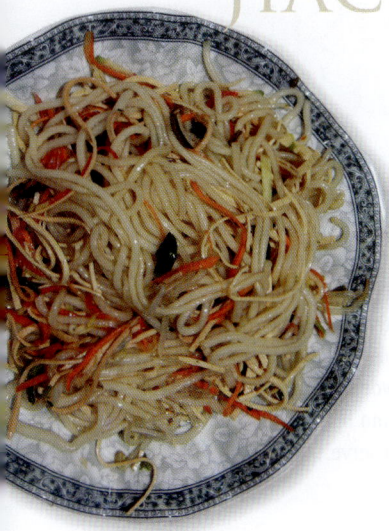

Ingredients:
Potato starch 500 g

Seasonings:
Alum 3 g, cucumber 50 g, mung bean sprout 50 g, soybean milk film 50 g, spinach 30 g, watermelon radish 50 g, red radish 50 g, Chinese prickly ash 3 g, vegetable oil 30 g, sesame oil 5 g table salt 5 g, vinegar 10 g, gourmet powder 3 g, green onion 5 g, garlic 5 g, fresh ginger 5 g

Preparation:
Preparation of fresh noodles made from potato starch:

1. Put 150 g of starch in a bowl with 250 g of boiling water and stir until it becomes a paste. Quickly put boiling water into the paste while stirring. After about 10 minutes, when the paste becomes transparent, transfer it to a big bowl with ground alum and mix well. Then add 350 g of starch and mix well with the paste, kneading it to soft dough.

2. Boil water in a cooking pot. Put the paste through a traditional Chinese noodle maker and let the noodles drop into the boiling water. Take them out when done and place in cool water, then place in a dish.

Preparation of sauce used to mix with the noodles:

1. Quick-boil the mung bean sprout and spinach. Remove and cool. Shred cucumber, watermelon radish, carrot and soybean milk film. Put all of them into the dish with the noodles.

2. Fry Chinese prickly ash in oil, then remove and discard. Fry the minced green onion, garlic and ginger in the wok, then add to the dish. Mix with sesame oil, salt, vinegar and gourmet powder.

Vegetarian: ✓ Muslim: ✓

Potato noodles with needle mushrooms
Malingshu Fensi Jinzhengu

Ingredients:
Potato starch noodles 50 g, needle mushroom 200 g, dried dark edible fungus 100 g

Seasonings:
Wet starch 10 g, refined salt 5 g, garlic 5 g, minced green scallion 10 g, Chinese prickly ash 3 g, ginger 5 g, soy sauce 5 g, chicken essence 3 g, sesame oil 5 g, vegetable oil 20 g

Preparation:
1. Marinate potato starch noodles for 20 minutes, then boil until they become soft. Warp the noodles into small bunches and place on a plate.
2. Quickly stew the cleaned needle mushroom and put on the potato starch noodles.
3. Cut dark edible fungus into pieces. Heat oil over high heat and fry the Chinese prickly ash until it smokes, then remove and discard. Fry the minced green scallion, ginger ash and garlic ash until they give off aroma. Then stir-fry with dark edible fungus. Add water and bring to a boil. Add a little refined salt, soy sauce and gourmet powder. Thicken soup with wet starch, add sesame oil and remove to a dish. Sprinkle the minced scallion and serve.

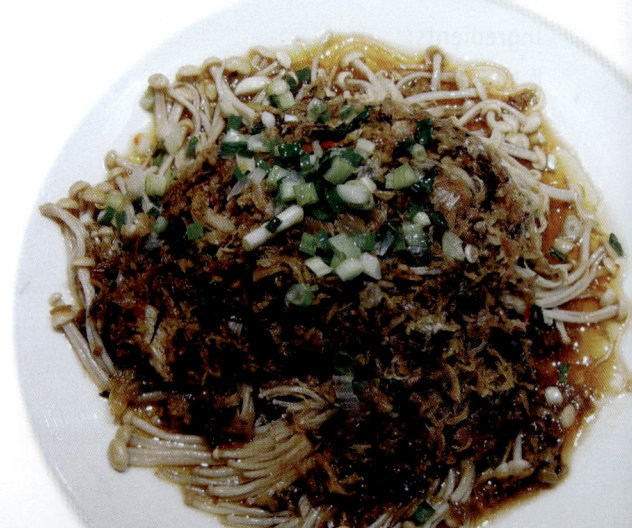

Vegetarian: ✗   Muslim: ✓

Potato Pie
Malingshu Gao

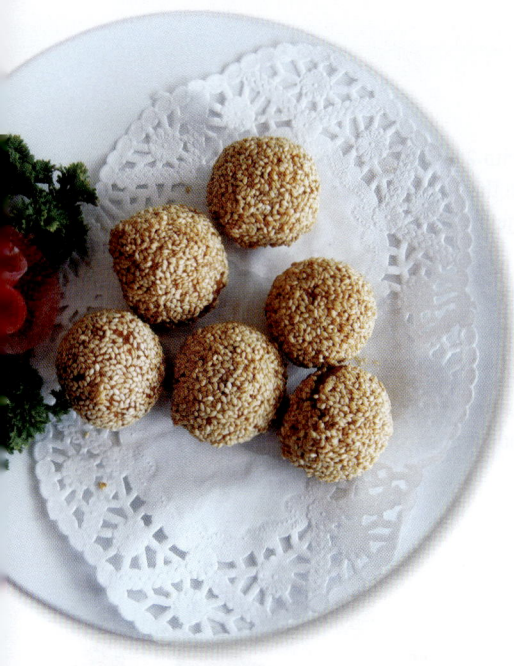

Preparation:

1. Peel and mash the cooked potatoes. Put into a basin.
2. Put sesame seeds in the frying pan and fry over low heat. Set aside.
3. Peel cleaned apples, removing seeds and skin, and mash. Mix the apple mash, white sugar and honey together with soy sauce. Add the prepared potatoes and stir evenly. Knead the potato paste into several identical-size small balls.
4. Heat linseed oil in a pan until medium-hot, then add the balls and deep-fry until they turn golden brown. Remove and coat the balls with sesame seeds.

Ingredients:

Potato 500 g, flour 150 g, white sugar 100 g, sesame seed 50 g, apple 100 g

Seasonings:

Honey 5 g, soy sauce 5 g

Vegetarian: ✓ Muslim: ✓

Potato pot-stickers
Malingshu Guotie

Ingredients:
Potato 800 g, oat flour 150 g, starch 100 g, leek 150 g, carrot 100 g

Seasonings:
Refined salt 5 g, Chinese prickly ash 3 g, gourmet powder glutamate 3 g, chicken essence 3 g, soy sauce 5 g, sesame oil 5 g, linseed oil 20 g

Preparation:
1. Peel and shred potatoes and carrots, cut leek into pieces and put in a bowl together with refined salt, Chinese prickly ash, gourmet powder, chicken essence, soy sauce, sesame oil, and linseed oil. Mix well and put aside to use as filling.
2. Peel 500 g of cooked potatoes and mash. Put a bowl, adding starch and oat flour to make dough. Divide the dough into four portions and roll into long rolls, then cut each into 25 pieces. Flatten each piece and roll into 2 inches (5 cm) pot-sticker wrapper. Put fillings on the wrappers, then fold and pinch the edges together tightly.
3. Heat the pan, add a little oil and fry the pot-stickers until the bottom turns golden brown. Then add half a cup of water, cover the pot, turn to medium heat and stew for two minutes until the soup evaporates.
4. Add linseed oil, cover the pot again, and fry until the bottom side is crisp, then serve.

Vegetarian: ✗   Muslim: ✓

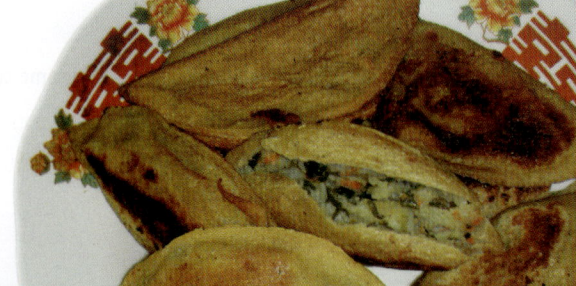

Potato strings with lichen
Dipicai Malingshu Si

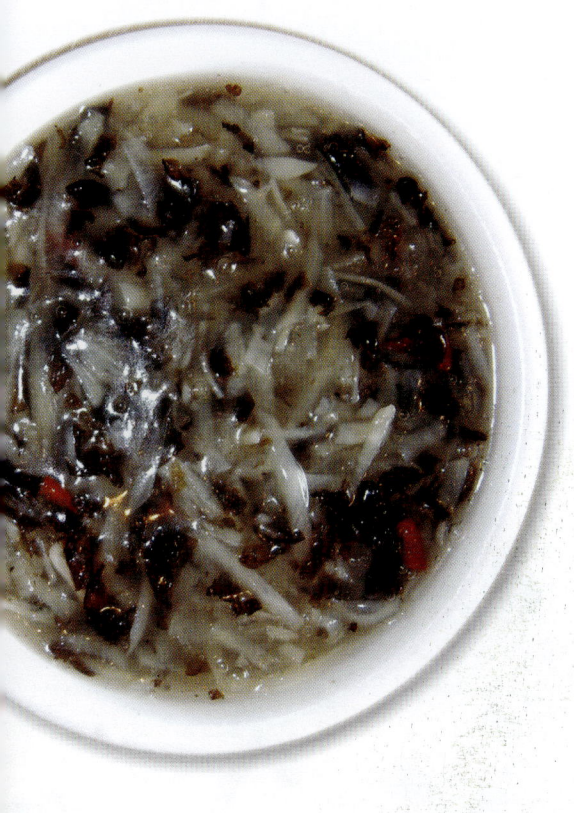

Ingredients:
Lichen 100 g, potato 300 g, vegetable oil 30 g

Seasonings:
Chili 3, garlic 5 g, Chinese prickly ash 1 g, table salt 5 g

Preparation:
1. Clean lichen and drain water. Peel potatoes and slice into strings, then put them into clean water. Chop red pepper into pieces.

2. Fry Chinese prickly ash in a wok over high heat. Remove when black. Put the chili and green and red pepper in the wok and stir-fry, then add the lichen, garlic and red pepper and stir-fry them.

3. Add water, some table salt and the potato strings. Then add some gourmet powder, cook to a boil and serve.

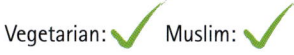

Vegetarian: ✓   Muslim: ✓

Potato strips with Japanese rhodea
Wannianqing malingshu Tiao

Ingredients:
Potato 300 g, Japanese rhodea 150 g, tofu 300 g, vegetable oil 20 g

Seasonings:
Green onion 10 g, ginger 5 g, garlic 5 g, gourmet powder 5 g, sesame oil 5 g, refined salt 5 g

Preparation:
1. Peel potatoes and cut into strips, cut Japanese rhodea into sections, cut tofu into strips, mince green onion and ginger, and slice garlic.
2. Heat oil, then add onion, ginger, garlic and water. After it boils, add the potato strips, Japanese rhodea and bean curd and stew for 10 minutes. Then add gourmet powder, sesame oil and salt. Remove and serve.

Vegetarian: ✓   Muslim: ✓

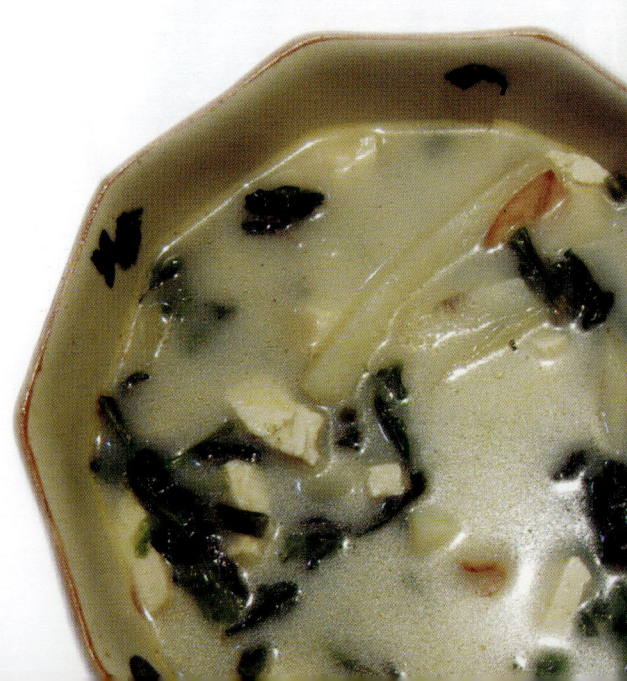

Potato-Oat Flour Made Fishlike Noodles
Xiangjian Tudou Roujuan

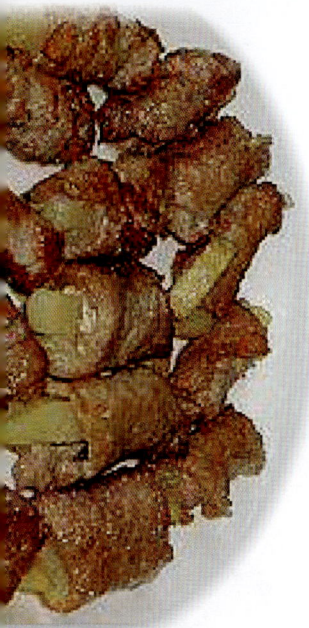

Preparation:

1. Slice pork fillet into thin slices, then add salt, soy sauce, chicken essence and rice wine to pickle the pork for a while. (Add a little starch to make the pork more tender.)

2. Peel potatoes and cut them into strips. Boil the strips for 1 minute then remove.

3. Put water starch on the pork pieces and lay two or three potato strips on each piece and make into a roll.

4. Heat oil in a wok and fry the pork rolls until they turn brown.

5. Keep oil in the wok and use soup stock, soy sauce, salt and gourmet powder to make thick sauce, then spread on the fried pork rolls.

Ingredients:

Potato 300 g, pork fillet 500 g

Seasonings:

Peanut oil, soy sauce, starch, salt, chicken essence and rice wine

Vegetarian: ✗ Muslim: ✗

Roasted potato
Kao Malingshu

Ingredient:
Potato 500 g

Seasonings:
Brined vegetable 100 g, salty vegetable 100 g, pickled vegetable 50 g

Preparation:
1. Clean the potatoes. Drain off excessive water.
2. Places potatoes in the oven and roast about 90 minutes at 220°C.
3. Potatoes are done when they become golden brown and crispy. Serve with brined, salty, or pickled vegetables.

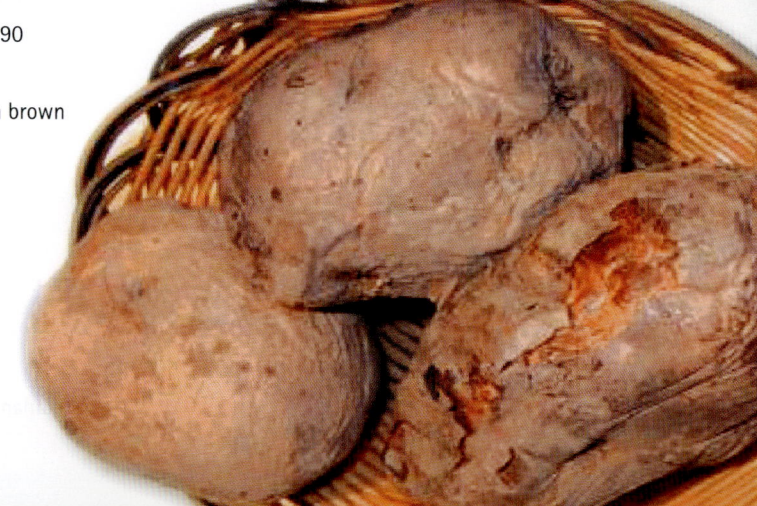

Vegetarian: ✓   Muslim: ✓

Roasted potato slices
Kao Malingshu Pian

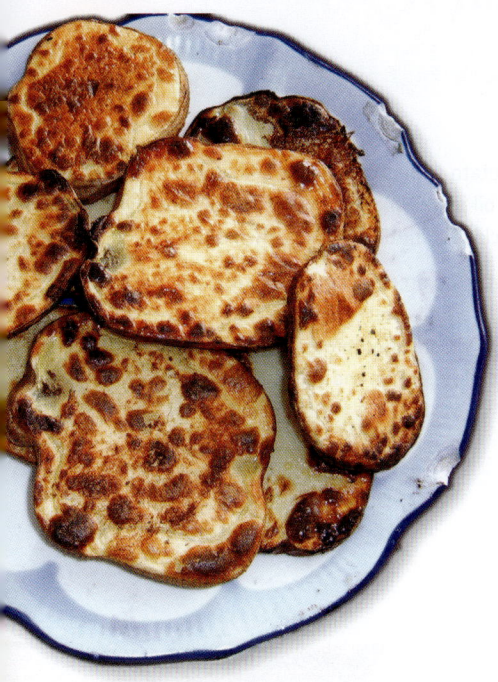

Preparation:

1. Peel and slice potato, then put in water to remove starch. Remove and drain.

2. Heat the pan, add oil and fry the potato slices. When potato slices turn yellow, add a little water, cover the pan, reduce to medium heat and stew for 2 minutes.

3. Sprinkle the potatoes with linseed oil, cover the pan and fry the other side of potato pieces until golden brown. Serve with brined, soy-pickled or pickled vegetables.

5. Keep oil in the wok and use soup stock, soy sauce, salt and gourmet powder to make thick sauce, then spread on the fried pork rolls.

Ingredients:

Potato 300 g, linseed oil 20 g

Seasonings:

Brined vegetable 100 g, soy-pickled vegetables 100 g, pickled vegetable 50 g

Vegetarian: ✓   Muslim: ✓

Shredded potato and wild vegetables in vinegar and spices
Malingshu Si Ban Yan Kucai

Ingredients:
Potato 100 g, pickled wild vegetables 300 g

Seasonings:
Chinese prickly ash 3 g, vegetable oil 20 g, sesame oil 5 g, table salt 5 g, vinegar 10 g, gourmet powder 3 g, green onion 5 g, garlic 5 g

Preparation:
1. Pickling wild vegetables: Clean the wild vegetables and boil, removing quickly when done.. Cool the vegetables, then put in a jar and add some millet soup. The pickled wild vegetables will be ready within 48 hours.

2. Potato preparation: Clean and peel potatoes and cut them into strings. Put the potato strings in water to remove starch. Then boil the potato strings until cooked. Remove and cool down.

3. Place the potato strings and wild vegetables on a plate. Heat oil in a frying pan over high heat and fry Chinese prickly ash until it smokes, then discard.

4. Lightly stir-fry the green onion, then put it and the oil on the potato strings and vegetables. Mix the sesame oil, table salt, vinegar, gourmet powder and garlic and put on the potato strings and vegetables, then serve.

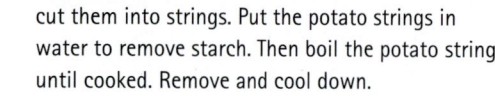
Vegetarian: ✓   Muslim: ✓

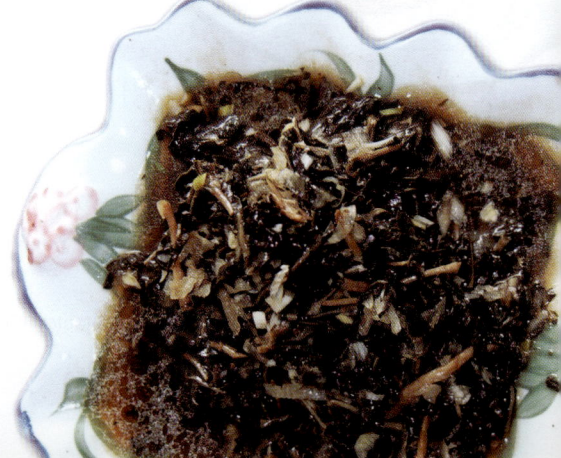

Shredded potato with sow thistle
Malingshu Si Ban Kucai

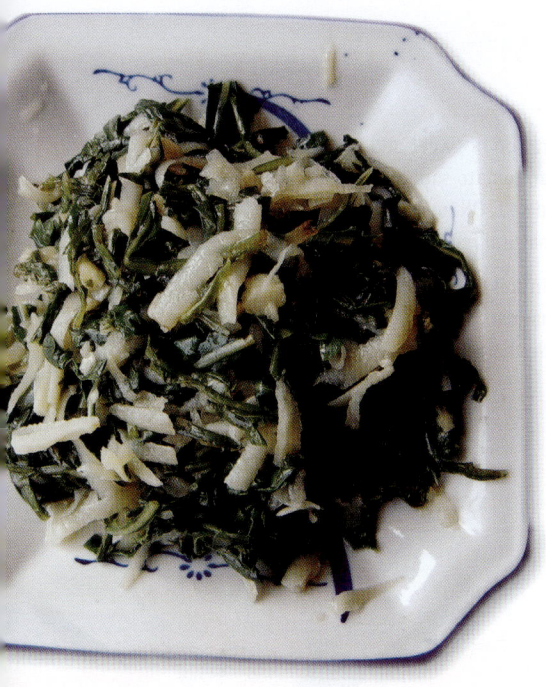

Ingredients:
Potato 200 g, sow thistle 300 g

Seasonings:
Linseed oil 20 g, onion 5 g, ginger 5 g, garlic 5 g, Chinese prickly ash 3 g, salt 5 g, gourmet powder 2 g, vinegar 5 g, sesame oil 5 g

Preparation:
1. Peel potatoes and shred with a grater, then put in water to remove starch. Cut the sow thistle into sections and put potato strings and sow thistle into boiling water to quick-boil. Remove, cool down and place on a dish.

2. Heat oil in wok over high heat and fry Chinese prickly ash until it smokes, then discard. Stir-fry the minced green onion, ginger and garlic until it gives off aroma, then put on dish with potato strings and sow thistle. Mix evenly with refined salt, gourmet powder, vinegar and sesame oil.

Vegetarian: ✓   Muslim: ✓

Silver boat carries the valuables
Yinzhou Zaibao

Ingredients:
Potato 1,000 g, sweetened bean paste 1,500 g

Seasonings:
Salt 10 g, salad oil 1,500 g, white vinegar 1,000 g, tomato sauce 200 g, sweet and sour plum 40 g, sugar bar 600 g, refined salt 20 g, OK juice 1/4 bottle, a little natural red food coloring

Preparation:
1. Peel potatoes, boil or steam, then make mashed potatoes. Add a little salt.
2. Wrap the sweetened bean paste with mashed potatoes, and knead the potato balls into Yuanbao (an ancient Chinese hard currency) shape about 6 cm in length. Put the pieces on a plate and set aside.
3. Heat the oil and fry the Yuanbao potatoes until brown, then remove.
4. Preparation of sweet and sour juice: Mix white vinegar, tomato sauce, sweet and sour plum, sugar, refined salt, OK juice (sour and sweet fruit juice) and a little natural red food coloring in a bowl.
5. Fold tin foil to make a boat and use it as a plate. Place the Yuanbao potatoes in the tin foil boat, then sprinkle them with sweet and sour juice to taste and serve.

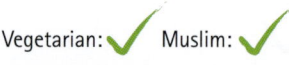

Vegetarian: ✓   Muslim: ✓

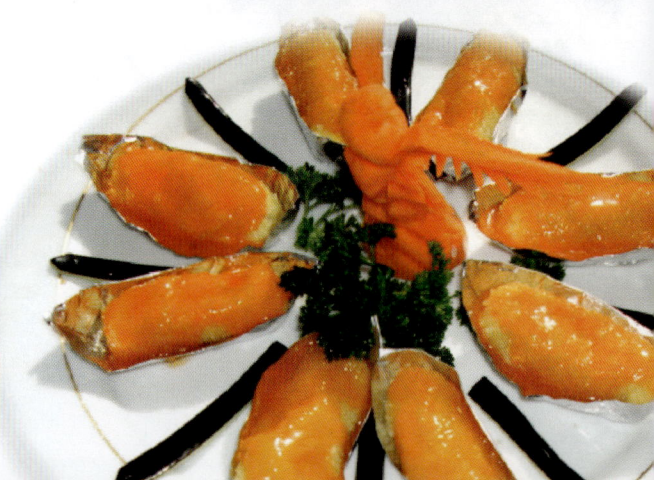

Soft-shell turtle encircled with small potatoes
Xiao Tudou Jiayu

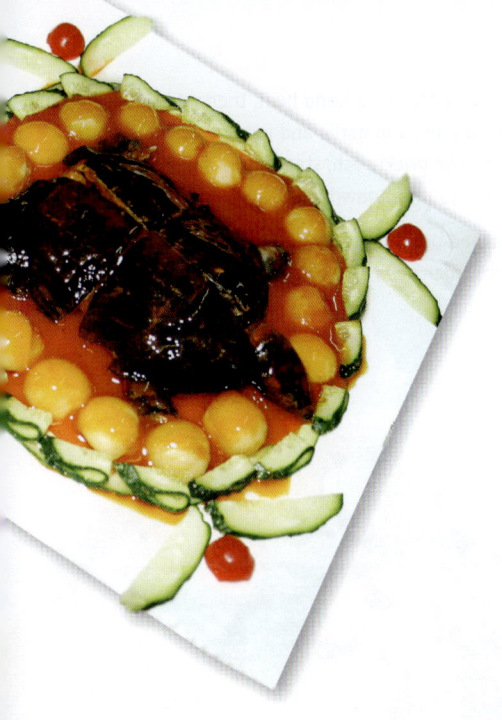

Ingredients:
Soft-shelled turtles 600 g, potato 200 g,

Seasonings:
Hot pepper, thick bean sauce, hot sauce, salt to taste

Preparation:
1. Remove harslet in soft-shell turtle, clean thoroughly and chop into pieces. Peel potatoes and make it into small potato balls.
2. Put turtle pieces and potato balls in a wok with hot pepper, thick bean sauce and hot sauce to fry until they give off aroma.
3. Put into pressure cooker with soup stock to stew for 7–8 minutes over medium heat.

Vegetarian: ✗ Muslim: ✗

Spareribs with Chinese sauerkraut and mashed potatoes
Paigu Suancai Malingshu Ni

Ingredients:
Potato 400 g, spareribs 200 g, Chinese sauerkraut 200 g, pakchoi 100 g, lard (refined) 30 g

Seasonings:
Green onion 20 g, ginger 15 g, garlic 10 g, Chinese prickly ash 3 g, star anise 5 g, salt 10 g, gourmet powder 5 g, cooking wine 5 g

Preparation:
1. Steam the potatoes, then peel and mash. Cut the Chinese sauerkraut into strips. Clean the pakchoi, cut into strips and blanch in boiling water until cooked.
2. Cut the spareribs into pieces about 5 cm in length. Slice the ginger and garlic and cut the green onion into strips. Blanch the spareribs in boiling water, and rinse off the froth.
3. Put some oil in a frying pan and heat, then add the green onion, ginger, and garlic and lightly stir-fry. Add the soup, Chinese prickly ash, star anise, cooking wine, salt and gourmet powder and stew until cooked.
4. Mix the mashed potatoes, Chinese sauerkraut, pakchoi and spareribs, then serve.

Vegetarian: ✗   Muslim: ✗

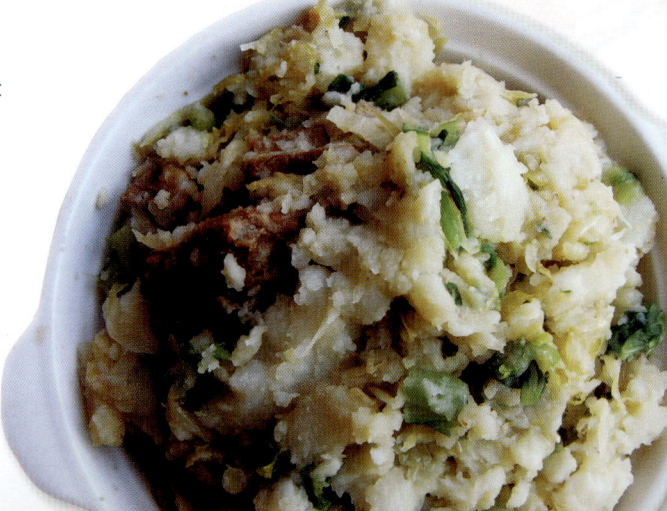

Spicy diced potatoes I
Xiangla Malingshu Ding

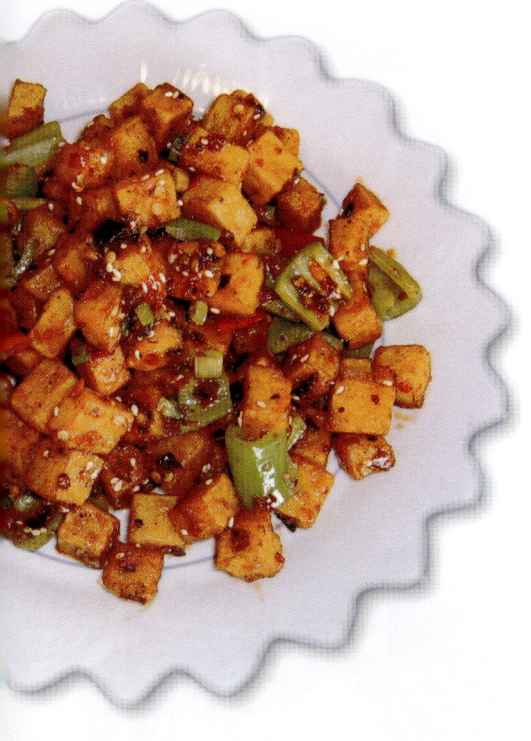

Ingredients:
Potato 300 g, green pepper 20 g, red pepper 5 g, minced dried pepper 20 g, sesame seed 3 g, linseed oil 200 g

Seasonings:
Minced green onion 5 g, salt 3 g, gourmet powder 2 g, chili powder 3 g

Preparation:
1. Peel and dice potatoes and put in clear water to remove starch, then drain. Fry potato pieces until crisp and golden brown, then remove, drain excess oil and set aside. Dice green and red peppers.

2. Heat oil in wok over high heat stir-fry minced dried pepper and minced green onion until it gives off aroma. Then add diced potatoes, green hot pepper and red hot pepper and stir-fry. Season with salt, gourmet powder, chili powder and sesame seed, then serve.

Vegetarian: ✓   Muslim: ✓

Spicy shredded potatoes
Xiangla Tudou Si

Ingredient:
Potato 700 g

Seasonings:
Oil 1,000 g, dried red pepper 20 g, green onion 20 g, cilantro 10 g, salt, gourmet powder and Chinese prickly ash powder

Preparation:
1. Peel potatoes and cut them into thick strips. Shred dried red pepper and green onion. Cut cilantro into sections.

2. Heat oil and fry the shredded potatoes. Remove once they turn brown. Fry the shredded dried pepper until brown and crisp, then remove and discard.

3. Mix the shredded potatoes with cilantro sections, shredded green onion, salt gourmet powder and Chinese prickly ash powder and stir well.

Vegetarian: ✓   Muslim: ✓

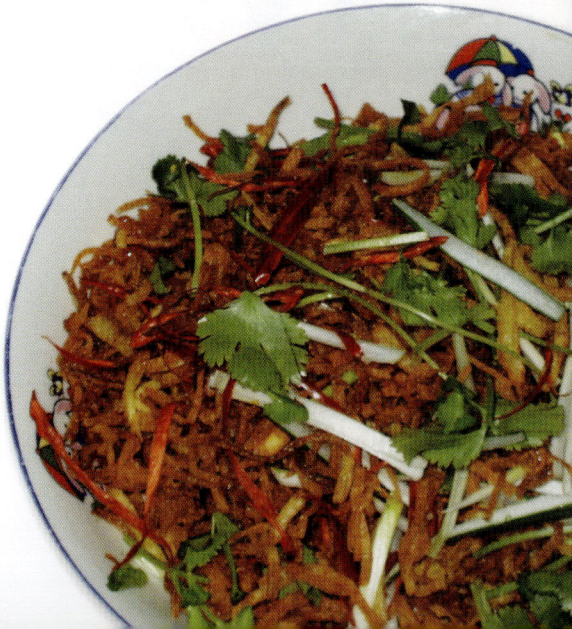

Steamed abalone-shaped potato pie
Su Bao Pai Fan

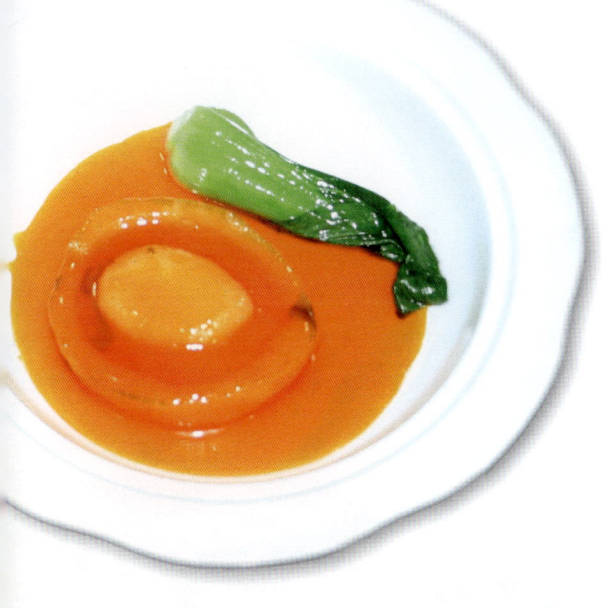

Ingredients:
Potato 500 g, abalone juice 150 g

Preparation:
1. Carve potatoes into abalone shape and steam in a steamer. Be aware of not overcooking. Add seasonings.
2. Spread abalone juice over the potato and serve with rice.

Vegetarian: ✗ Muslim: ✓

Steamed buns with potato and Chinese chive filling
Tudou Jiucai Baozi

Ingredients:
Wheat flour 500 g, potato 500 g, Chinese chives 250 g

Seasonings:
Green onion, refined salt, gourmet powder, soy sauce, Chinese prickly ash, aniseed powder, vegetable oil

Preparation:
1. Peel, clean and dice potatoes, mince Chinese chives, add green onion, refined salt, gourmet powder, soy sauce, ginger powder, Chinese prickly ash, aniseed powder and vegetable oil, and mix well, then set aside.

2. Ferment wheat flour and knead well. Roll the dough with a rolling pin into a column shape, then divide into several sections. Roll the sections into dumpling wrappers with a diameter of 5 cm and wrap the filling. Steam the dumplings for 20 minutes.

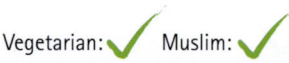
Vegetarian: ✓ Muslim: ✓

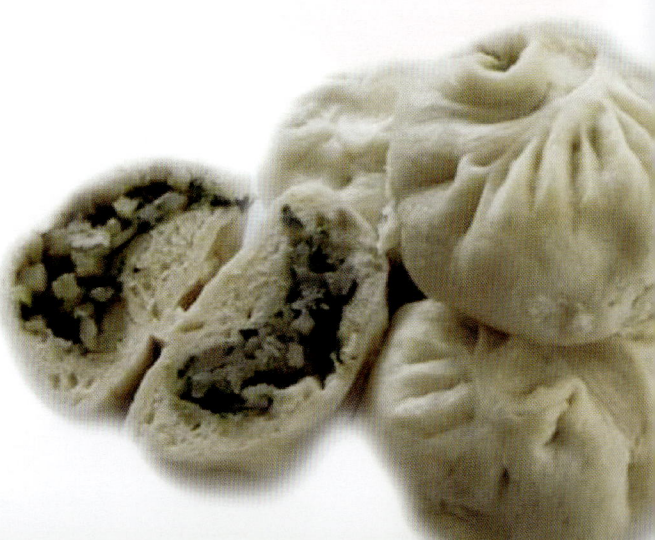

Steamed Dumplings
Zheng Jiao

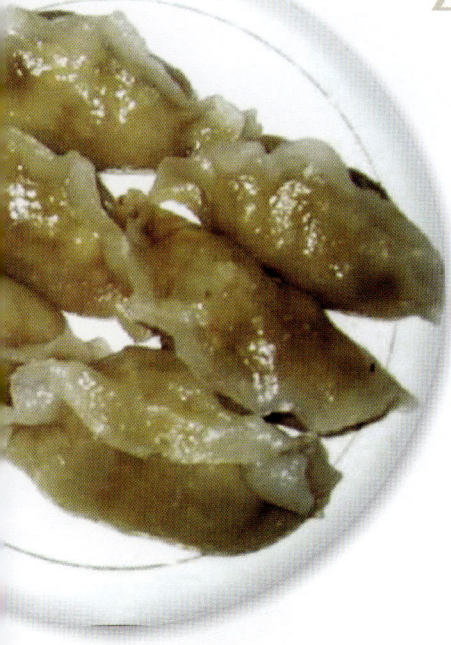

Preparation:

1. Put starch in a bowl, add boiling water and stir well. Then add oat flour, knead and set aside.

2. Mix pork filling with green onion, refined salt, gourmet powder, soy sauce, ginger powder, Chinese prickly ash, aniseed powder and vegetable oil. Peel and dice potatoes, then add pork filling and stir well, then set aside.

3. Place the well-kneaded dough on a bread board and roll the dough with a rolling pin into a column shape, then divide into several sections. Roll the sections into dumpling wrappers about 5 cm in diameter and wrap the pork filling, then steam for 20 minutes.

Ingredients:

Oat flour 250 g, starch 250 g, potato 400 g, pork filling 100 g

Seasonings:

Green onion to taste, refined salt, gourmet powder, soy sauce, ginger powder, Chinese prickly ash, aniseed powder, vegetable oil

Vegetarian: ✗   Muslim: ✗

Steamed fish-shaped oat noodles
Youmian Zheng Yu

Ingredients:
Potato 1,000 g, oat flour 200 g

Seasonings:
Adjusted according to individual taste

Preparation:
1. Clean the potatoes and boil in water. Remove, peel and mash, then add oat flour. Knead the dough into fish-shape dumplings about 4 cm long.
2. Steam for 8 minutes. Serve with seasonings to taste.

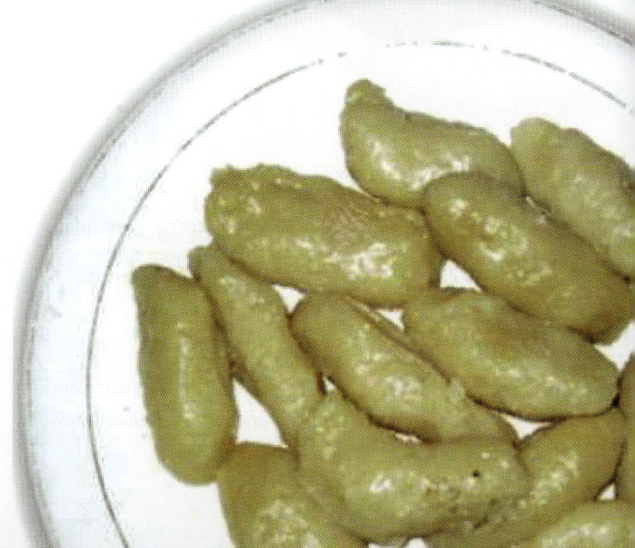

Vegetarian: ✓ Muslim: ✓

Steamed fish-shaped potatoes with Chinese sauerkraut
Suancai Malingshu Yu

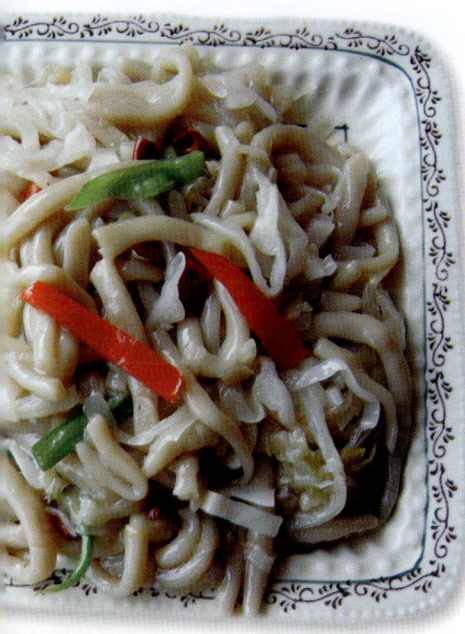

Seasonings:

A little red pepper, green and red paprika 20 g, table salt 5 g, chicken essence 3 g, Chinese prickly ash 3 g, green onion 10 g, garlic 5 g, fresh ginger 5 g, vegetable oil 20 g

Preparation:

1. Fish-shaped potatoes: Steam the potatoes, peel and mash them. Mix the plain flour, starch and potatoes and knead them into dough. Divide the dough into small portions and knead each into a fish shape, then steam for about 10 minutes.

2. Cut the Chinese sauerkraut into pieces. Heat oil in frying pan over high heat and fry Chinese prickly ash until it smokes, then discard. Quick-fry red pepper, green and red paprika, green onion, ginger and garlic. Add the Chinese sauerkraut pieces and potato dough and stir-fry. Season with table salt and gourmet powder, then serve.

Ingredients:

Potato 500 g, plain flour 125 g, starch 125 g, Chinese sauerkraut 200 g

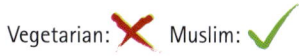

Steamed oat rolls with potato and eggplant
Malingshu Men Qiezi

Ingredients:
Potato 300 g, oat flour 200 g, eggplant 150 g, pork 200 g, lard (refined) 30 g, onion 15 g, green pepper 25 g

Seasonings:
Green onion 10 g, onion 15 g, ginger 5 g, garlic 10 g, soy sauce 5 g, vinegar 5 g, Chinese prickly ash 3 g, star anise 5 g, salt 10 g, chicken essence 5 g, cooking wine 5 g

Preparation:
1. Add boiled water to oat flour and make a slightly hard dough. Make small dumplings from the dough and roll on a smooth marble cooking-board. Put the rolls on a steamer tray one by one to form a honeycomb shape. Steam for 10 minutes.
2. Slice pork, peel potatoes and cut into pieces, dice onion and green pepper, slice ginger and garlic, and cut green onion into sections.
3. Heat oil and fry green onion, ginger and garlic until it gives off aroma, then add the pork and stir-fry. Add soy sauce and vinegar and fry slightly.
4. Add water, Chinese prickly ash, star anise, cooking wine, salt and chicken essence and stew until almost done, then add potatoes and eggplant and stew on medium heat to make the sauce. Put the cooked soup on steamed oat rolls and sprinkle with onion and green pepper.

Vegetarian: ✗ Muslim: ✗

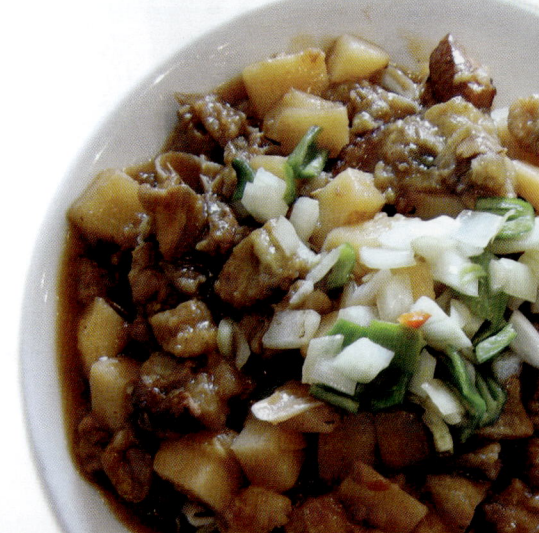

Steamed potato balls
Tudou Wanzi

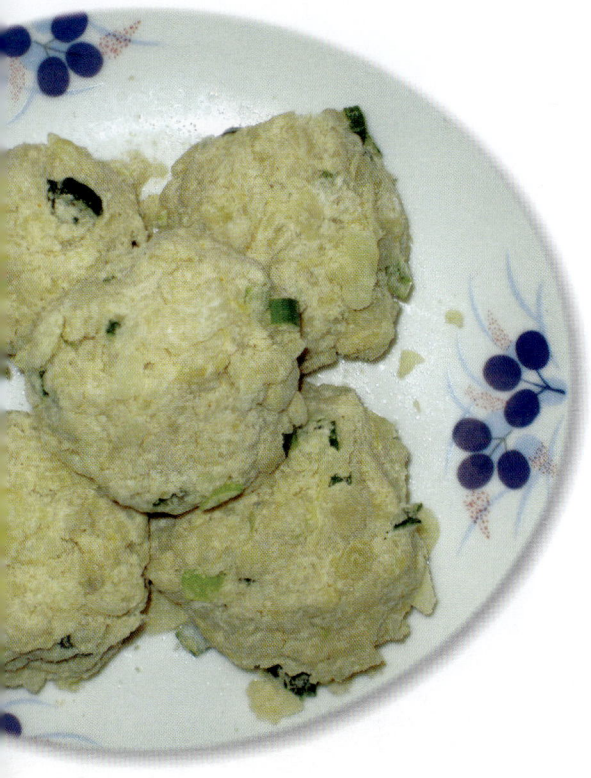

Ingredients:
Potato 500 g, oat flour 200 g

Seasonings:
Minced green onion 10 g, refined salt 5 g, gourmet powder 1 g, Chinese prickly ash 1 g

Preparation:
1. Clean and boil potatoes, then peel while hot and mince with a grater.
2. Mix oat flour, refined salt, minced green onion and Chinese prickly ash together with the potatoes.. Knead the mixture into dough, then put on a steamer tray and set aside.
3. Boil 500 g of water in the steamer over high heat, then steam the dough for about 6 minutes, remove from the steamer, and serve.

Vegetarian: ✓ Muslim: ✓

Steamed potato cake
Zheng Malingshu Yangz[i]

Ingredients:
Potato 400 g, oat flour 250 g

Seasonings:
Refined salt 3 g, Chinese prickly ash 3 g, sliced green onion 10 g, gourmet powder 1 g, linseed oil 10 g

Preparation:
1. Peel and shred potatoes, then wash in water to remove starch.
2. Mix oat flour, refined salt, Chinese prickly ash, minced green onion, gourmet powder and linseed oil with the potatoes to make potato dough. Roll the dough into several cake-like circles, braise in a steamer for 15 minutes.

Vegetarian: ✓ Muslim: ✓

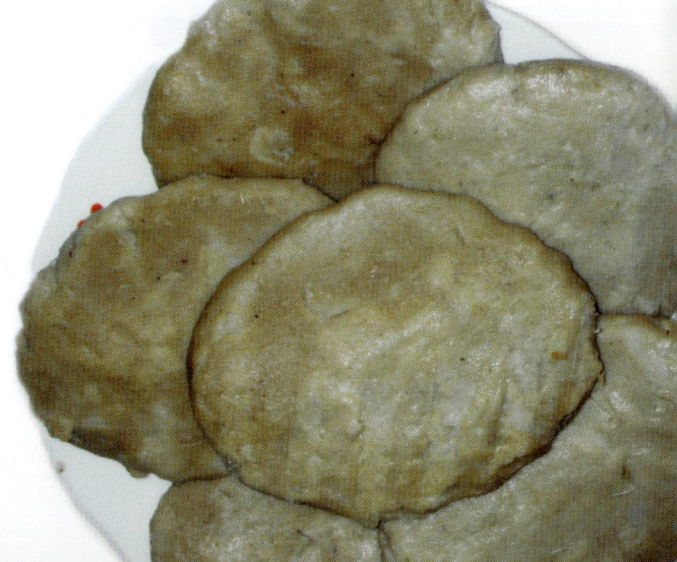

Steamed potatoes and pork balls
Jing Wan Wan

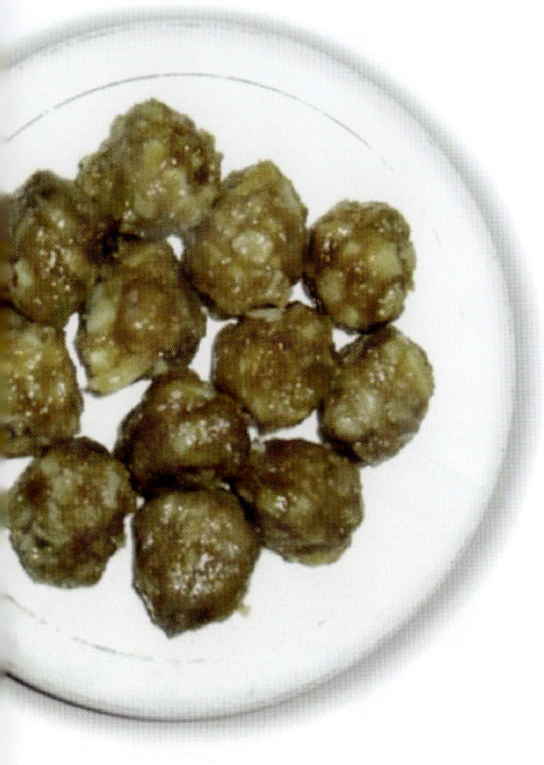

Ingredients:
Oat flour 250 g, starch 250 g, potato 400 g, pork filling 100 g

Seasonings:
Green onion, refined salt, gourmet powder, soy sauce, ginger powder, Chinese prickly ash, aniseed powder, vegetable oil

Preparation:
1. Put minced pork in a bowl and add green onion, refined salt, gourmet powder, soy sauce, ginger powder, Chinese prickly ash, aniseed powder and vegetable oil. Mix evenly.

2. Peel potatoes, clean and dice, and mix with the pork filling. Add starch and mix evenly, then shape into balls and steam for 15 minutes.

Vegetarian: ✗   Muslim: ✗

Steamed potatoes I
Zheng Malingshu

Ingredient:
Potato 500 g

Seasonings:
Brined vegetable 100 g, soy-pickled vegetables 100 g, pickled vegetable 50 g

Preparation:
1. Peel and slice potatoes, then put on the steamer tray to steam.
2. Serve with brined, soy-pickled or pickled vegetables.

Vegetarian: ✓　Muslim: ✓

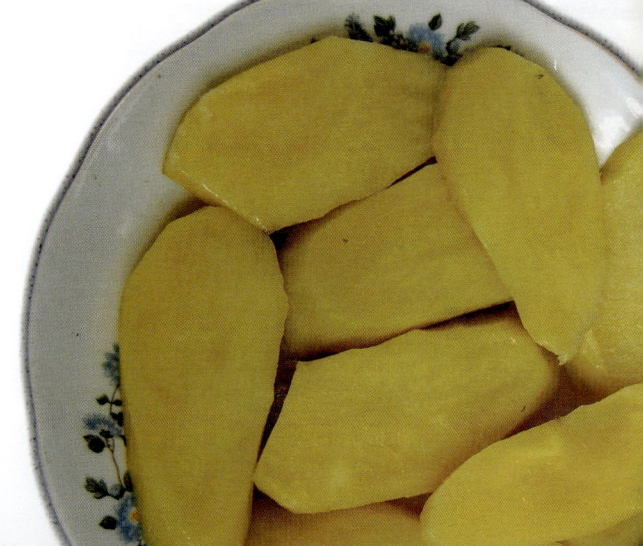

Stewed chicken with potato
Malingshu Dun Xiaoji

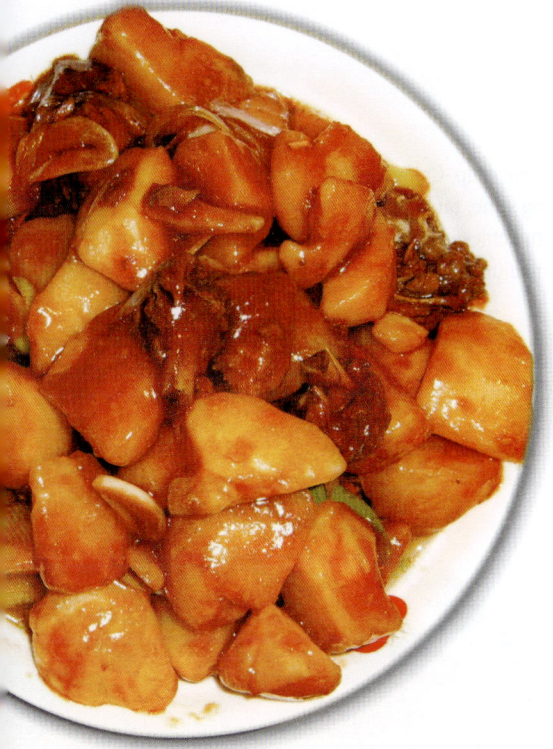

Seasonings:

Vegetable oil 200 g, scallion 10 g, ginger 10 g, garlic 10 g, soy sauce 15 g, white sugar 10 g, Chinese prickly ash 3 g, star anise 5 g, small red pepper 2 g, salt 10 g, chicken essence 3 g, cooking wine 5 g

Preparation:

1. Chop the chicken and blanch in boiling water. Remove and drain water.

2. Peel and clean potatoes, then dice them irregularly. Deep-fry in hot oil until golden brown then remove. Cut the ginger, garlic and scallion into sections.

3. Put a little oil in the wok and heat. Fry white sugar to black-red, then stir-fry the sliced chicken until brown.

4. Add water and all seasonings (except chicken essence) to the chicken then stew until it boils. Cook over low heat until chicken is done, then discard the star anise and add the potatoes. When almost cooked, add chicken essence and remove to a dish.

Ingredients:
Chicken 300 g, potato 300 g

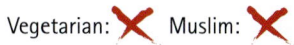

Stewed chicken with potato and tofu
Malingshu Tofu Dun Jiaji

Ingredients:
Potato 400 g, tofu 400 g, chicken 200 g, vegetable oil 30 g

Seasonings:
Green onions 20 g, ginger 15 g, garlic 10 g, Chinese prickly ash 3 g, star anise 5 g, table salt 10 g, gourmet powder 5 g, cooking wine 5 g

Preparation:
1. Peel and dice potatoes. Dice tofu.
2. Chop ginger and garlic into slices and green onion into pieces.
3. Blanch the chicken in hot water and rinse away froth.
4. Heat cooking oil in a pan and stir-fry the green onion and ginger, then add the chicken and stir-fry.
5. Add some soup, Chinese prickly ash, star anise, cooking wine, table salt and gourmet powder and stew the chicken together with the potatoes and tofu over medium heat until done.

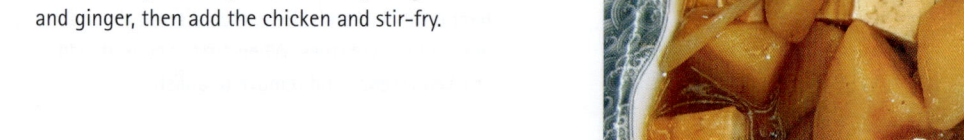

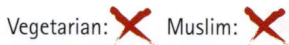

Vegetarian: ✗   Muslim: ✗

Stewed pork bones with potato and squash
Malingshu Wogua Dun Gutou

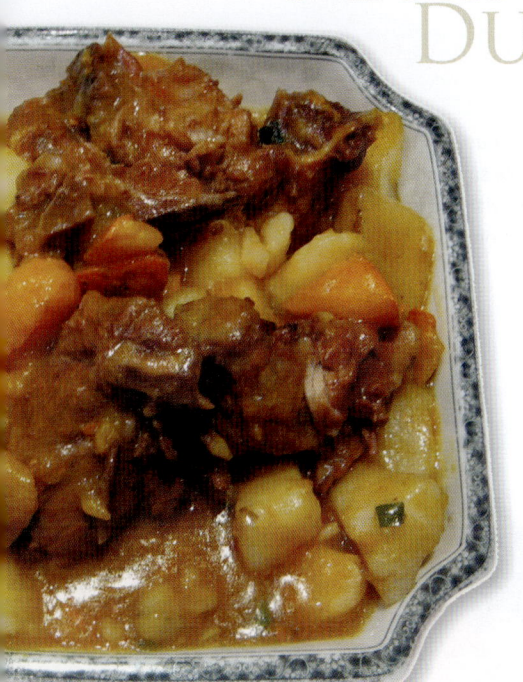

Seasonings:
Green onions 20 g, ginger 15 g, Chinese prickly ash 3 g, star anise 5 g, table salt 10 g, gourmet powder 5 g, cooking wine 5 g

Preparation:
1. Peel and dice potatoes. Dice squash and slice ginger and green onion into pieces.
2. Blanch the pork bones in boiling water and rinse away the floating froth.
3. Heat some cooking oil and stir-fry the green onion and ginger, then add the pork bones and stir-fry.
4. Add some soup, Chinese prickly ash, star anise, wine sauce, table salt and gourmet powder; then stew the bones along with the potatoes and squash over medium heat until done.

Ingredients:
Potato 400 g, squash 300 g, pork bones 200 g, lard oil (refined) 30 g

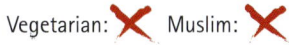

Vegetarian: ✗ Muslim: ✗

Stewed Pork Ribs with Potato and Squash
Malingshu Wogua Dun Paigu

Ingredients:
Potato 400 g, squash: 300 g, pork ribs 200 g, lard oil 30 g

Seasonings:
Green onions 20 g, ginger 15 g, Chinese prickly ash 3 g, star anise 5 g, table salt 10 g, gourmet powder 5 g, cooking wine 5 g

Preparation:
1. Cut the ribs into small pieces about 5 cm long. Peel and dice the potatoes. Dice the squash and chop ginger and garlic into slices. Cut the green onion into small pieces.
2. Blanch pork bones in boiling water and rinse out the floating froth.
3. Stir-fry the ribs in vegetable oil together with green onion, ginger and garlic.
4. Add some soup, Chinese prickly ash, star anise, wine sauce, table salt and gourmet powder; then stew the ribs along with the potatoes and squash over medium heat until done.

Vegetarian: ✗   Muslim: ✗

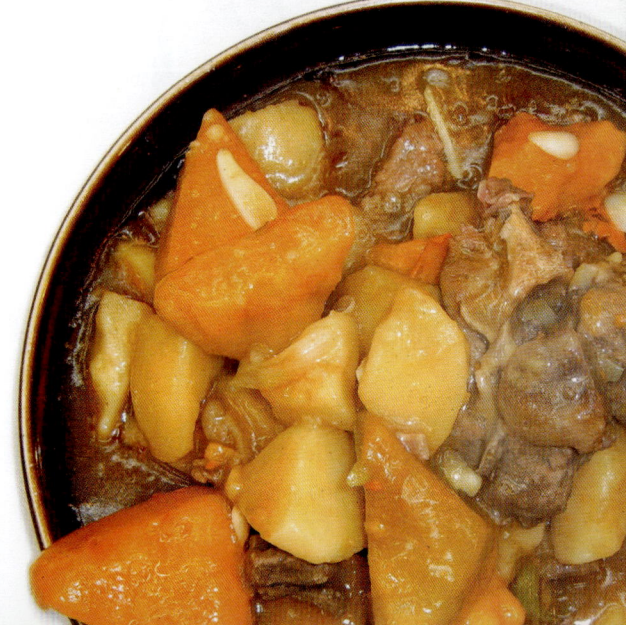

Stewed potatoes with chicken
Xiaoji Dun Tudou

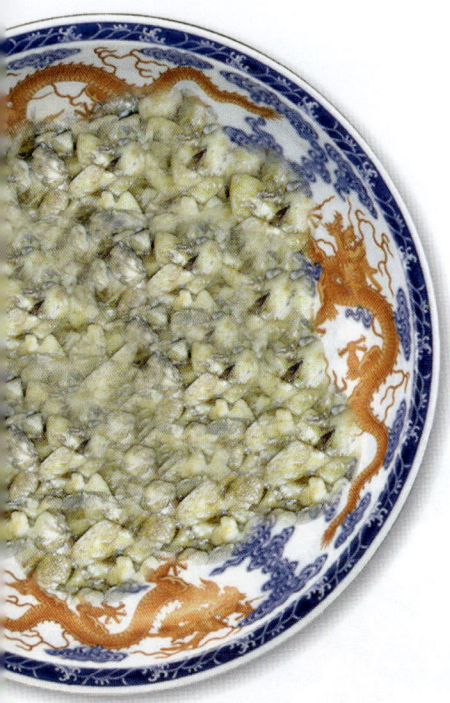

Seasonings:

Beer 50 g, white granulated sugar 15 g, salt 5 g, soy sauce 15 g, potatoes (yellow skin) 500 g, gourmet powder 2 g, chicken essence 2 g, star anise 5 g, dried orange peel 3 g, green onion 10 g, ginger 10 g, soybean oil 50 g

Preparation:

1. Cut chicken and blanch in boiling water, then remove and drain excess water.
2. Peel potatoes and cut into irregular pieces, put in hot oil and fry until golden brown.
3. Put oil in wok, add white granulated sugar and fry to deep red. Add chicken pieces to stir-fry before the color changes. Add all seasonings except gourmet powder and boil, then stew over low fire. Remove green onion, ginger, aniseed and dried orange peel, and add potatoes to stew until they are well-cooked. Add gourmet powder, then remove stew from the wok and put in a bowl, sprinkle coriander and serve.

Ingredients:

Chicken 1,000 g, potatoes (yellow skin) 500 g. cilantro 15 g

Vegetarian: ✘   Muslim: ✘

Stewed potatoes with eggplant
Malingshu Men Qiezi

Ingredients:
Potato 200 g, eggplant 200 g, 50 g

Seasonings:
Soy sauce 5 g, salt 5 g, Chinese prickly ash 3 g, chicken essence 2 g, garlic 15 g, green scallion 10 g, ginger 5 g, linseed oil 20 g

Preparation:
1. Peel and cut potatoes and eggplant. Cut pepper to strips.
2. Heat oil in wok and fry Chinese prickly ash until it smokes, then discard. Add sliced garlic and ginger and stir-fry. Then add potatoes and stir-fry, followed by soy sauce and eggplant, and stir-fry again for a moment Add water and boil over high heat, then change to medium heat for stewing. When it is medium-done, add green and red pepper strips and salt. Stew over low heat, then remove, add chicken essence, and stir well.

Vegetarian: ✗   Muslim: ✓

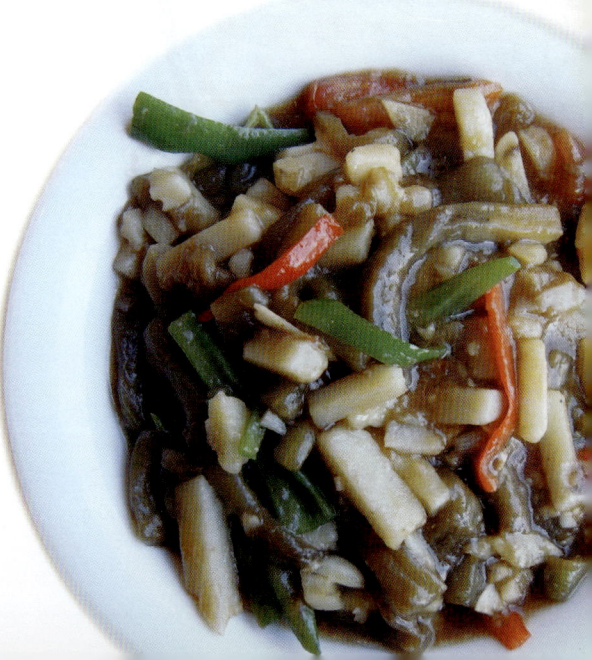

Stewed potatoes with pumpkin I
Malingshu Dun Wogua

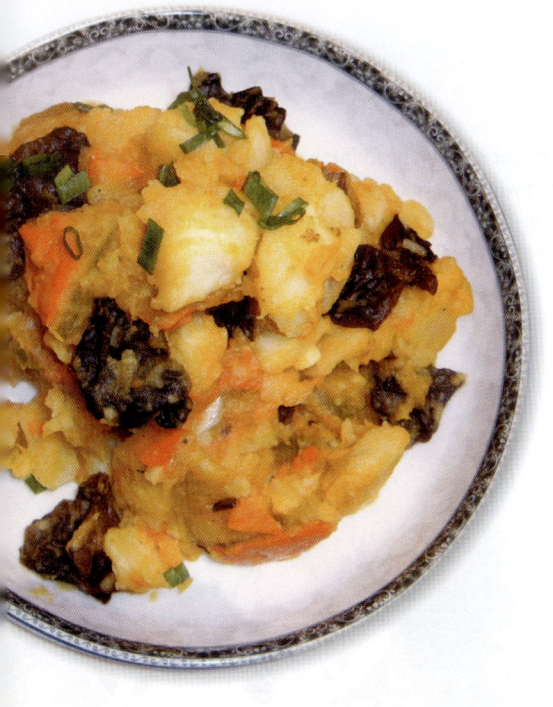

Ingredients:
Potato 300 g, pumpkin 300 g, dried agaric 50 g

Seasonings:
Onion 10 g, ginger 5 g, Chinese prickly ash 3 g, salt 5 g, gourmet powder 2 g

Preparation:
1. Peel and dice potatoes. Clean pumpkin and cut into sections; mince onion, ginger and garlic.

2. Heat oil and fry Chinese prickly ash until it smokes, then discard. Stir-fry onion, ginger and garlic until it gives off aroma, then add potato and pumpkin pieces and water and boil over high heat. Then add salt and gourmet powder and stew until soup thickens. Remove and serve.

Vegetarian: ✓   Muslim: ✓

Stewed spareribs with potato and frozen tofu
Malingshu Paigu Dong Tofu

Ingredients:
Potato 200 g, frozen tofu 200 g, pork spareribs 200 g

Seasonings:
Lard (refined) 30 g, scallion 20 g, ginger 15 g, garlic 10 g, Chinese prickly ash 3 g, star anise 5 g, salt 10 g, gourmet powder 2 g, cooking wine 5 g

Preparation:
1. Chop the spareribs into 5 cm-long section. Peel potatoes and cut potatoes and frozen tofu into pieces. Slice ginger, garlic and scallion.
2. Boil water in a wok and add spareribs. When cooked, rinse off the froth.
3. Heat oil in the wok and fry the scallion, ginger and garlic, then stir-fry with spareribs.
4. Add the cooking liquor, Chinese prickly ash, star anise, cooking wine, salt and gourmet powder, then cook to medium-done. Add potatoes and cowpeas and cook over medium heat.

Vegetarian: ✗   Muslim: ✗

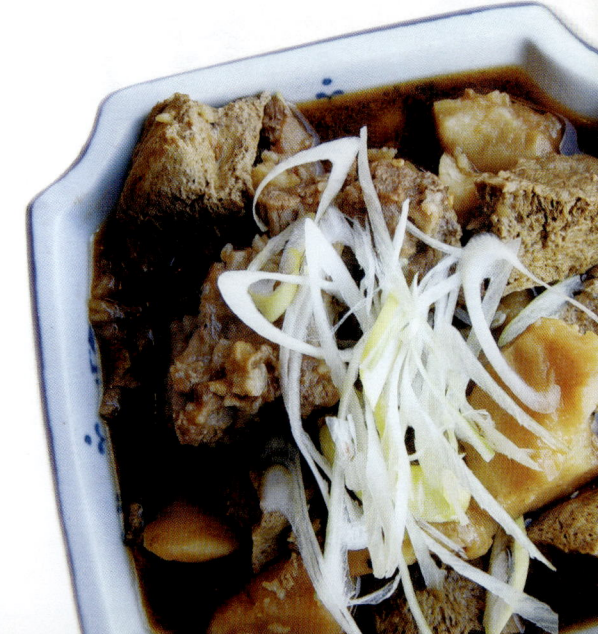

Stir-fried knife-sliced noodles with potato chips and fried pork fillet
Guoyourou Malingshu Pian Chao Daoxiaomian

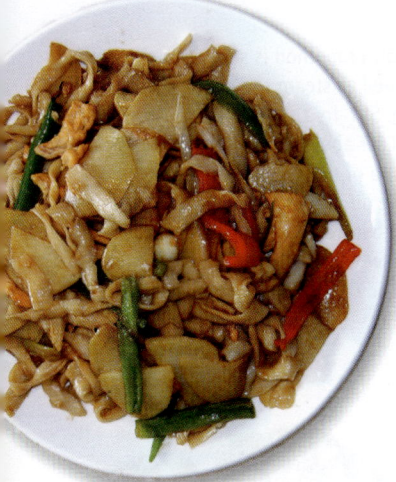

Ingredients:
Loin pork 200 g, potato 300 g, lard 500 g, flour 200 g

Seasonings:
Green pepper 25 g, red pepper 25 g, garlic 5g, vinegar 20 g, Chinese prickly ash water 5 g, green onion stalk 20 g, soybean sauce 15 g, fresh ginger 15 g, table salt 5 g, cooking wine 5 g, starch 50 g, gourmet powder 5 g, 1 egg

Preparation:
1. Put the flour into a big bowl and slowly add cold water and stir. Knead the dough into a relatively hard ball. Keep the dough standing for 30 minutes, covering it with a damp cloth.
2. Knead the dough into one thick lump. Use a knife to cut the dough into slices as quickly as possible directly into the boiling water. When the water boils again, take out the noodle slices and cool them down with cold water.
3. Slice the pork loin into fillets 2cm wide and 2cm long. Put fillets in a bowl and mix with some Chinese prickly ash water, soybean sauce, table salt, egg and starch. Marinate for 60 minutes. Deep-fry the fillets until golden brown, then remove.
4. Clean the potatoes and chop into chips the same size as the pork fillets. Fry the potato chips until golden brown. Slice green and red pepper, green onion and garlic. Finely minced the ginger.
5. Heat the lard in the frying pan and stir-fry the green onion, minced ginger and garlic. Add the fillets and some vinegar and cook for a little bit before adding the potato chips. Then add green and red pepper, the noodles and some cooking wine, gourmet powder and soybean sauce. Stir-fry a little bit and then serve.

Vegetarian: ✗   Muslim: ✗

Stir-fried mashed potatoes
Chao Malingshu Kuailei

Ingredients:
Potato 500 g, oat flour 300 g

Seasonings:
Linseed oil 30 g, green onion 10 g, garlic 5 g, table salt 5 g

Preparation:

1. Steam the mashed potatoes: Boil potatoes in a wok for about 30 minutes, then peel and mash. Add some oat flour and table salt, and knead together into small pieces. Then steam the mashed potatoes in a bamboo steamer for about 10 minutes. Take them out when you can smell the aroma.

2. Stir-fry the mashed potatoes: There are two different ways to stir-fry the mashed potatoes. One is to put some linseed oil in the wok, fry the minced onion and garlic, and when you can smell the aroma, add the steamed mashed potatoes, stir-frying them together over low heat for about 3 to 4 minutes. Then the dish is ready. The other method is similar to the first, but you do not need to steam the mashed potatoes before frying. Stir-fry the mashed potatoes in the wok without oil for about 10 minutes. When you can smell the aroma of oat flour, take the mashed potatoes out. Add some oil in the wok and stir-fry green onion and garlic before adding the mashed potatoes back into the wok and stir-fry them together. The dish is ready to serve once the mashed potatoes turn brown.

Vegetarian: ✓   Muslim: ✓

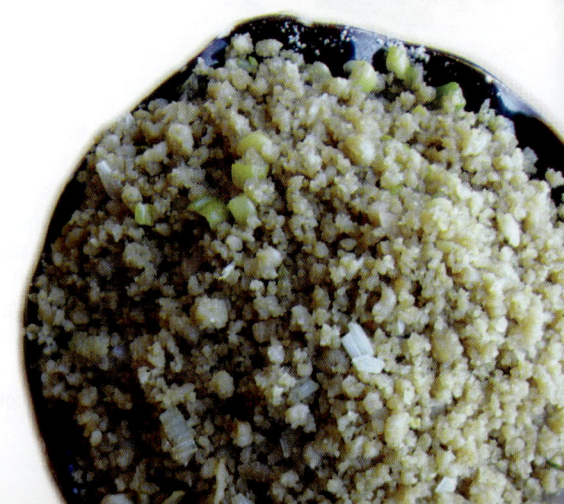

Stir-fried potato strips and shredded carrot
Malingshu Tiao Chao Huluobo Si

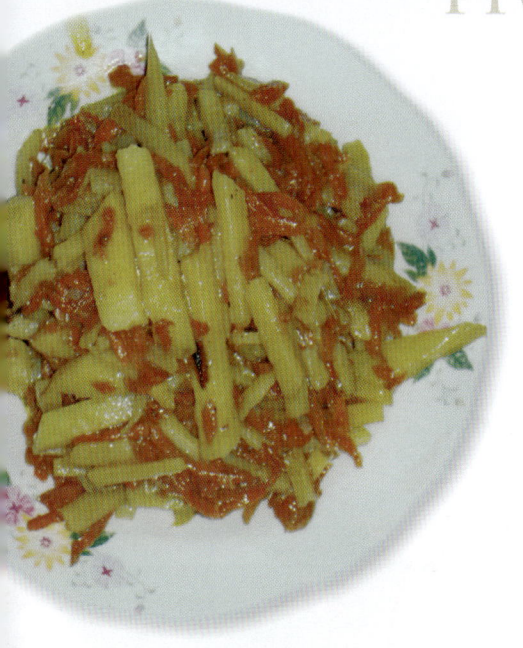

Ingredients:
Potato 300 g, carrot 100 g

Seasonings:
Salt 5 g, chicken essence 3 g, Chinese prickly ash 3 g, green onion 5 g, garlic 5 g, fresh ginger 5 g, vegetable oil 20 g

Preparation:
1. Clean potatoes and chop into strips. Clean and shred the carrots.

2. Heat the oil over high heat and fry the Chinese prickly ash until it smokes, then discard. Lightly stir-fry green onion, garlic and ginger, then add potato strips and carrot. Put water into the pot and stir-fry until it is cooked, then add chicken essence and table salt and serve.

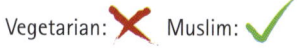

Vegetarian: ✗   Muslim: ✓

Swan playing with water
Tian E Xishui

Ingredient:
Potato 500 g

Seasonings:
Salt to taste, gourmet powder, whisked egg

Preparation:

1. Peel potatoes and steam well. Remove from steamer and mash, then flavor the mashed potatoes and form into a swan shape with a soup spoon.

2. After basting with whisked egg, put into steamer and steam for 2 minutes. Remove and place on a plate with sea water-like juice, using vegetables to make the swan's wings, eyes and mouth.

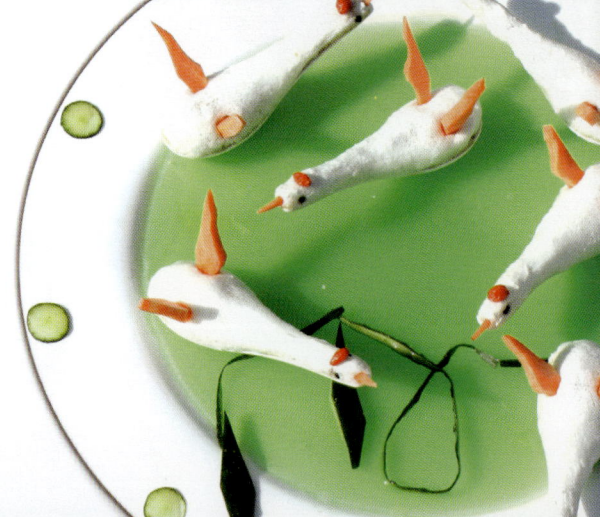

Vegetarian: ✗ Muslim: ✓

Tired bird returns to the nest
Juan Niao Gui Chao

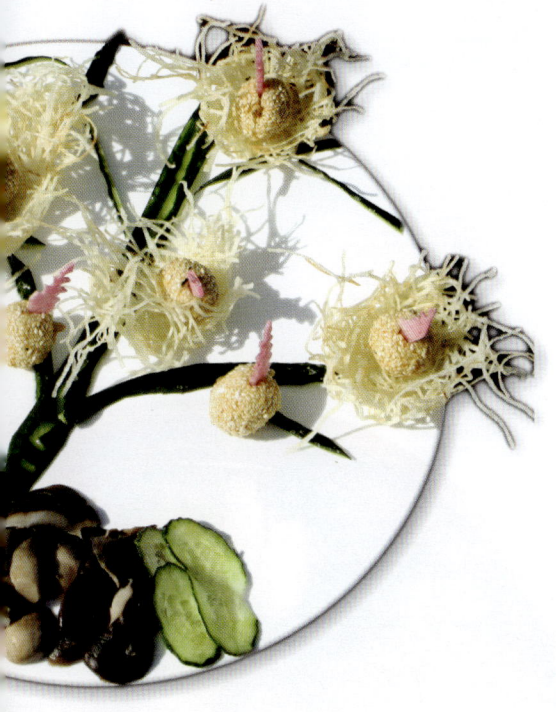

Ingredient:
Mashed potatoes 500 g

Seasonings:
Shredded potato, salt to taste, gourmet powder, chicken essence, sesame seeds, a little cooking wine, minced green onion and minced ginger

Preparation:
1. Season the mashed potatoes, sprinkle wheat flour, coat with whisked egg and sesame seeds, then put in wok and fry until well-done. Form into a bird shape and set aside.
2. Coat potato with wheat flour and deep-fry to form a nest shape. Place the nest on the cucumber branches and put the bird in the nest.

Vegetarian: ✗   Muslim: ✗

Tofu soup with potato and cabbage
Malingshu Baicai Tofu Tang

Ingredients:
Potato 300 g, small rape 100 g, tofu 300 g

Seasonings:
Gourmet powder 5 g, sesame oil 5 g, refined salt 5 g

Preparation:
Peel the potatoes and cut into strips, clean the small rape and cut into sections and cut tofu into strips. Put everything in a stockpot. After stewing on low heat for 10 minutes, add gourmet powder, sesame oil and refined salt. Remove from heat and serve.

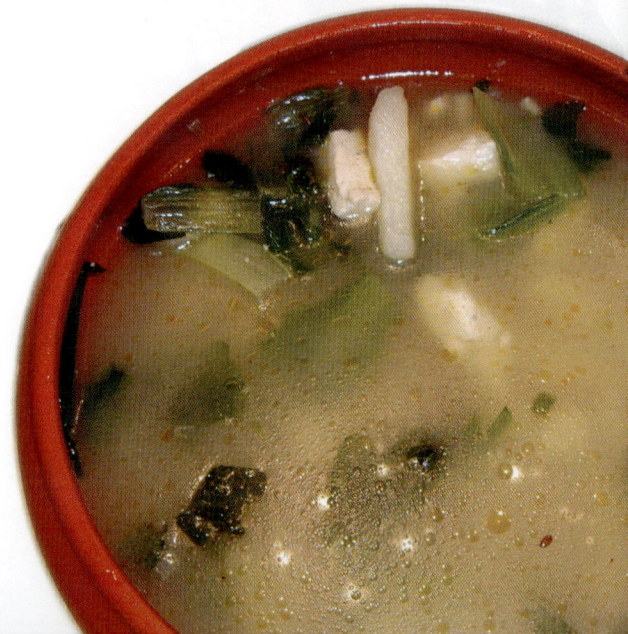

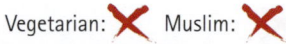

Translucent dumplings
Boli Jiaozi

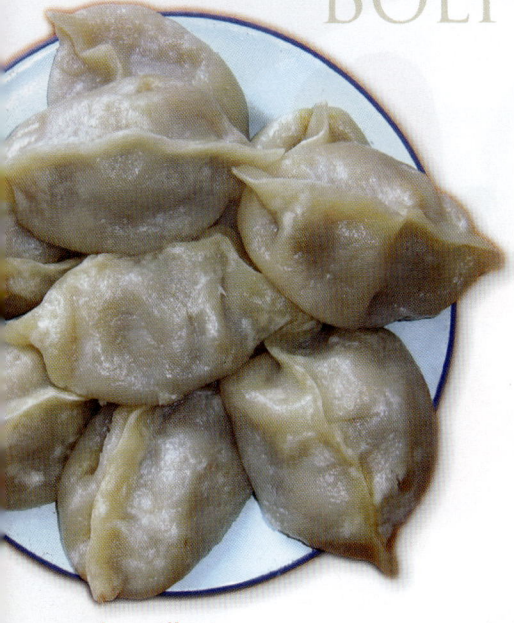

Preparation:

1. Finely mince the mutton, add some green onion, minced ginger and soybean sauce and mix. Gradually add prickly ash water and stir. Let mixture stand for 20 minutes.

2. Clean carrots, scrape into strings, add 3 g of table salt and mix.

3. Chop cilantro, squeeze the carrot strings a little bit to drain water and mix. Then add to mutton mixture together with some peanut oil and table salt.

4. Steam the potatoes, then peel and mash them. Add starch and mix them together into dough. Make dumpling wrappers from the dough and fill with mutton mixture. Steam the dumplings for about 13 minutes over high heat.

Ingredients:
Potato 500 g, starch 250 g, mutton 400 g, carrot 300 g, cilantro 50 g

Seasonings:
Green onion 20 g, ginger (chopped into granules) 20 g, prickly ash, soybean sauce 15 g, table salt 7 g, peanut oil 30 g, sesame oil 20 g

Vegetarian: ✗   Muslim: ✓

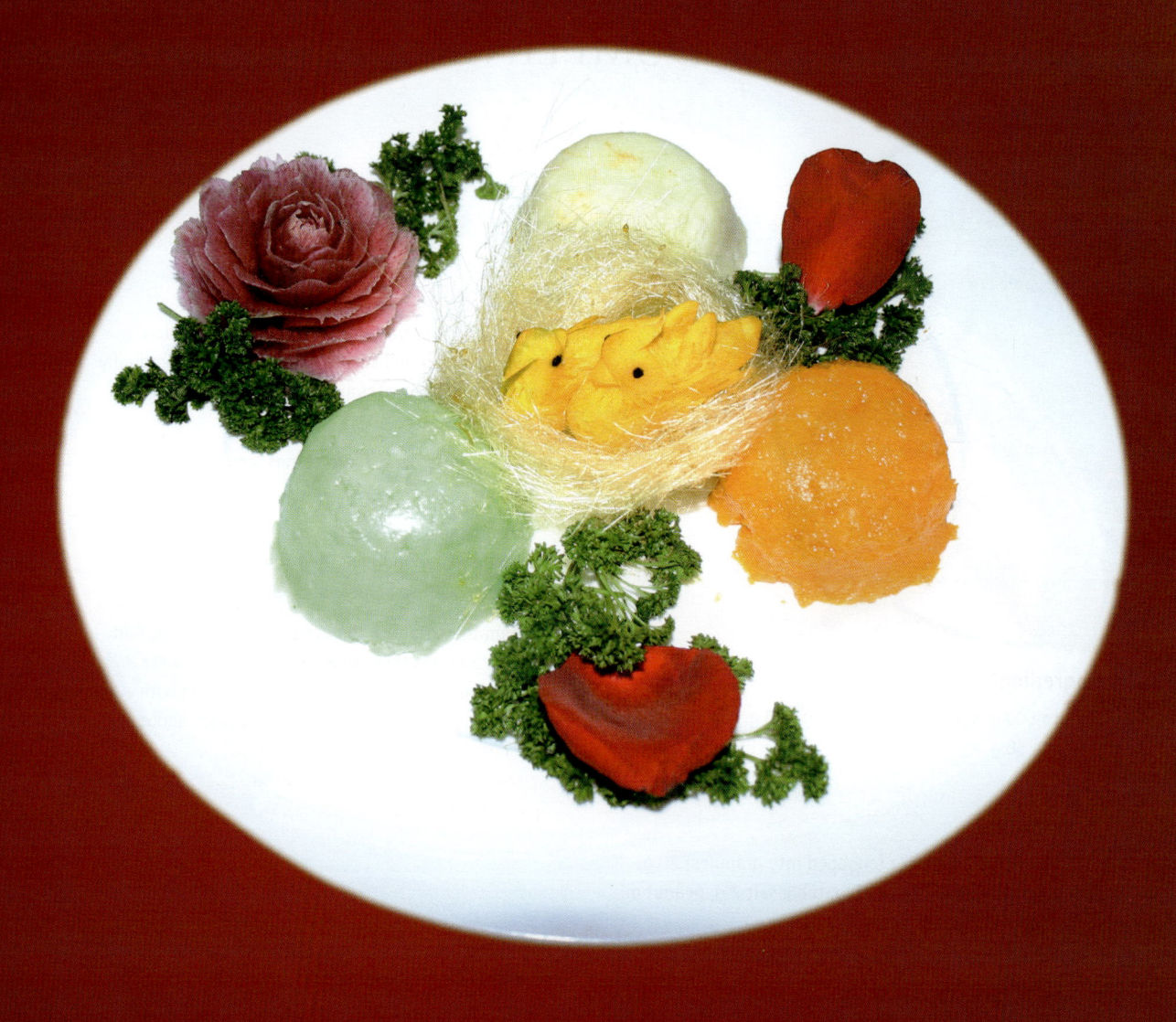

Tricolor mashed potatoes
Sanse Tudou Ni

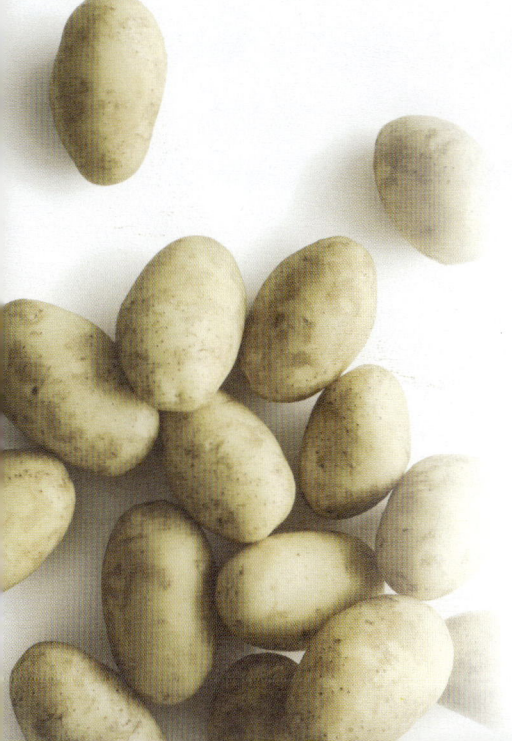

Ingredient:
Fresh potato 500 g

Seasonings:
Carrot juice 50 g, radish juice 50 g, white sugar 50 g, crisp peanuts

Preparation:
1. Make mashed potatoes, then add fried peanuts and fry over medium heat.
2. Put the fried potatoes in three different bowls with white sugar, carrot juice and radish juice, respectively. Turn bowls upside down on the same plate and serve.

Note:
1. Avoid high oil temperature when frying potato mash.
2. Divide the fried mashed potatoes and place in three separate bowls, then add sugar, carrot juice and radish juice in three bowls, respectively.

Vegetarian: ✓   Muslim: ✓

Potato Recipes from Northwest China

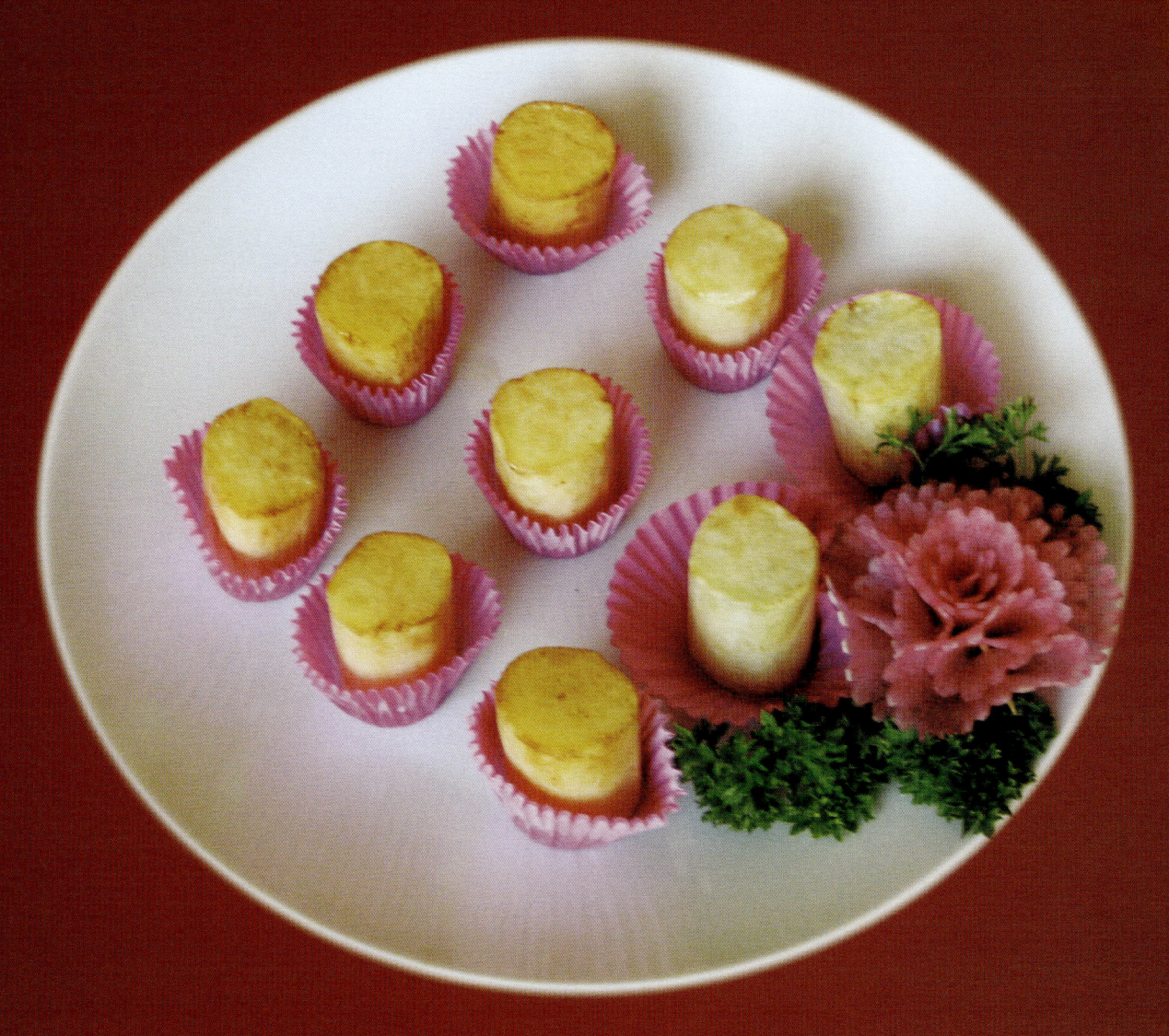

Baked potatoes
Kao Tudou

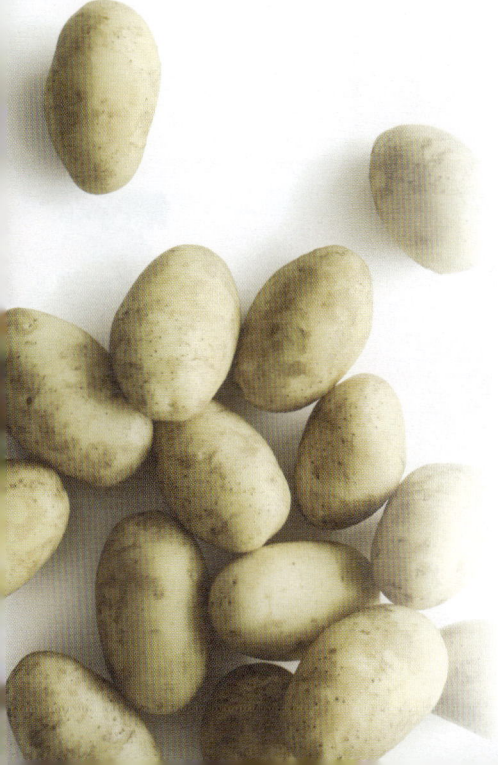

Ingredient:
Potato 400 g

Preparation:
Peel potatoes and cut them into columns, then put them into oven, bake for 20 minutes and serve.

Vegetarian: ✓   Muslim: ✓

Baked potato cake with red bean filling
Tudou Dousha Bing

Ingredients:

Potato, red bean filling

Seasonings:

Glutinous rice flour to taste

Preparation:

Peel potatoes and steam. Then mash the potato, add glutinous rice flour and roll into small cakes. Wrap the cakes around the red bean filling, then bake in the oven for 5 minutes.

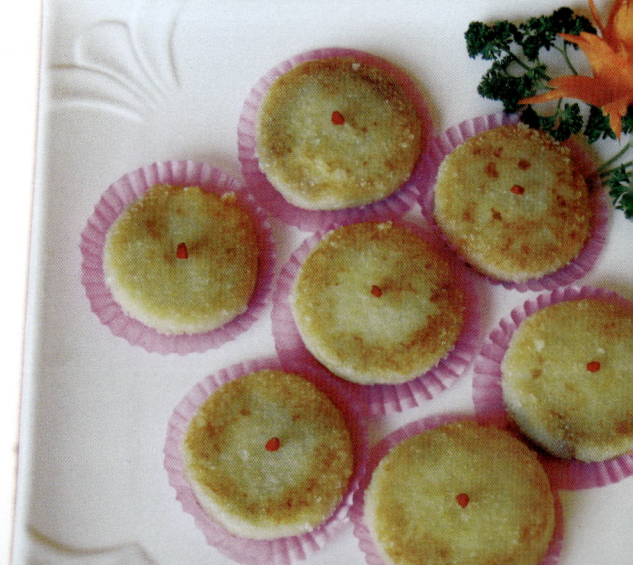

Vegetarian: ✓   Muslim: ✓

Black Beauty Potato Slices
Hei Meiren Yangyu

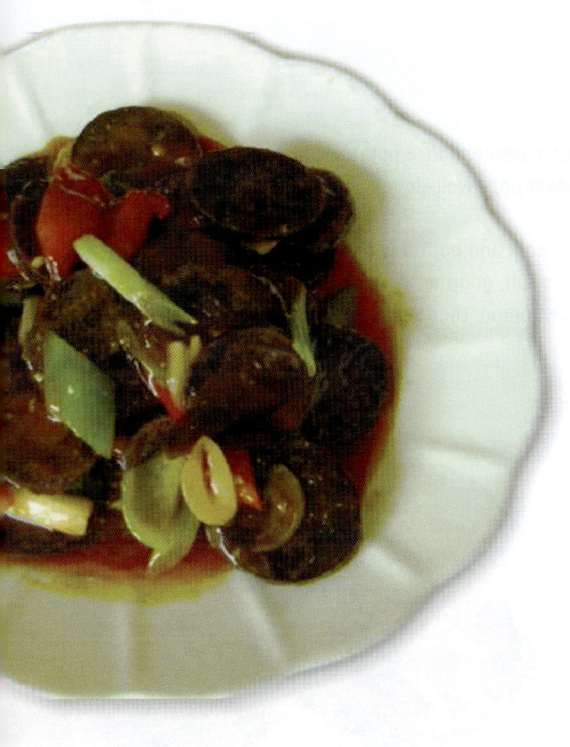

Ingredient:
Black beauty potato 500 g

Seasonings:
Vegetable oil 30 g, 1 green pepper, 1 red pepper, 2 pieces of ginger, Chinese prickly ash 10 g, 1 onion, 2 garlic pieces, salt 5 g, chicken essence 2 g

Preparation:
1. Peel and slice potatoes then set aside.

2. Heat vegetable oil and fry Chinese prickly ash and ginger it gives off aroma, then remove from heat. Fry potato slices and green and red pepper slices, then add garlic, salt, chicken essence and green onion and mix and fry until flavor is absorbed.

Vegetarian: ✗   Muslim: ✓

Braised assorted dishes, Yulin style
Yu Lin Da Huicai

Ingredients:
Potato 700 g, potato noodles 200 g, lean pork 500 g, frozen tofu 500 g, sauerkraut 200 g

Seasonings:
Peanut oil 50 g, soy sauce 5 g, chopped green onion 10 g, minced garlic 10 g, minced ginger 5 g, Chinese prickly ash 3 g, fennel powder 3 g, table salt 3 g, gourmet powder 1 g, coriander 10 g

Preparation:
1. Slice 500 g of lean pork into pieces that are 0.5 cm thick and 3 cm long. Fry the pieces until the meat is dry. Add soy sauce, chopped green onion, minced garlic, minced ginger, Chinese prickly ash, fennel powder, table salt and 500 ml of water, then braise in a pressure cooker until medium-well.

2. Clean, peel and dice potatoes; braise in pressure cooker until well-done.

3. Mix pork and potato with frozen tofu, sauerkraut, table salt, gourmet powder, coriander and chopped green onion, then serve.

Vegetarian: ✗ Muslim: ✗

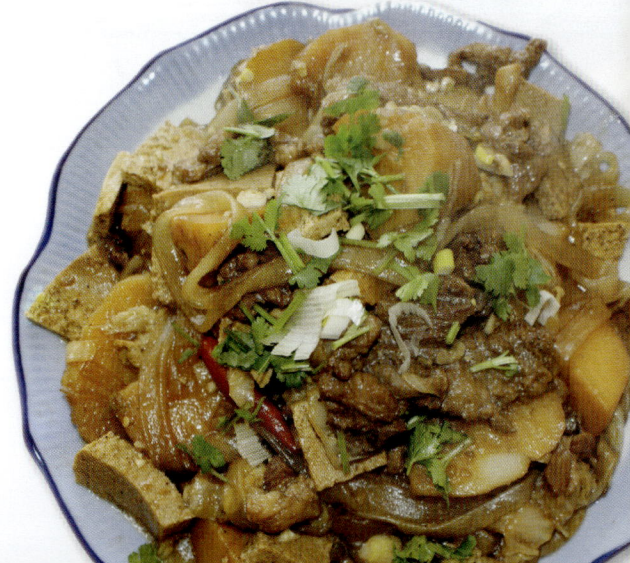

Braised chicken with potato and green pepper
Da Pan Ji

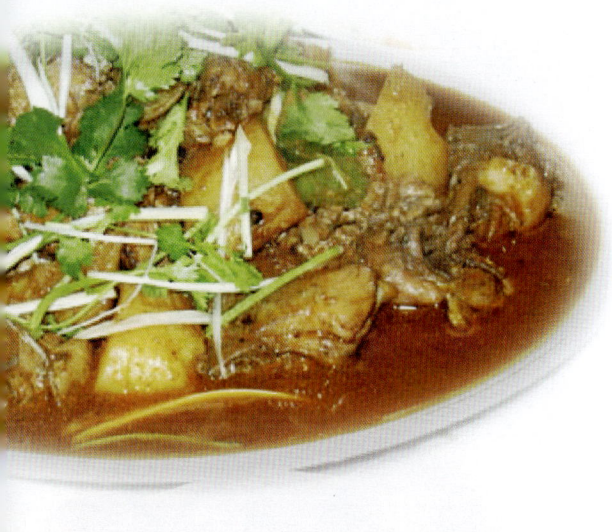

Ingredients:
Potato 500 g, chicken 500 g

Seasonings:
Peanut oil 50 g, Chinese prickly ash 3 g, ginger powder 3 g, green onion 3 g, crushed garlic 3 g, green pepper 10 g, soy sauce 2 g, sugar 2 g, table salt 3 g, cooking wine 3 g, gourmet powder 2 g

Preparation:
1. Fry Chinese prickly ash and green onion in hot oil until it gives off aroma, then add chicken and seasonings and stir-fry for 5 minutes. Add water and braise for about 30 minutes.
2. Add diced potato cook over light heat until the well-done.
3. Add the green pepper and stir-fry lightly, then serve.

Vegetarian: ✘   Muslim: ✘

Braised potatoes with mutton rack
Tudou Wei Yangpai

Ingredients:
Potato 500 g, mutton rack 250 g

Seasonings:
Salt 5 g, oil 2 g, sugar 5 g, gourmet powder 1 g, bay leaves 3 g, Chinese prickly ash 5 g, star anise 4 g

Preparation:
Cut potato into cubes. Chop the mutton into 6 cm sections and quick-boil in water. Then put in a pressure cooker, adding salt, oil, sugar, gourmet powder, bay leaves, Chinese prickly ash and star aniseed. Simmer for 15 minutes.

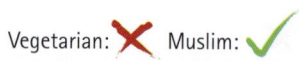

Vegetarian: ✗ Muslim: ✓

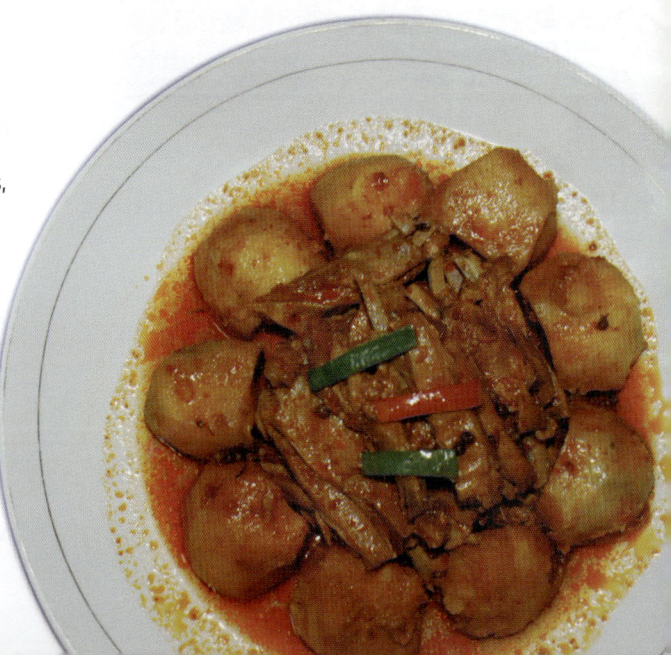

Braised potatoes with pumpkin
Dun Nangua Tudou

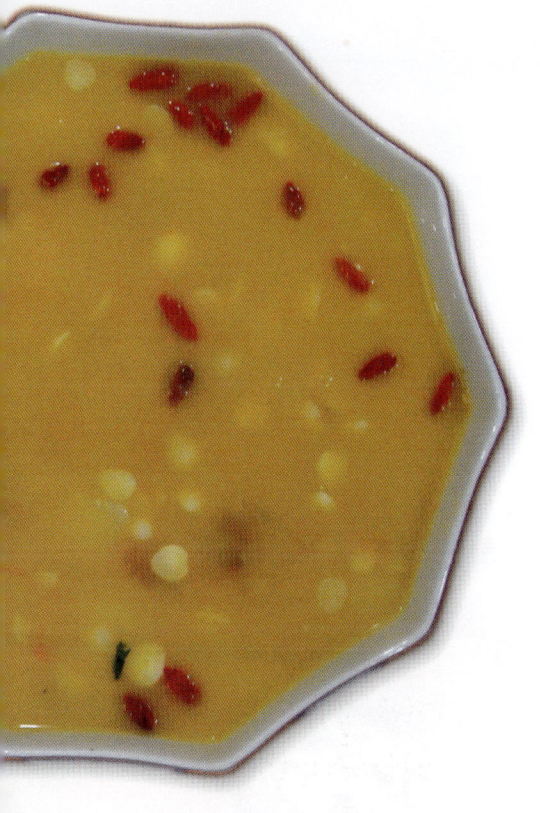

Ingredients:
Potato 400 g, almond 50 g, pumpkin 400 g

Seasonings:
Oil and salt to taste

Preparation:
Cut potato and pumpkin into cubes and quickly fry. Then add a little salt and stew with almond for 30 minutes over low heat.

Vegetarian: ✓   Muslim: ✓

Braised spareribs with potatoes
Tudou Dun Paigu

Ingredients:
Potato 500 g, spareribs 200 g

Seasonings:
Peanut oil 50 g, soy sauce 2 g, coriander 3 g, green onion 3 g, crushed garlic 3 g, ginger powder 3 g, Chinese prickly ash 3 g, fennel powder 2 g, table salt 2 g, gourmet powder 1 g

Preparation:
1. Stir-fry pork until it dries out. Add soy sauce, green onion, crushed garlic, ginger powder, Chinese prickly ash, fennel powder, salt and water. Put everything in a pressure cooker and braise until medium-well.

2. Clean and peel the potatoes and cut them into big pieces. Put the pieces in the pressure cooker and cook until well-done. Add gourmet powder, coriander, and green onion, then serve.

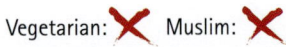
Vegetarian: ✗ Muslim: ✗

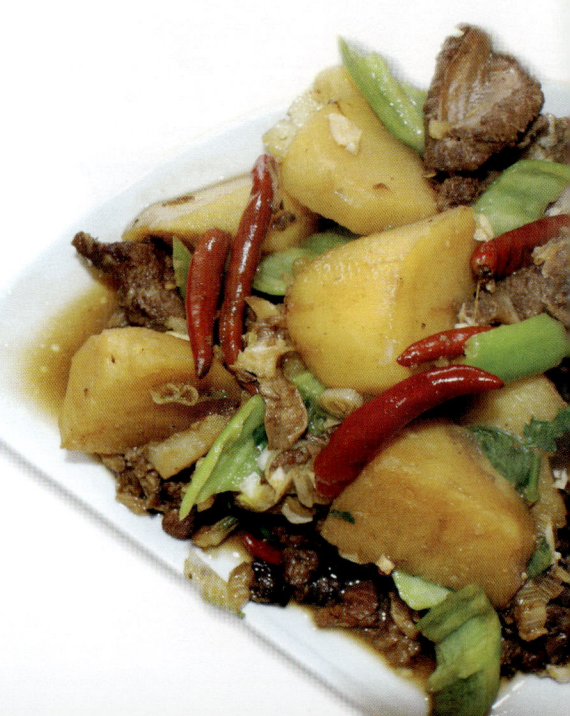

Braised tofu with pakchoi
Xiao Baicai Hui Tofu

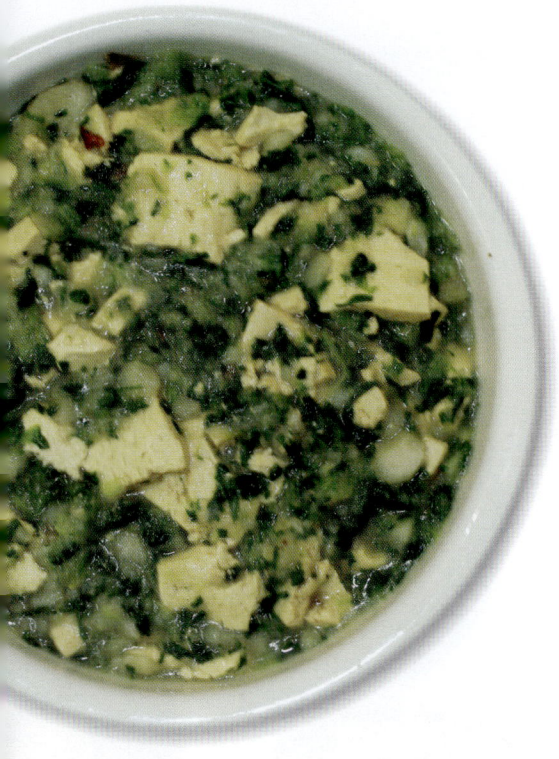

Ingredients:
Potato 500 g, tofu 200 g, pakchoi 200 g

Seasonings:
Peanut oil 50 g, green onion 3 g, ginger 2 g, Chinese prickly ash 2 g, table salt 1 g, gourmet powder 1 g

Preparation:
1. Dice the potatoes, slice the tofu, and cut the pakchoi into strings.
2. Heat oil and fry the green onion until it gives off aroma. Add potatoes and water, ginger powder, Chinese prickly ash and salt, and braise for about 10 minutes.
3. Add pakchoi and tofu. When the water has evaporated, add gourmet powder and serve.

Vegetarian: ✓   Muslim: ✓

CRISP POTATO BALLS COATED WITH SUGAR
YINZHUANG SUGUO

Ingredients:
Potato, starch noodles, shelled peanuts

Seasoning:
White sugar

Preparation:
Mash steamed potatoes, add shelled peanuts and form into a big ball. Use sugar to make sugar juice and coat the ball with it.

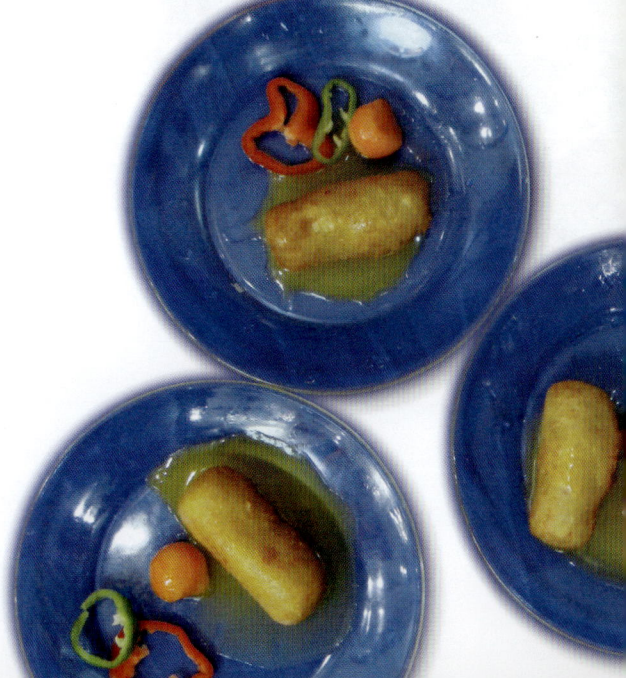

Vegetarian: ✓   Muslim: ✓

Crystal mashed potato roll
Yuni Shuijing Juan

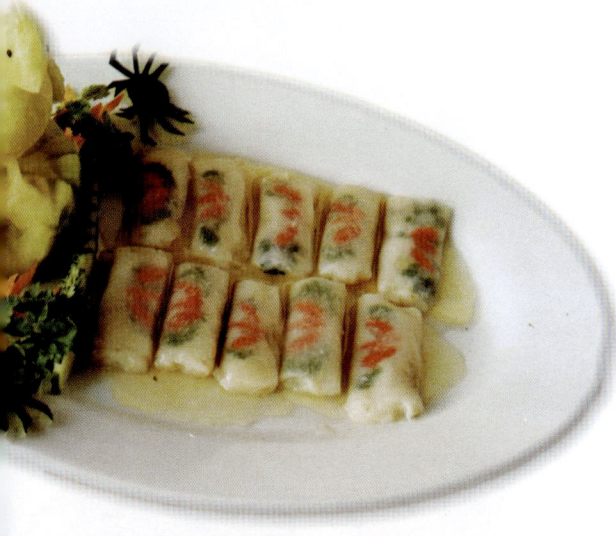

(Photo: by Dingxi Hotel)

Ingredients:
Potato 500 g, flour 50 g

Seasonings:
Candied fruit 20 g, sugar 20 g, water starch 15 g

Preparation:
1. Clean potatoes, steam for 30 minutes, then peel and mash. Mix evenly with flour and sugar. Make small rolls and put a little candied fruit on each roll.
2. Steam the potato rolls for 10 minutes then remove to a dish. Add sugar and water starch to thicken the soup, then sprinkle onto the potato rolls before serving.

Vegetarian: ✓   Muslim: ✓

Cucumber with potato noodles
Huanggua Fenpi

Ingredients:
Potato noodles 300 g, cucumber 200 g

Seasonings:
Coriander 2 g, vinegar 2 g, sesame oil 1 g, chili oil 1 g, table salt 1 g, minced ginger 1 g, mustard oil 0.5 g, gourmet powder 1 g

Preparation:
1. Stew 250 g of potato noodles in hot water for 5 minutes. Cut 250 g of cucumber into slices. Place noodles and cucumber on a dish.

2. Add coriander, vinegar, sesame oil, chili oil, table salt, minced ginger, mustard oil and gourmet powder, then serve.

Vegetarian: ✓ Muslim: ✓

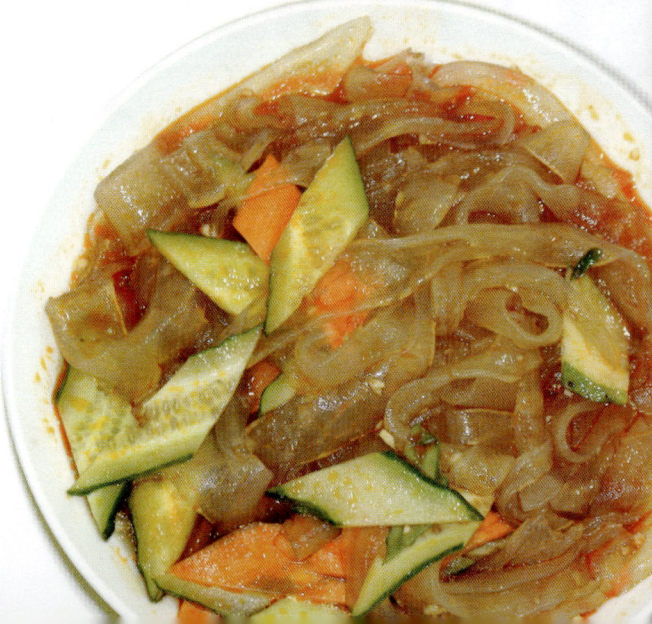

Dark steamed potato balls
Heilengleng

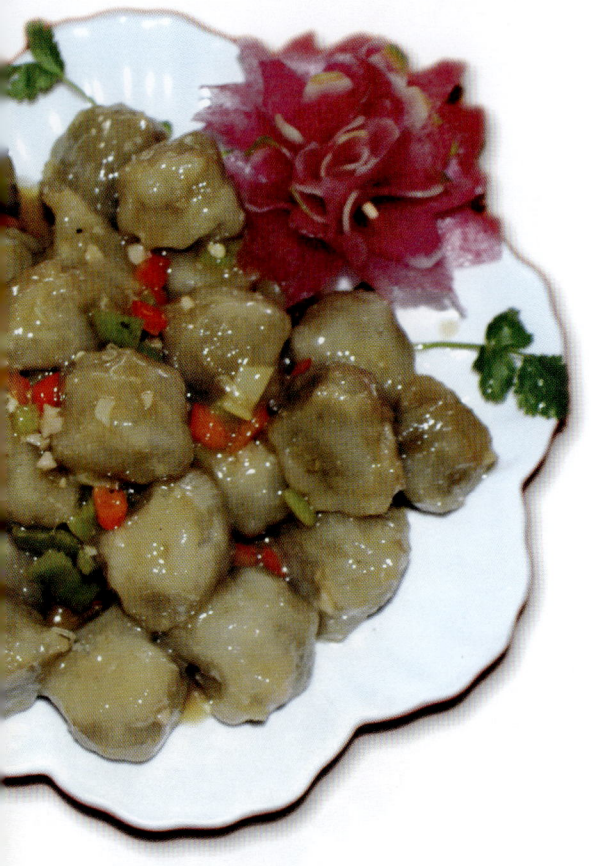

Ingredients:
Potato 500 g, potato starch 50 g

Seasonings:
Linseed oil 50 g, chopped green onion 10 g, Chinese prickly ash 3 g, minced ginger 5 g, table salt 3 g, tomato paste 10 g

Preparation:
1. Clean and peel potatoes. Drain off water and mash them into paste, squeezing the water out with a piece of gauze. Mix with starch and pinch to form into balls. Steam for 15 minutes and place the steamed balls on a plate.
2. Heat the peanut oil and add chopped green onion, Chinese prickly ash, minced ginger, table salt, tomato paste, a little water and a little starch, and mix with steamed Heilengleng in a dish.

Vegetarian: ✓   Muslim: ✓

Deep-fried potato balls covered in sesame seeds
Tudou Matuan

Ingredients:
Potato 100 g, sesame seed 10 g

Seasonings:
White sugar 20 g, starch 10 g

Preparation:
1. Peel and steam potatoes, mash them, add white sugar and starch, and form into balls.
2. Coat the ball with sesame seeds and deep-fry for 5 minutes.

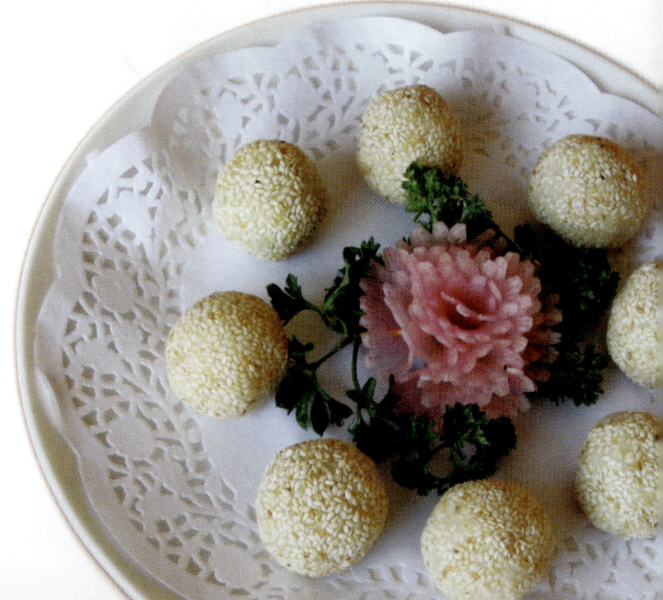

Vegetarian: ✓   Muslim: ✓

Dongxiang county potato chips
Dongxiang Tudou Pian

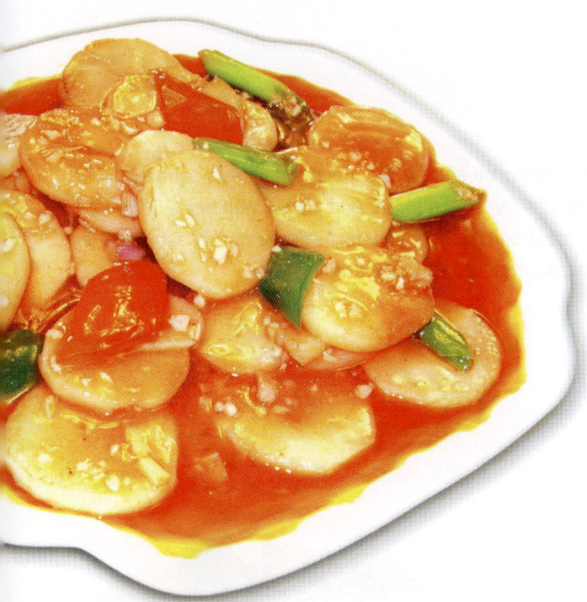

Preparation:

1. Peel potatoes and cut into 5cm cubes, then slice into 4.5cm-long column, slice the columns into 3cm-thick pieces.
2. Simmer potato pieces in chicken soup, and then fry until golden brown in the wok with cooking oil.
3. Put a little salad oil in the wok, add minced green onion and garlic piece and fry until it gives off aroma. Then add ketchup, salt, gourmet powder, chicken essence, chili oil, flavor spices and a little chicken soup. Use water starch to thicken the soup, then add the fried potato chips and sprinkle with a little sesame oil.

Ingredient:
Potato 600 g

Seasonings:
Green pepper 10 g, red pepper 10 g, garlic sprout 5 g, salt 5 g, gourmet powder 3 g, chicken essence 2 g, flavor spices 15 g, ketchup 3 g, chili oil 4 g, cosmetic 8 g, garlic 2 g, ginger 1 g, minced onion 1 g, sesame oil 1 g, chicken soup to taste, sesame oil 5 g

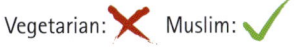

Fried meatballs
Zha Ge Wanzi

Ingredients:
Potato 500 g, potato starch 150 g, potato jelly 200 g, side pork 500 g, cabbage 100 g

Seasonings:
Peanut oil 50 g, fennel powder 3 g, ginger powder 3 g, Chinese prickly ash 3 g, table salt 2 g, gourmet powder 2 g, soy sauce 2 g, 3 eggs

Preparation:
1. Grind the side pork and the potatoes, and add potato starch, fennel powder, ginger powder, Chinese prickly ash, table salt, gourmet powder, soy sauce and eggs, and mix together. Knead the mixture into small balls and fry the balls in hot oil until golden yellow.
2. Stew potato jelly for about 10 minutes. Slice the cabbage.
3. Heat some oil and fry the green onion. Add cabbage and stir-fry for 1 minute. Add potato noodles, 250 g of meat balls, ginger powder, Chinese prickly ash, salt, and gourmet powder and stir-fry.

Vegetarian: ✗   Muslim: ✗

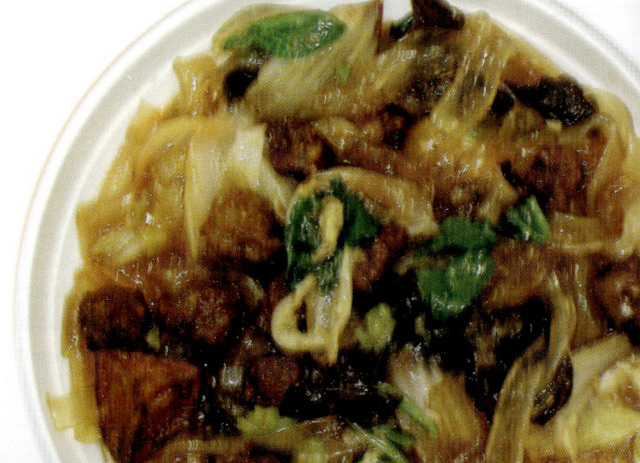

Fried pork liver with potato
Zhugan Tudou Tiao

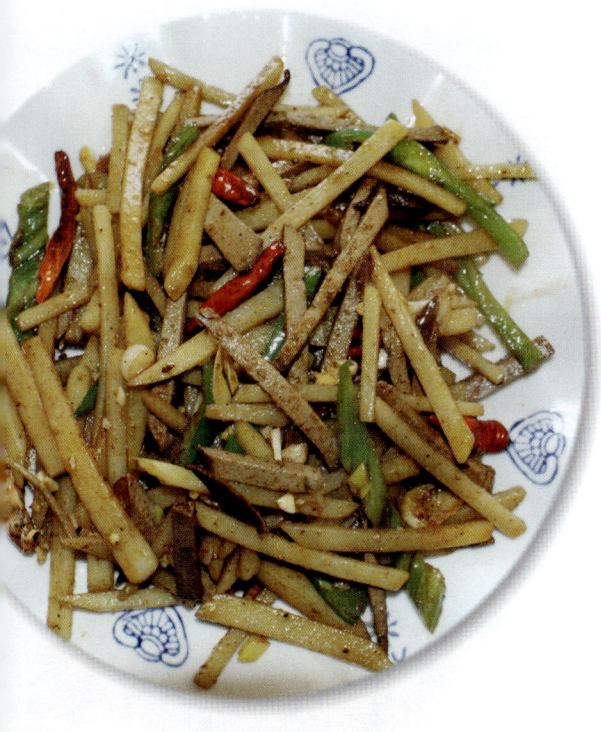

Ingredients:
Potato 300 g, cooked pork liver 150 g

Seasonings:
Peanut oil 50 g, green onion 3 g, red pepper 2 g, crushed garlic 3 g, ginger powder 2 g, Chinese prickly ash 2 g, table salt 1 g, gourmet powder 1 g

Preparation:
1. Dice potatoes and put them into cool water to remove starch, then drain. Cut the pork liver into pieces.
2. Heat oil and fry green onion and red pepper. Add potato pieces and seasonings and stir-fry for about 3 minutes. Add pork liver and stir-fry for about 2 minutes, then serve.

Vegetarian: ✗ Muslim: ✗

Fried pork slices with potato
Tudou Chao Rou Pian

Ingredients:
Side pork 1,300 g, potato 50 g, pumpkin 400 g, a little green pepper and red pepper, boiled oil 50 g

Seasonings:
Green onion 5 g, ginger 5 g, garlic 5 g, a little salt, gourmet powder, chicken essence, soy sauce

Preparation:
1. Slice potato into thin pieces, clean and soak in water for 10 minutes, then remove.
2. Heat oil and fry sliced side pork in wok until half medium-done. Add soy sauce and fry, then add green onion, ginger and garlic and stir-fry.
3. Add potato pieces and fry together. Add salt chicken essence and stir-fry before removing to the plate and serving.

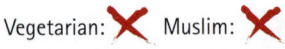
Vegetarian: ✗ Muslim: ✗

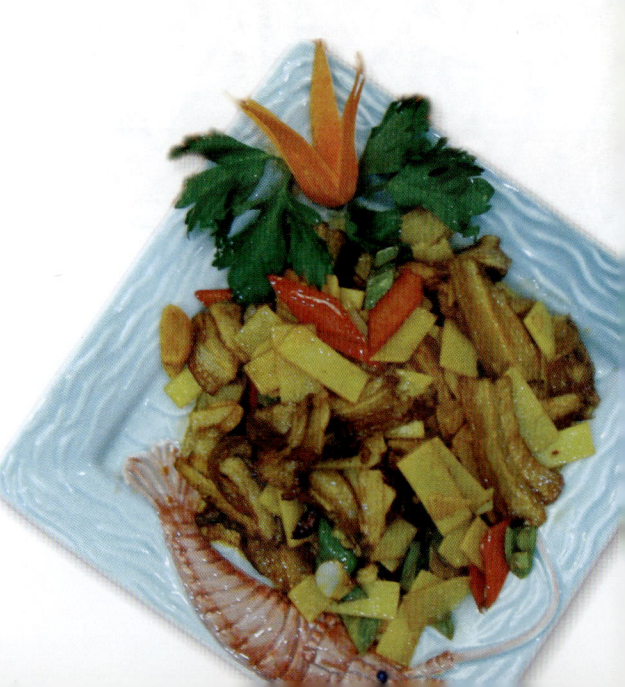

Fried Potato Cake III
Tudou Jianbing

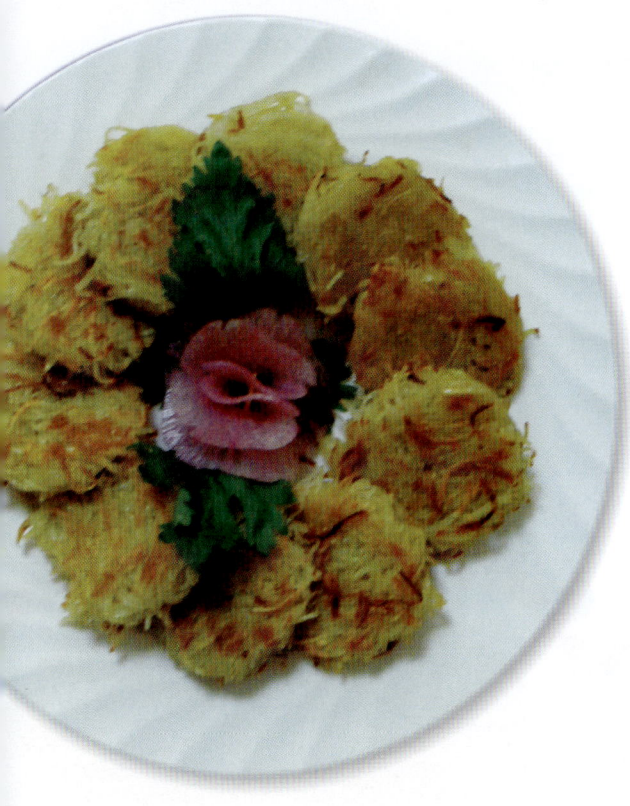

Ingredient:
Potato 1,000 g

Seasonings:
Salt 5 g, chicken essence 2 g, gourmet powder 1 g, starch 5 g

Preparation:
1. Shred potatoes; add salt, chicken essence, gourmet powder and starch to make a raw cake.
2. Steam the cake, then deep-fry in a wok until both sides are golden brown.

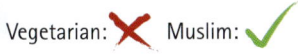

Fried shredded potato cake II
Tudou Tanbing III

Ingredients:
Potato 500 g, starch 50 g

Seasonings:
Salt 5 g, minced green onion 10 g, sesame seed 5 g, gourmet powder 2 g, vegetable oil 50 g

Preparation:
1. Peel and shred potatoes and clean them. Mix with starch, salt, minced green onion, and gourmet powder.
2. Heat oil in a wok and add flavored potatoes. Fry until golden brown, sprinkle with sesame seeds and, then remove to a dish and serve.

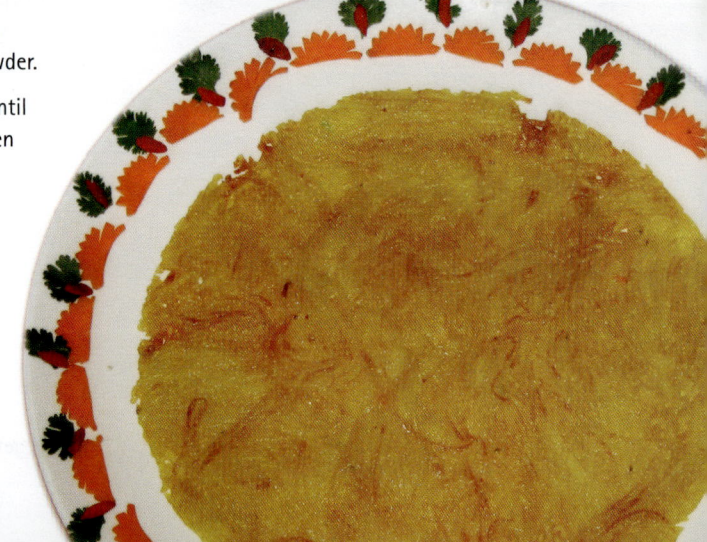

Vegetarian: ✓   Muslim: ✓

Fried Shredded Potatoes with Vinegar
Culiu Yangyu Si

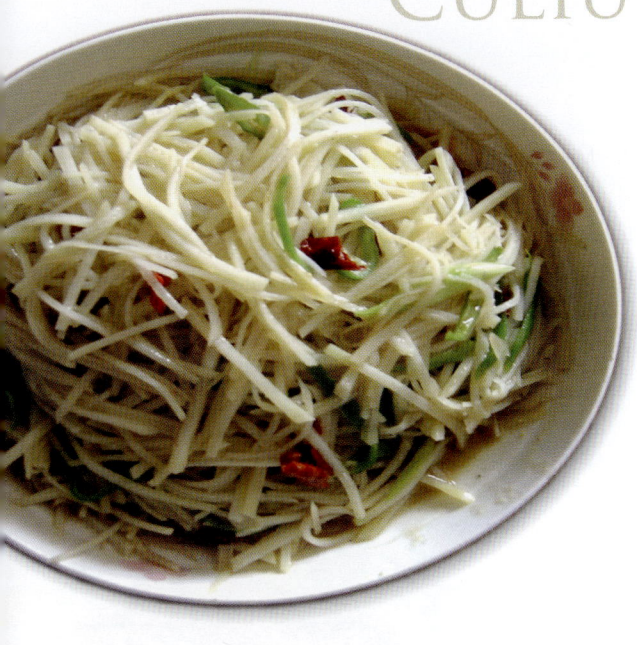

Ingredient:
Potato 500 g

Seasonings:
Vegetable oil 20 g, green pepper 1, 3 pod peppers, 2 pieces of ginger, Chinese prickly ash 10 g, 1 onion, salt 5 g, vinegar 10 g, chicken essence 2 g

Preparation:
1. Peel and shred the potatoes.

2. Heat vegetable oil in wok and fry Chinese prickly ash and ginger until it gives off aroma, then set aside.

3. Add potato strings, green pepper, pod peppers, salt, vinegar, chicken essence and green onion; stir-fry until the flavor is absorbed.

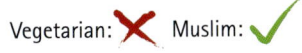

Fried stick-shaped mutton-potato mash
Tu Yang Jiehe Bang

Ingredients:
Mutton 250 g, potato 300 g

Seasonings:
Minced ginger to taste, 2 pieces of ginger, 1 star anise, 1 garlic segment, starch, 2 egg whites, salt, sugar, gourmet powder, liquor, light soy sauce, dark soy sauce and oil

Preparation:
1. Boil three big potatoes in water for about 40 minutes. Once well-cooked, peel and mash while hot.
2. Finely mince the mutton.
3. Put the minced mutton into a bowl, add minced ginger, 1/2 tsp salt, 1/2 tsp gourmet powder, 2 tsps of liquor, 2 tsps light soy sauce, starch to taste, 2 egg whites and a little water; mix evenly. Put the mixture in the refrigerator for 15 minutes to coagulate slightly.
4. Mix the mashed potatoes with the minced mutton and form into several sticks.
5. Steam the sticks for 10 minutes in steamer.
6. Heat oil in wok and deep-fry the potato and mutton sticks until golden. Remove and drain off excess oil.
7. Put the meat sticks on a plate. Mix water starch with sesame oil, minced onion and ginger to make a thick soup, then put on meat.

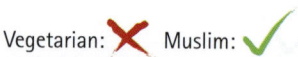

Vegetarian: ✗ Muslim: ✓

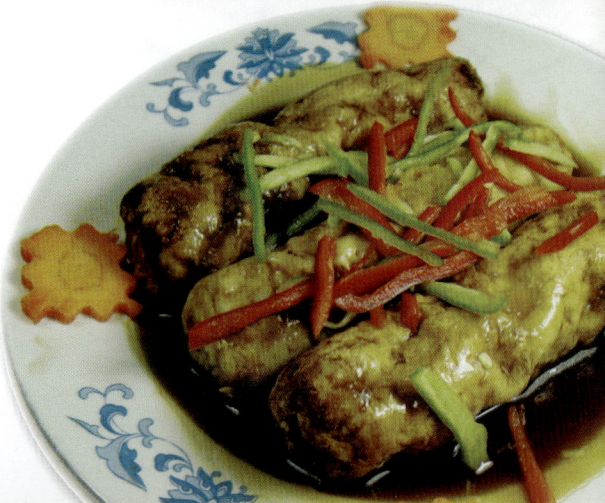

Fried Tofu and Potatoes with Green and Red Pepper
Jin Yu Man Tang

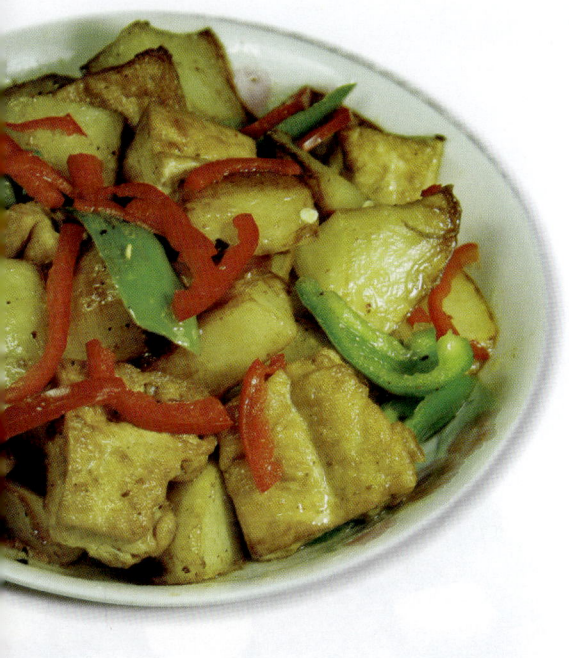

Ingredients:
Tofu 150 g, potato 1,500 g, green pepper 125 g

Seasonings:
Minced green onion 10 g, black pepper 1 g, refined salt 6 g, gourmet powder 1 g, fresh soup 250 g, sesame oil 10 g

Preparation:
1. Slice tofu into pieces about 2.5 cm × 2.0 cm × 0.7 cm, and quick-boil. Remove and add refined salt, then put tofu in oil to deep-fry until golden. Dice potatoes and green peppers.
2. Heat oil in wok over medium heat and add drained tofu pieces, diced potato, green peppers, fresh soup, refined salt, black pepper, and gourmet powder to cook together until they boil. Add wet starch to thicken soup, sprinkle with minced green onion and sesame oil, then serve.

Vegetarian: ✓   Muslim: ✓

Golden shredded potato nest
Jin Quechao

Ingredient:
Potato 500 g

Seasonings:
Green onion, spiced salt and gourmet powder to taste, several boiled eggs

Preparation:
1. Shred potatoes and cut green onion into sections.
2. Rinse the shredded potato to remove excess starch on the surface and drain.
3. Heat oil over medium heat, then put potato strings in a colander to fry, forming a nest shape.
4. Cut boiled egg and remove egg white. Put the egg yolk in the fried potato string nest.
5. Sprinkle evenly with spiced salt and gourmet powder and serve.

Vegetarian: ✗   Muslim: ✓

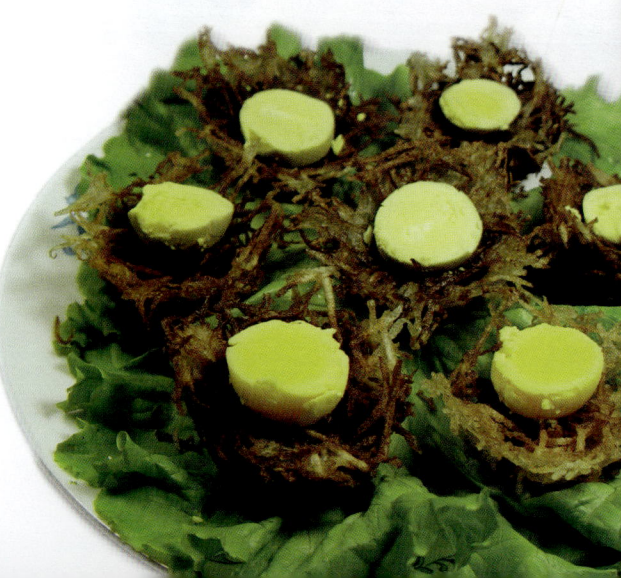

Golden thread with lotus
Jinsi Wang Lian

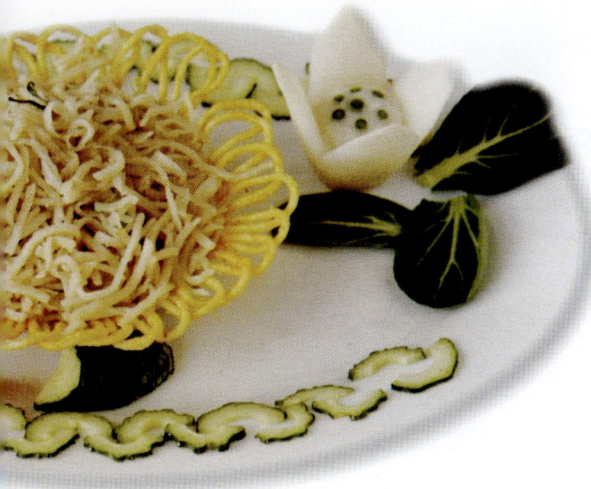
(Photo: by Dingxi Hotel)

Ingredients:
Potato 500 g, flour 250 g

Seasonings:
Vegetable oil 15 g, salt 10 g, ginger powder 3 g, Chinese prickly ash 2 g

Preparation:
1. Peel potatoes and shred into thin strips with a grater in a bowl. Add flour and mix well with salt, ginger powder and Chinese prickly ash.
2. Steam in a steamer for 15 minutes.
3. Heat vegetable oil in a wok stir-fry the steamed potatoes. Remove to a dish and serve.

Vegetarian: ✗   Muslim: ✗

Goulash with potato
Tudou Shao Niurou

Ingredients:
Potato 300 g, beef 200 g

Seasonings:
Peanut oil 50 g, Chinese prickly ash powder 3 g, ginger powder 3 g, table salt 2 g, gourmet powder 1 g, soy sauce 1 g, fennel powder 3 g, Chinese cinnamon 2 g, sugar 2 g, green onion 3 g, red and green paprika 20 g

Preparation:
1. Dice beef into 2 cm cubes.
2. Put the beef in boiling water and then remove and rinse off blood and froth.
3. Heat oil and add green onion, then stir-fry with the beef. Add soy sauce, star anise, Chinese cinnamon, sugar and salt. Then add enough water to cover the beef and cook over high heat.
4. Cover the pot and stew about one hour. Add diced potato stew for about 10 minutes. Add red and green paprika and stir-fry. Remove and add gourmet powder, then serve.

Vegetarian: ✗   Muslim: ✓

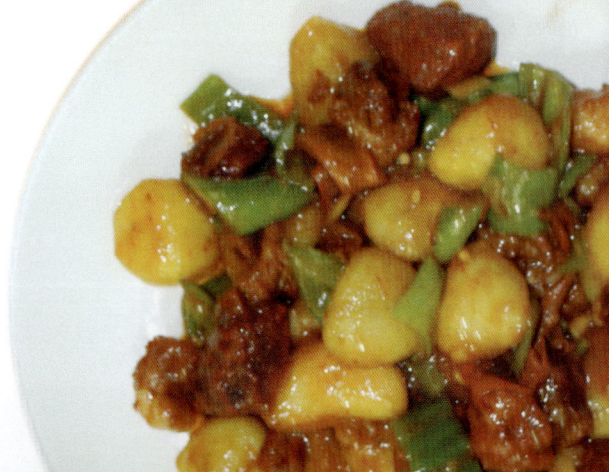

Grape-Shaped Potato Dish
Fengshou Putao

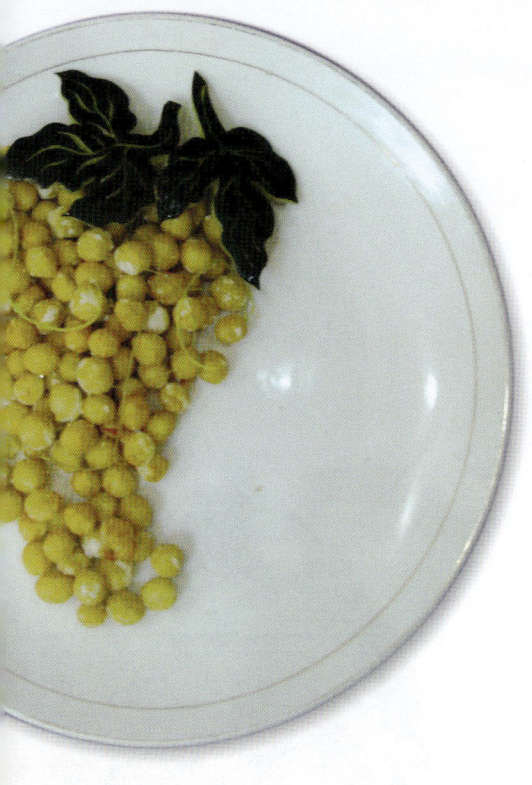

Ingredient:
Potato 500 g

Seasoning:
White sugar 4 g

Preparation:
Steam the potatoes and mash them. Add white sugar and form the potato mash into small balls. Heat oil and fry the balls. Remove and lay out in grape shapes

Vegetarian: ✓   Muslim: ✓

Mashed potatoes with pakchoi
Hua Cai

Ingredients:
Potato 500 g, pakchoi 200 g

Seasonings:
Peanut oil 50 g, green onion 3 g, table salt 1 g, gourmet powder 1 g, ginger powder 3 g, sesame 5 g, red pepper 2 g

Preparation:
1. Clean the potatoes and put in 200 ml of water. Boil over a medium heat until water is boiling. Turn off heat and simmer the potatoes about 10 minutes. Peel and mash the potatoes.
2. Put the pakchoi in the boiling water and remove immediately. Cut into strings.
3. Heat some oil and add green onion and red pepper until it gives off aroma. Then mix in mashed potato, pakchoi and seasonings..

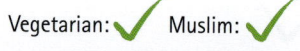
Vegetarian: ✓   Muslim: ✓

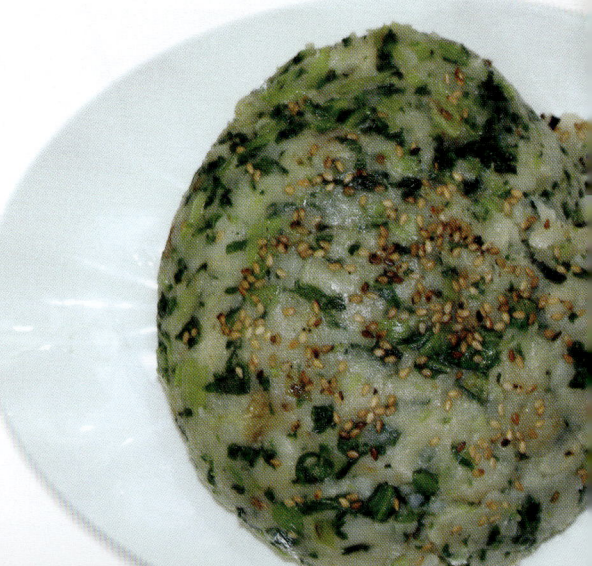

Pear-shaped potato
Xiang Sheng Li

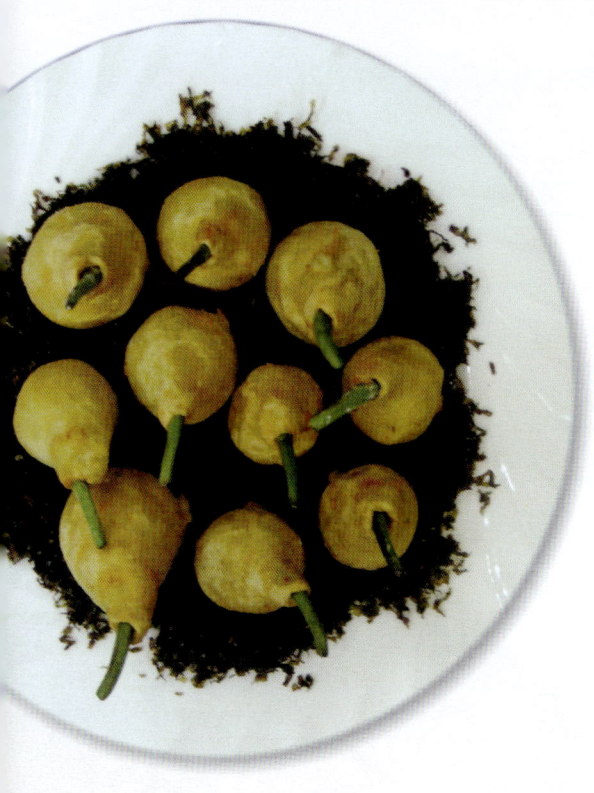

Ingredients:
Potato, five kernels filling

Seasonings:
Green pepper peduncle, vegetable oil

Preparation:
Steam potato and mash. Add five kernels filling and form into a pear shape. Put in the wok and deep-fry until the skin is crispy. Remove to a dish and put the green pepper peduncle on it.

Vegetarian: ✓   Muslim: ✓

Potato and buckwheat pancakes
Malingshu Jianbing

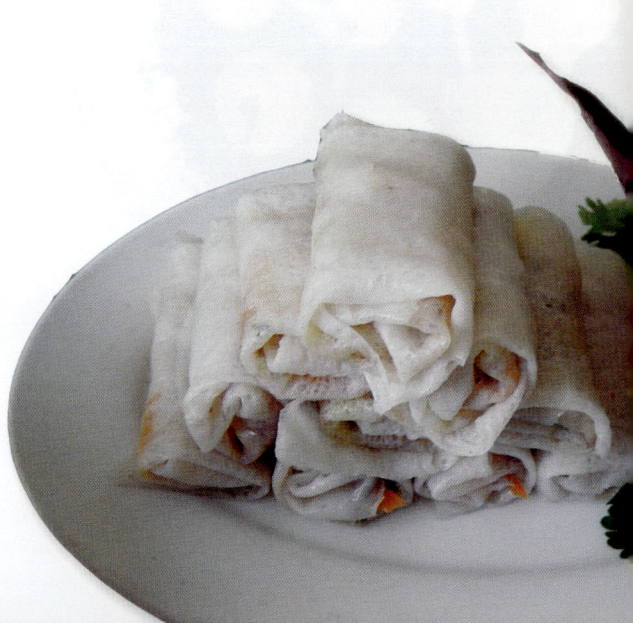

Ingredients:
Potato starch 500 g, buckwheat flour 100 g, pork strings 100 g, mung bean sprout 200 g

Seasonings:
Peanut oil 50 g, dried chili 3 g, table salt 1g, paprika 3 g, ginger powder 3 g, gourmet powder 1 g, chopped green onion 3 g

Preparation:

1. Blend potato starch and buckwheat flour with cool water until it is a smooth, viscous pastry.

2. Heat a pan, apply a little oil, then add a spoonful of pastry (about 25 g). Shake the pan in a circled curve to make sure that the pastry spreads around the pan. Take the pancake out after 1 minute.

3. Stir-fry the pork strings and mung bean sprouts with seasonings until they are done. Stuff pancakes with filling and roll up to eat.

Vegetarian: ✗   Muslim: ✗

Potato and Oat Pancakes
Tudou Bing IV

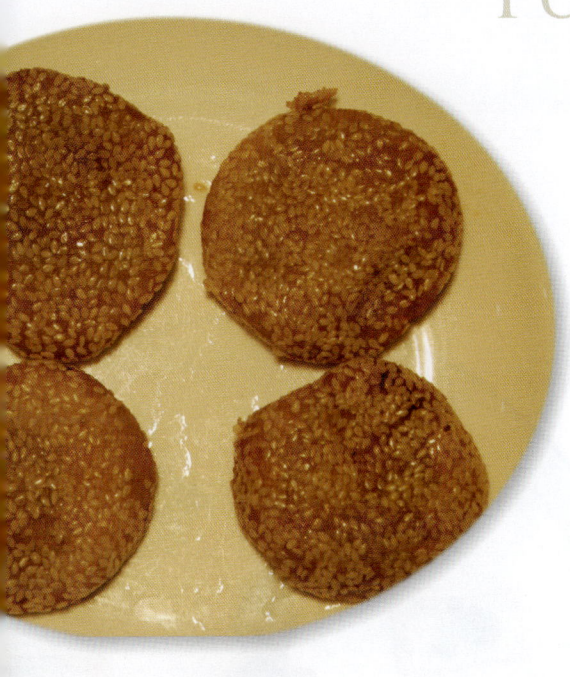

Ingredients:
Potato 500 g, oat flour 100 g

Seasonings:
Sesame 300 g, linseed oil 50 g, table salt 3 g

Preparation:
1. Boil potatoes in 100 ml of water over medium heat. Turn off the oven after the water boils and simmer for 10 minutes.

2. Cool, peel and mash the potatoes. Mix with oat flour and knead into a pan shape.

3. Sprinkle with sesame seeds, table salt and linseed oil, then bake with a little oil in the pan until it turns golden brown.

Vegetarian: ✓ Muslim: ✓

Potato and pumpkin sandwich
Baihua Tudou He

Ingredients:
Potato 500 g, pumpkin 1,000 g, beef 250 g, carrot 500 g, dried mushroom 250 g

Seasoning:
Salt 5 g

Preparation:
Slice potatoes and steam. Carve pumpkin to make small match-sized boxes. Fry beef, mushroom and carrot with salt, then fill pumpkin boxes with them. Put mashed potatoes on the top and garnish with vegetable flowers.

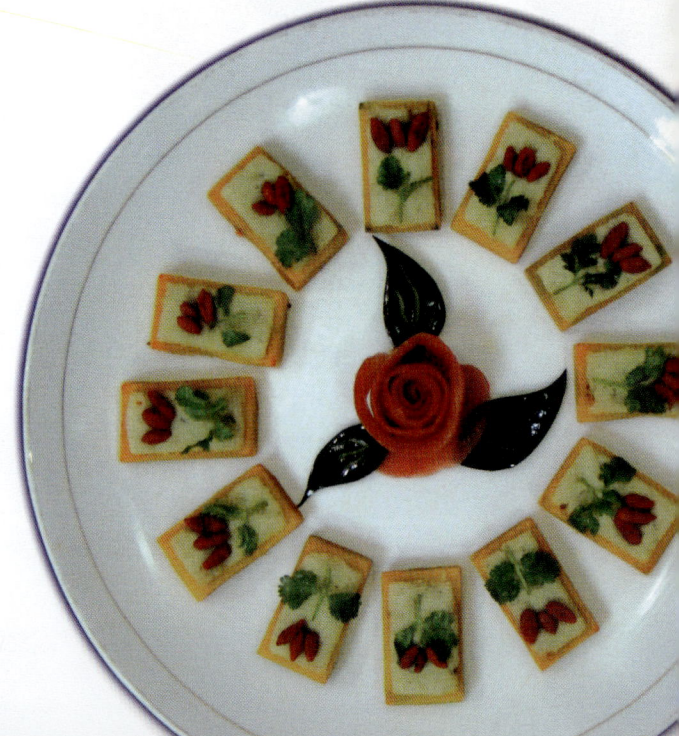

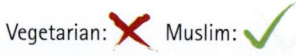

Potato and shiitake mushroom cake
Tudou Xianggu Bing

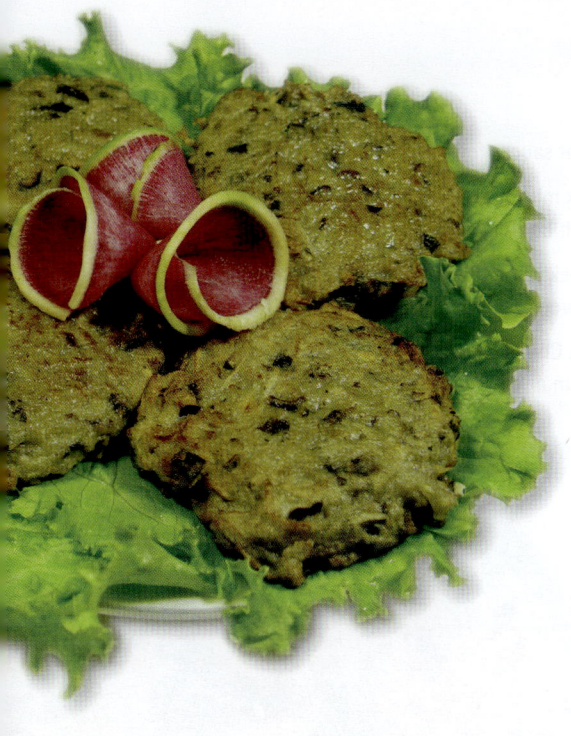

Ingredients:
Potato 300 g, shiitake mushroom 50 g

Seasonings:
Refined salt 3 g, soybean oil 15 g

Preparation:
1. Peel potato and soak in water. Use a grater to mash the potato, then put into cold water to be shaken with sieve. Change water twice, and then wait for starch to wash away; drain the left-over potato in the sieve.
2. Soak shiitake mushrooms in lukewarm water until they become soft, then mince.
3. Mix potato starch, sediment, shiitake mushroom and refined salt evenly to make a raw cake; set aside.
4. Heat oil in a pan and fry the raw cake until both sides turn brown. Remove to a dish and serve.

Vegetarian: ✓   Muslim: ✓

Potato Bula
Yangyu Bula

Ingredients:
Potato 300 g, flour 150 g

Seasonings:
Refined salt 2 g, minced garlic 3 g, chili powder 5 g, minced green onion or garlic sprout 50 g, Chinese chives 50 g, diced pork 100 g

Preparation:
1. Peel potatoes, cut into about 4–5 cm long strips.
2. Add flour and salt and mix evenly with potato strips by hand.
3. Put onto a plate and then put the plate in a steamer for 20 minutes. Mix with sauce and serve.

Different sauces for serving with potato Bula:
1. Mix minced garlic, chili powder and salt, and sprinkle with hot oil.
2. Quickly stir-fry minced green onion (or fragrant-flowered garlic) and chili powder with salt in a wok.
3. Cut Chinese chives into 7–10 mm sections and quick-fry in a wok, adding salt to taste.

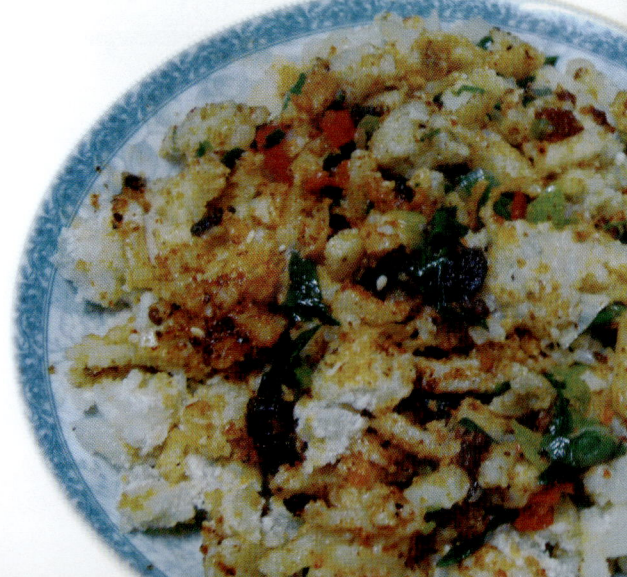

Vegetarian: ✗ Muslim: ✗

Potato cake III
Tudou Gao

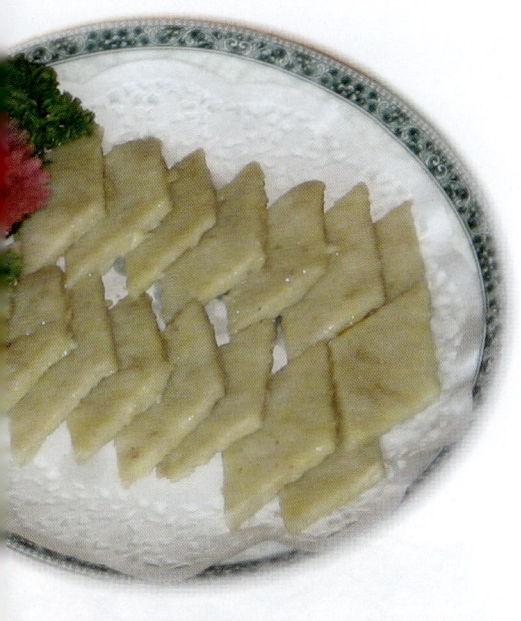

Ingredient:
Potato 100 g

Seasonings:
Cheese powder, salt 3 g, flavor spices 1 g, starch 5 g, oil 500 g

Preparation:
Shred wash potatoes. Fry potato strings in oil with cheese powder, salt, flavor spices and starch until it forms a cake, then serve.

Vegetarian: ✓   Muslim: ✓

Potato chicken egg soup
Tudou Jidan Geng

Ingredients:
3 egg (about 200 ml), 1 or 2 potatoes, raisins 20 g, Chinese matrimony vine 20 g, a few carrots

Seasonings:
Soy sauce, salt and chicken essence to taste

Preparation:
1. Dice potatoes and cut carrot into strips or small pieces. Combine with raisins and Chinese matrimony-vine in a bowl. Set aside.
2. Whisk eggs in a bowl; stop before eggs start to foam.
3. Add 400 ml water, soy sauce, chicken essence and a little salt.
4. To improve the taste, filter egg fluid with a colander.
5. Steam the bowl for about 7 minutes.
6. Remove bowl and sprinkle with cilantro as well as a few drops of sesame oil, serve.

Vegetarian: ✘   Muslim: ✓

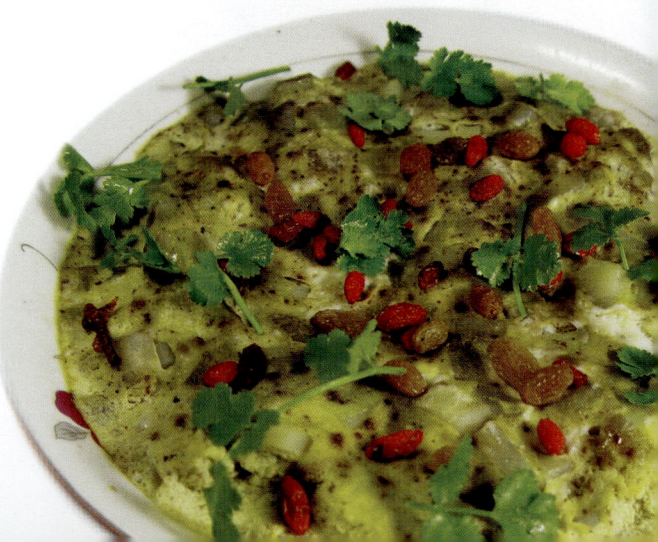

Potato Noodles
Yangyu Mian

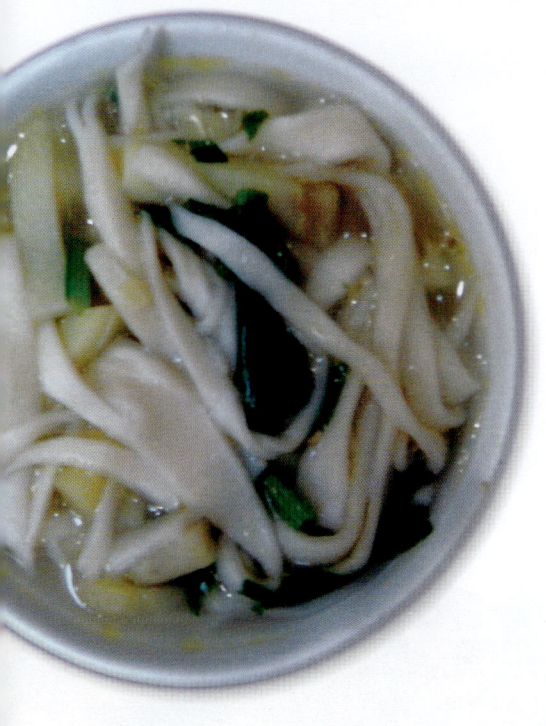

Ingredients:
Potato, wheat flour, spinach

Seasonings:
Salt to taste, minced green onion

Preparation:
1. Make wheat flour into dough, then knead it into hand-made noodles.
2. Cut potatoes into strips. Fry minced green onion, then add potato strips and spinach and stir-fry. Add water and stew to make a thick sauce.
3. Cook the noodles, remove to the bowl and serve with the sauce.

Vegetarian: ✓   Muslim: ✓

Potato nut cake
Malingshu Ganguo Gao

Ingredients:
Potato 200 g, apricot kernels, raisins and walnut kernels, 2 eggs

Seasonings:
Salt to taste, sugar, gourmet powder, oil, lettuce and tomato

Preparation:
1. Boil three big potatoes for about 40 minutes until well-cooked, then peel and mash while hot.
2. Mince apricot and walnut kernels.
3. Mix the mashed potatoes and minced nuts in a bowl. Add 2 egg whites and a little water and mix evenly.
4. Form the mashed potato mixture into several sticks.
5. Fry the sticks until yellow, then remove and drain oil.
6. Put the potato-nut sticks on a plate and serve with lettuce and tomato.

Vegetarian: ✗ Muslim: ✓

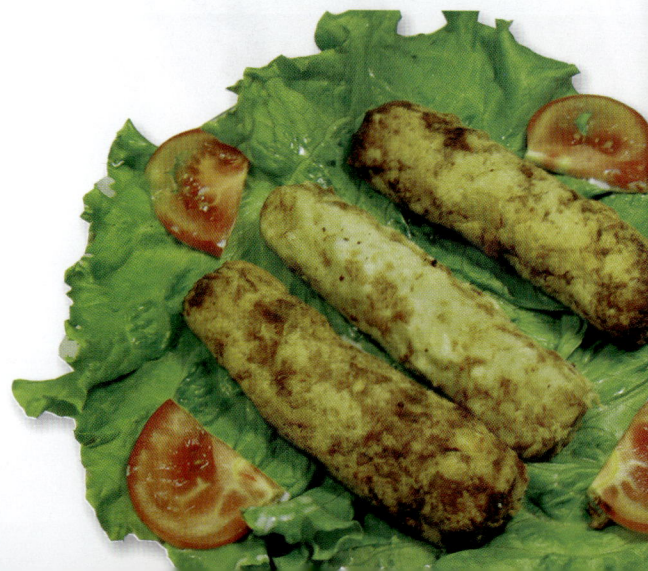

Potato Salad
Tudou Shala

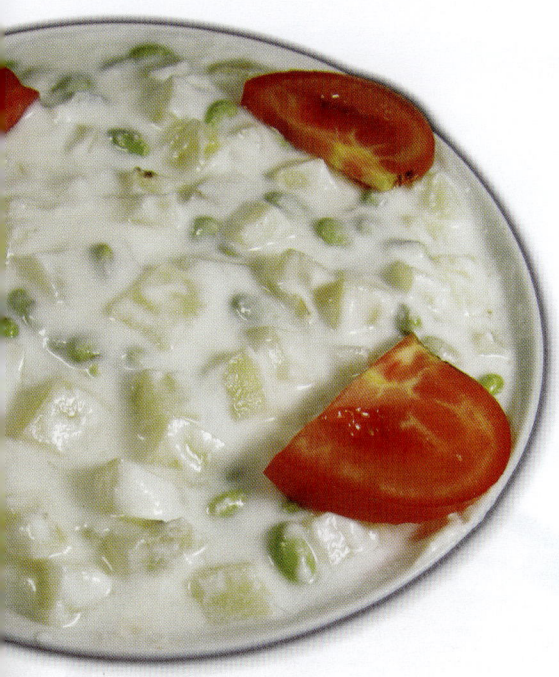

Seasonings:

Salad dressing, yogurt

Preparation:

1. Dice potatoes and boil with green beans in wok over medium heat for 10–15 minutes. Then remove and drain.
2. Mince carrot and onion. The carrot is to add color, the onion for seasoning,
3. Separate the boiled egg yolk and white. Add the yolk to the potatoes. Mince the egg white and set aside.
4. Combine the minced onion, carrot and egg white in a bowl with the potato and green beans. Add some yogurt, ground white pepper and salt, as well as salad dressing. Stir well. The preparation is quite simple and this dish is popular among children. It is also healthy for them because it contains vegetables that most children do not like to eat.

Ingredients:

Potato, green beans, onion, carrot, ground white pepper, boiled egg

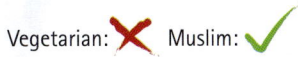

Potato starch jelly
Malingshu Liangfen

Ingredient:
Potato starch 500 g

Seasonings:
Chinese leek 10 g, coriander 10 g, table salt 3 g, vinegar 3 g, sesame oil 1 g, mustard oil 0.5 g, chili oil 0.5 g, gourmet powder 0.5 g

Preparation:
1. Blend potato starch with 1,000 ml of water. Slowly put the mixture into boiling water while stirring the starch paste. Boil, then reduce to low heat and stir until it is well-done and thick.
2. Wait until it cools down and slice.
3. Add Chinese leek, coriander, table salt, vinegar, sesame oil, mustard oil, chili oil and gourmet powder before serving.

Vegetarian: ✓   Muslim: ✓

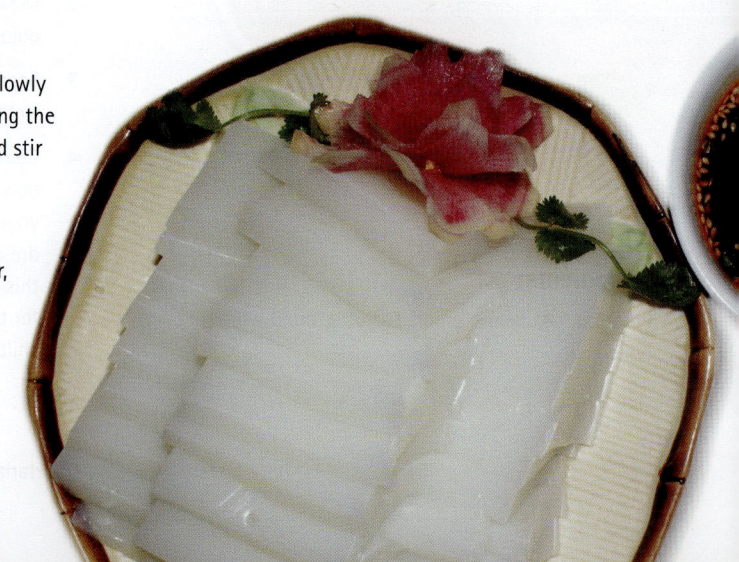

Potato-wrapped Beef Rolls
Tudou Niurou Juan

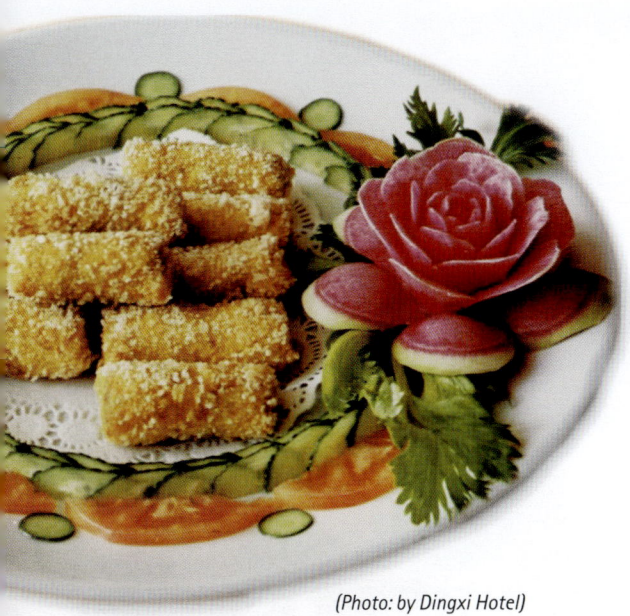

(Photo: by Dingxi Hotel)

Ingredients:
Potato 1,000 g, beef 250 g

Seasonings:
Vegetable oil 500 g, flour 50 g, salt 10 g, ginger powder 3 g, Chinese prickly ash 2 g

Preparation:
1. Clean potatoes and steam for 30 minutes. Peel and mash the potatoes, then mix evenly with flour and set aside.
2. Add salt, ginger powder and Chinese prickly ash to the minced beef to make the filling. Wrap the beef filling with the potato mash and coat with flour. Heat vegetable oil in a wok and deep-fry beef rolls until golden.

Vegetarian: ✗   Muslim: ✓

Rolls with potato and beef filling
Tudou Niurou Bing

Ingredients:
Potato 300 g, beef 100 g, wheat flour 200 g

Seasonings:
Salt, flavor spices, gourmet powder and chicken essence

Preparation:
Add boiling water to wheat flour to make dough. Roll the dough into a cake. Flavor cooked beef and potatoes with salt, flavor spices, gourmet powder and chicken essence, then use as filling. Stuff the cake with the filling, then steam for 20 minutes.

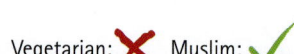
Vegetarian: ✗   Muslim: ✓

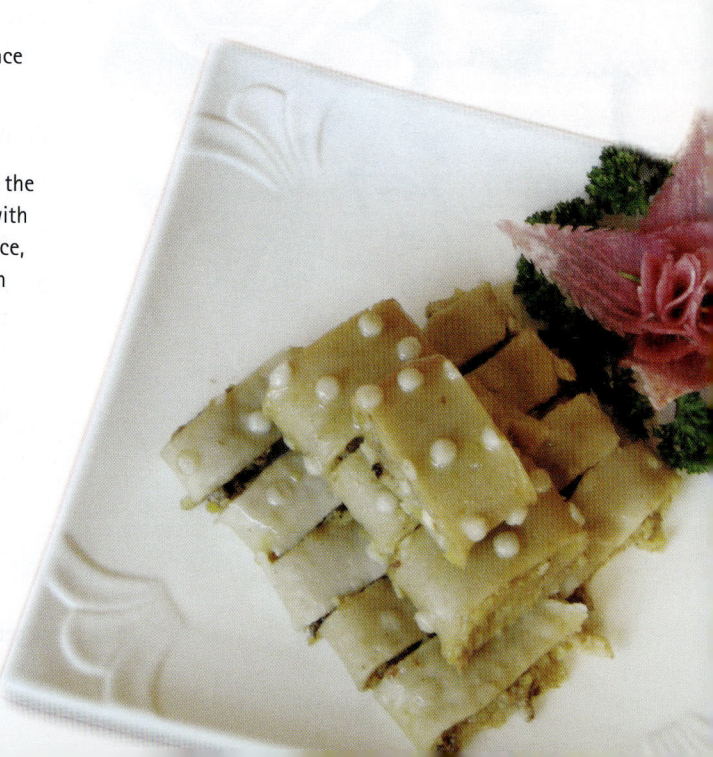

San Zha Wu Pin

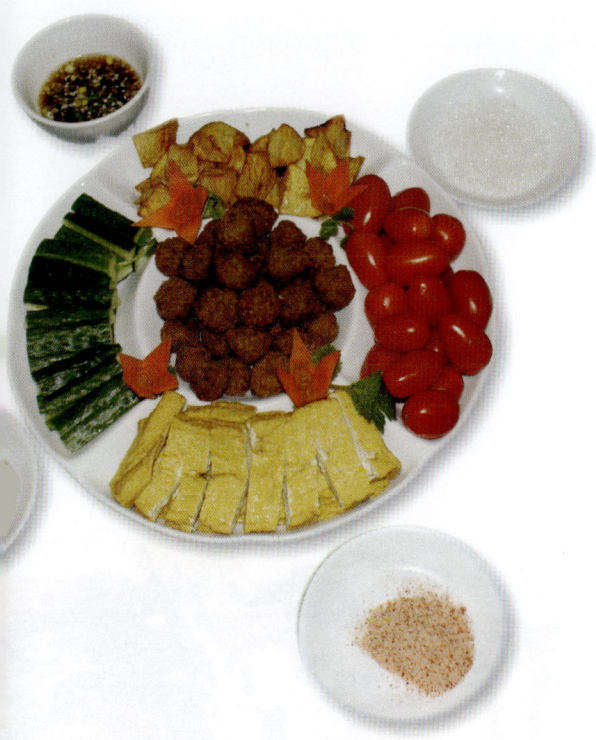

Seasonings:

Fennel powder 3 g, minced ginger 3 g, Chinese prickly ash 3 g, table salt 2 g, gourmet powder 2 g, soy sauce 2 g, Chinese chives 2 g, coriander 2 g, vinegar 2 g, sesame oil 1 g, chili oil 2 g, spiced salt 4 g, 3 eggs

Preparation:

1. Peel and clean 250 g of potatoes. Cut into pieces and fry until golden.

2. Grind 200 g of streaky pork and 200 g of potatoes. Mix well with 60 g of potato starch, fennel powder, minced ginger, Chinese prickly ash, table salt, gourmet powder, a little soy sauce and an egg. Form mixture into balls and fry in hot oil until golden, then remove.

3. Fry 250 g of tofu slices in hot oil until golden.

4. Cut cucumbers into several pieces and combine with cherry tomatoes, fried potato chips, meet balls and Tofu in a dish.

5. Mix with Chinese chives, coriander, vinegar, sesame oil, chili oil, gourmet powder and soy sauce, then serve.

Vegetarian: ✗ Muslim: ✗

Ingredients:

Potatoes 450 g, streaky pork 200 g, potato starch 150 g, tofu 250 g, cucumber 250 g, cherry tomato 250 g

Shredded potatoes with sweet and sour sauce
Yuxiang Tudou Si

Ingredient:
Potato 500 g

Seasonings:
Vegetable oil 30 g, 2 pieces of ginger, 1 green onion, 2 cloves of garlic, broad bean paste 20 g, soy sauce 5 g, sugar 2 g, vinegar 2 g, chicken essence 2 g

Preparation:
1. Peel and shred potatoes.
2. Heat vegetable oil in wok and fry minced ginger, onion, garlic and broad bean paste until it gives off aroma. Add potato strips, soy sauce, sugar, vinegar and chicken essence and fry, then serve.

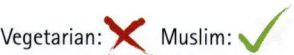
Vegetarian: ✗ Muslim: ✓

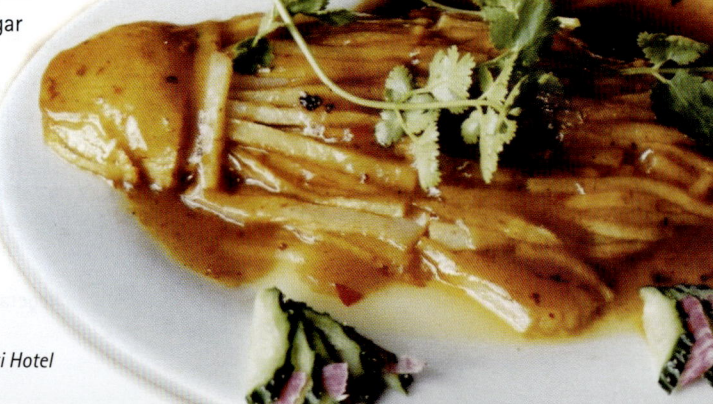
Photo: by Dingxi Hotel

Soft potato cake
Yangyu Langao

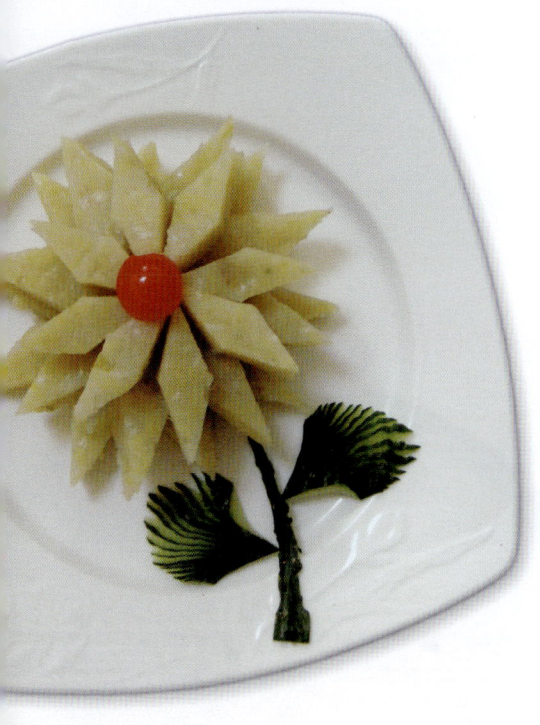

Ingredient:
Potato 500 g

Seasonings:
Corn starch 3 g, salt 5 g

Preparation:
Cut potato into thin strips with a grater. Add corn starch and salt and steam. Slice cake and serve with sauce.

Vegetarian: ✓   Muslim: ✓

Steamed potato and lichen dumplings
Tudou Diruan Baozi

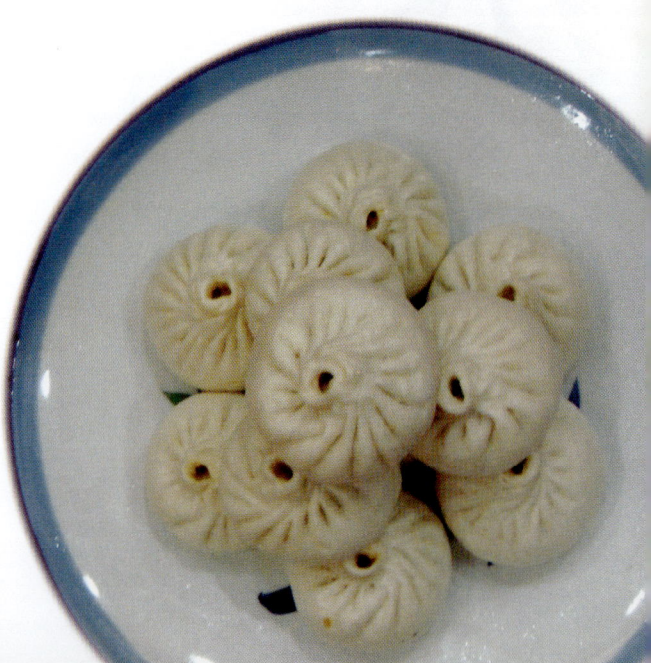

Ingredients:
Cooked potato 150 g, lichen 300 g, wheat flour 500 g, yeast 5 g

Seasonings:
Minced green onion 20 g, diced chili 30 g, noodles 30 g, green onion oil 20 g, a little salt and gourmet powder, baking powder 5 g, shortening 3 g

Preparation:
1. Peel and dice potatoes, mince lichen, add green onion, salt, gourmet powder, green onion oil and diced chili, and mix well. Use as filling.

2. Ferment wheat flour, add baking powder and shortening and knead well. Roll the dough with a rolling pin into a column shape, then divide into several dumplings. Roll the small dumplings into wrappers with a diameter of 5 cm and wrap the filling. Put into steamer and steam for 20 minutes.

Vegetarian: ✓   Muslim: ✓

Steamed potato flakes mixed with flour
Yangyu Caca

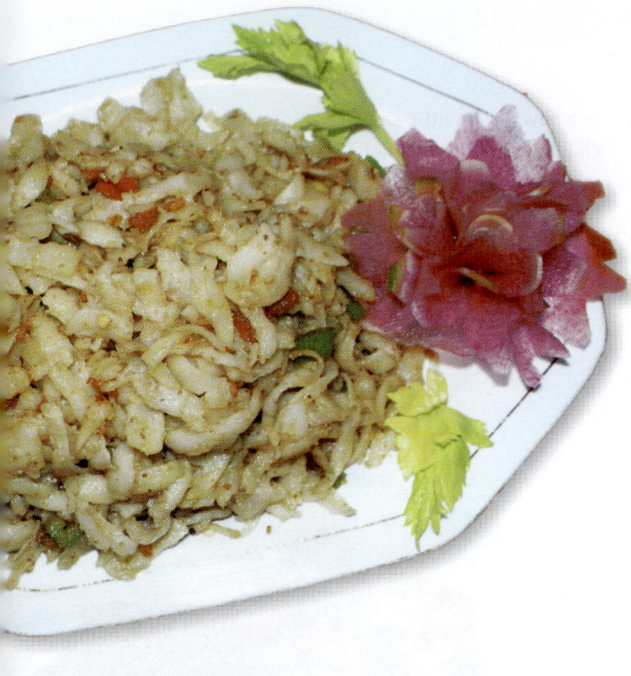

Ingredients:
Potato 500 g, flour 80 g

Seasonings:
Linseed oil 100 g, chopped green onion 10 g, Chinese prickly ash 2 g, minced ginger 5 g, table salt 3 g, diced celery 10 g, diced green pepper 10 g

Preparation:
1. Clean and peel potatoes. Slice with a grater and mix with flour. Steam for 15–20 minutes.
2. Heat oil and stir-fry the steamed potatoes with chopped green onion, Chinese prickly ash, minced ginger, table salt, diced celery and green pepper for 1 minute.

Vegetarian: ✓   Muslim: ✓

Steamed potato jelly
Yangyu Jinjin

Ingredients:
Potato 400 g, flour 100 g

Seasonings:
Salt 4 g, ginger powder 1/2 tsp, mashed garlic and chili powder to taste, minced green onion or garlic sprout 50 g, Chinese chives 50 g, diced pork 100 g, vegetable oil 30 g, soy sauce, vinegar, sesame oil to taste.

Preparation:
1. Peel potatoes, then use a grater to shred the potatoes into paste.
2. Add flour, salt and ginger powder, then put the mixture into water and stir to form a thick paste. Spread on a bamboo steamer to form a big 1 cm-thick cake. Steam for 20 minutes, remove and cut into strips, then serve.
3. In a bowl, mix a little salt with garlic mash and chili powder, then add hot oil, soy sauce, vinegar and sesame oil to make sauce.
4. Use sauce for dipping or pour over the potatoes and serve with vegetables.

Vegetarian: ✗   Muslim: ✗

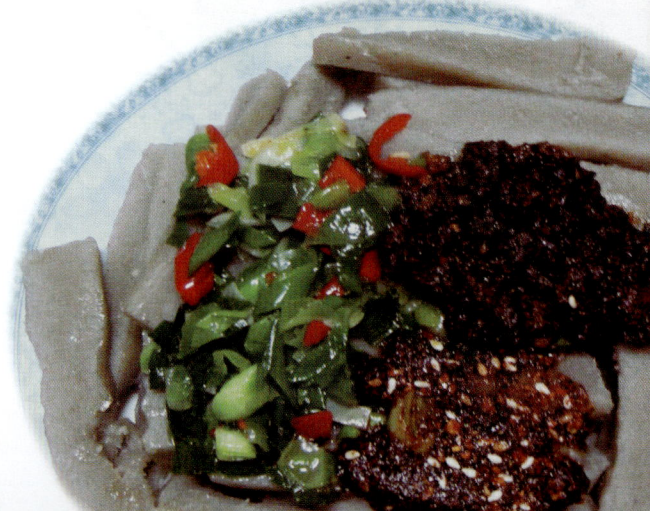

Steamed potatoes II
Zheng Tudou

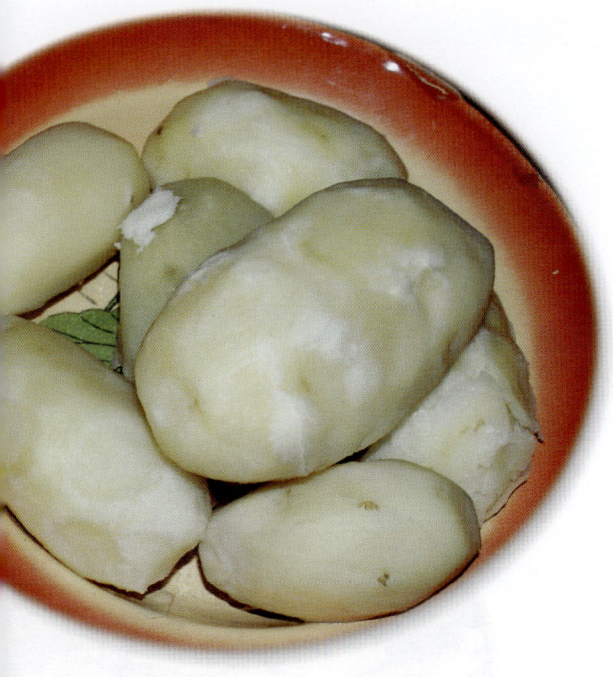

Ingredient:
Potato 500 g

Seasonings:
Chinese pickled vegetables 200 g

Preparation:
1. Clean and peel potatoes. Steam the potatoes for 15 to 20 minutes.

2. Add Chinese pickled vegetables and serve.

Vegetarian: ✓   Muslim: ✓

Steamed potatoes with chicken
Tudou Zheng Ji

Ingredients:
Potato 200 g, chicken 500 g, wheat flour 100 g

Seasonings:
Salt to taste, gourmet powder, flavor spices and minced green onion to taste

Preparation:
1. Cut up the chicken and marinate in salt, gourmet powder, flavor spices and minced green onion.
2. Dice potatoes. Add boiling water to the wheat flour and make dough. Roll the dough into a big cake, then spread the diced potatoes on the cake together with the chicken pieces and steam for 40 minutes.

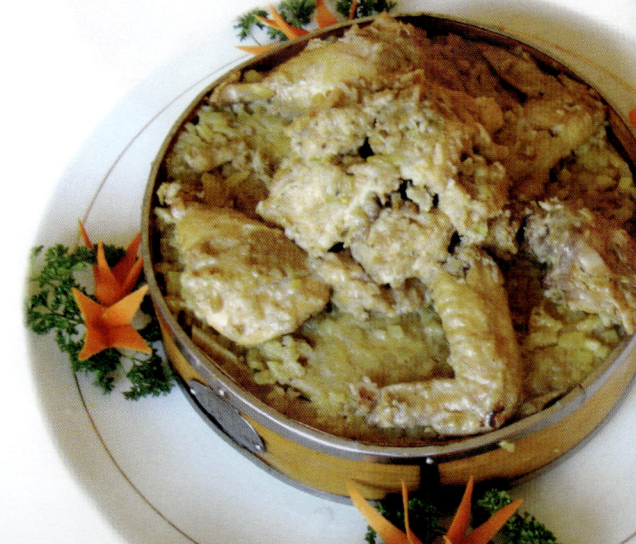

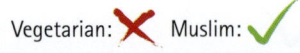

Stewed potatoes
Men Tudou

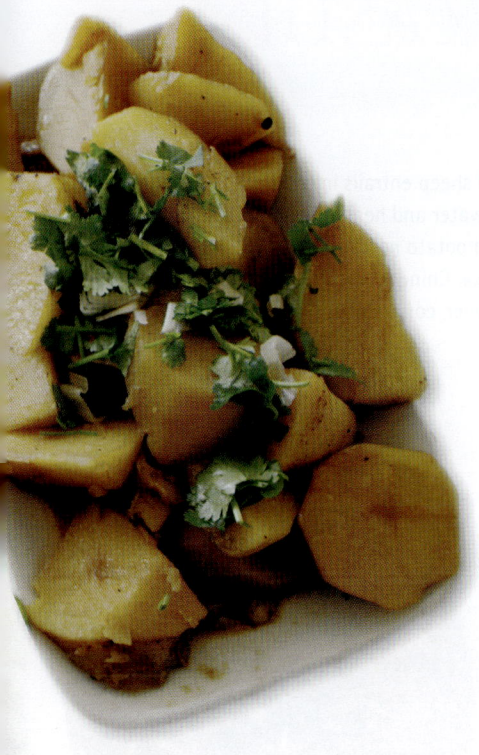

Ingredient:
Potato 500 g

Seasonings:
Peanut oil 50 g, green onion 3 g, red pepper 2 g, soy sauce 2 g, ginger powder 2 g, Chinese prickly ash 2 g, table salt 1 g, gourmet powder 1 g

Preparation:
1. Dice potatoes.
2. Heat oil and lightly fry green onion and red pepper until it gives off aroma. Add diced potatoes and soy sauce and stir-fry until brown. Add water, ginger powder, Chinese prickly ash and salt and stew for 15 minutes. Add gourmet powder and serve.

Vegetarian: ✓   Muslim: ✓

Stewed sheep entrails with potato noodles
Yu Lin Yang Zasui

Ingredients:
Potato noodles 500 g, fried potato strings 200 g, fried tofu 200 g, sheep entrails 200 g

Seasonings:
Minced green onion 10 g, sliced fresh ginger 10 g, minced ginger 3 g, pepper 5 g, Chinese prickly ash 3 g, dry chili 5 g, paprika 2 g, table salt 3 g, ground pepper 2 g, gourmet powder 2 g, coriander 10 g

Preparation:
1. Clean and boil sheep entrails in water with chopped green onion, sliced fresh ginger, pepper granules, dry chili and table salt until well-done. Remove and shred.
2. Shred tomatoes and tofu, then fry in hot oil until golden. Steam potato noodles.
3. Put shredded sheep entrails into the meat soup with 2,500 ml of water and heat. After it boils, add potato noodles, fried potato noodles, fried tofu, minced ginger, paprika, Chinese prickly ash, table salt, gourmet powder, coriander and chopped green onion, then serve.

Vegetarian: ✘ Muslim: ✓

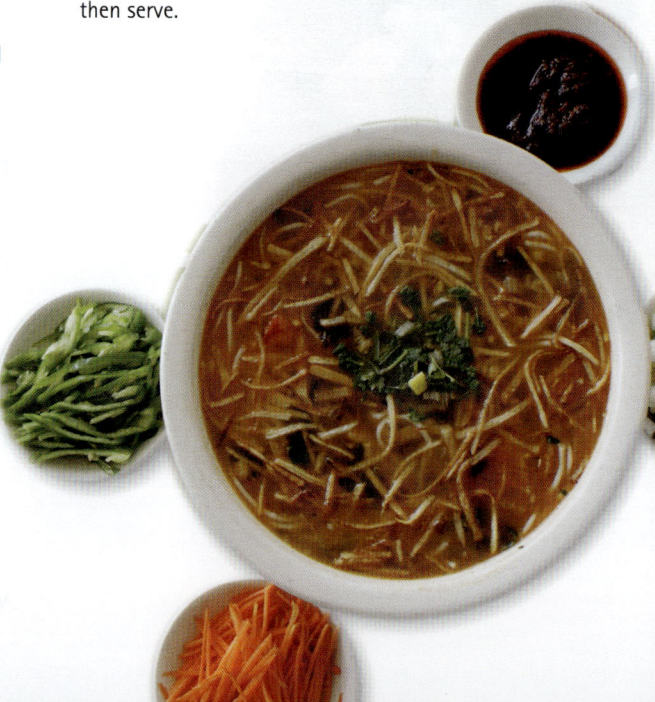

Stir-fried beef with potato noodles
Niurou Chao Fen

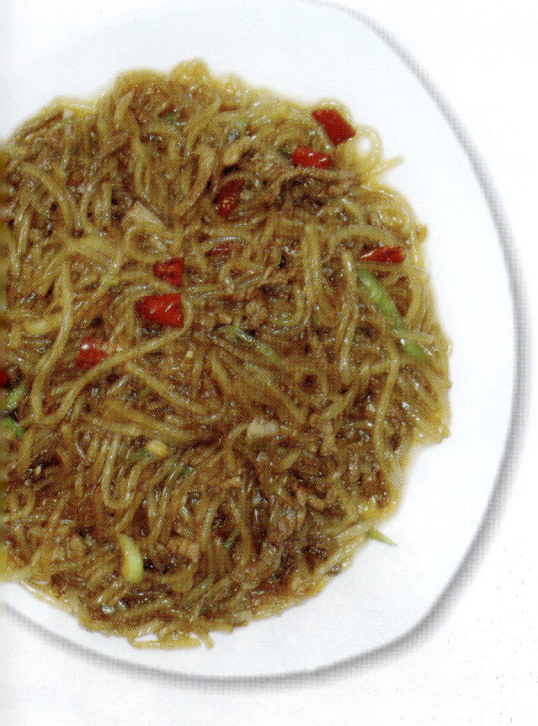

Ingredients:
Potato noodles 500 g, beef 100 g

Seasonings:
Peanut oil 50 g, soy sauce 2 g, green onion 3 g, crushed garlic 3 g, ginger powder 3 g, Chinese prickly ash 2 g, fennel powder 2 g, table salt 1 g, gourmet powder 1 g

Preparation:
1. Slice beef. Stew potato noodles.
2. Stir-fry the beef until it is dry. Add soy sauce, green onion, minced garlic, ginger powder, Chinese prickly ash, fennel powder and salt. When the beef is almost well-done, add noodles and stir-fry for 3 minutes.

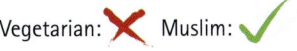

Stir-fried pork with potato noodles
Zhurou Qiao Ban Fen

Ingredients:
Potato noodles 500 g, lean pork 100 g

Seasonings:
Peanut oil 50 g, soy sauce 2 g, green onion 3 g, crushed garlic 3 g, ginger 3 g, Chinese prickly ash 2 g, fennel powder 2 g, table salt 1 g, gourmet powder 1 g

Preparation:
1. Cut 100 g of pork into slices. Put the potato noodles in boiling water and braise about 10 minutes.
2. Stir-fry the pork slices until they are dry, and then add soy sauce, green onion, crushed garlic, ginger powder, Chinese prickly ash, fennel powder and salt. When the pork is almost well-done, add the noodles and stir-fry them about 3 minutes.

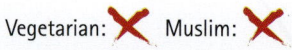

Vegetarian: ✗   Muslim: ✗

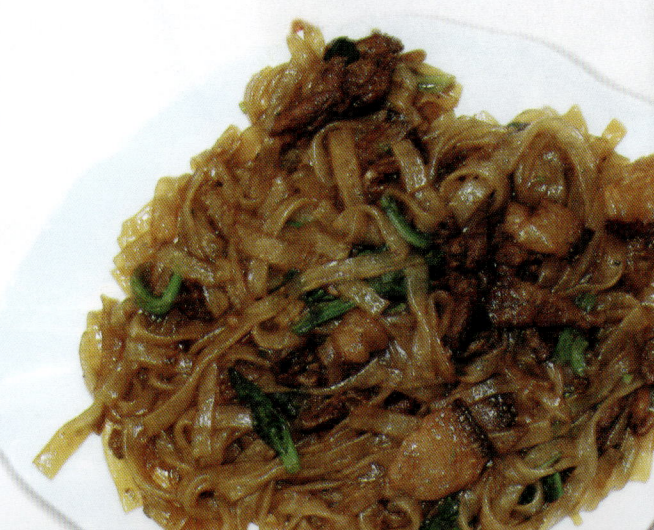

Strawberry-filled Mashed Potato Cake
Caomei Yuni Su

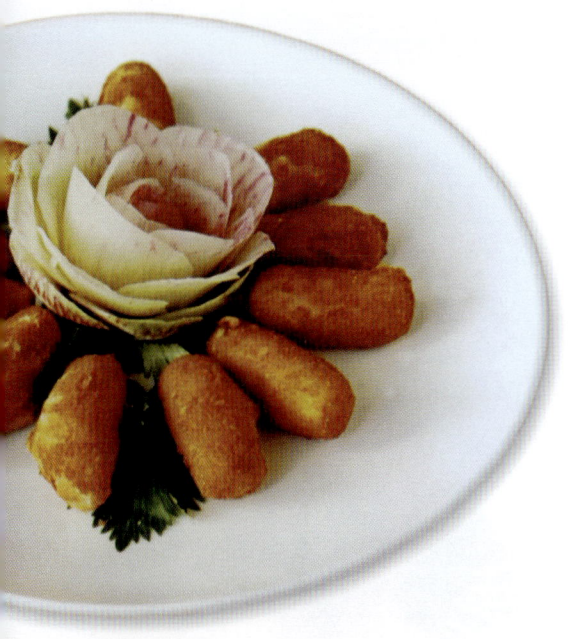

Photo: by Dingxi Hotel

Ingredients:
Potato 1,000 g, strawberry jam 300 g

Seasonings:
Vegetable oil 500 g, bread flour 50 g

Preparation:
1. Clean potatoes and steam for 30 minutes, then peel and mash. Mix evenly with bread flour. Fill the potato balls with strawberry jam and set aside.
2. Heat vegetable oil in wok and deep-fry potato-strawberry balls until brown, then remove and serve.

Vegetarian: ✓   Muslim: ✓

Sweet fried potato chips
Huanying Tudou Pian

Ingredient:
Potato 500 g

Seasoning:
White sugar to taste

Preparation:
Select potatoes of about the same size. Finely slice them and deep-fry. Sprinkle the chips with white sugar before serving.

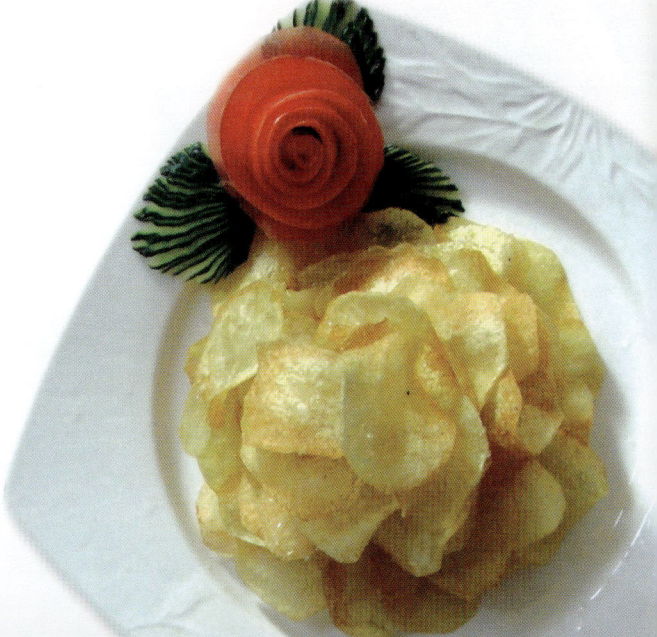

Vegetarian: ✓   Muslim: ✓

Three Kinds of Stewed Vegetable Balls
Shao San Yuan

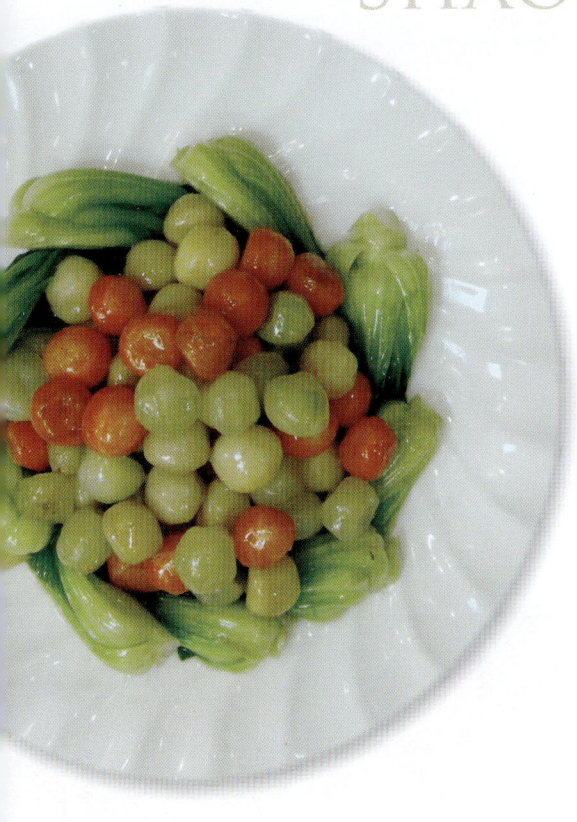

Ingredients:
Potato, green asparagus, carrot

Seasoning:
Salt 3 g

Preparation:
Make potatoes, green asparagus and carrot into small balls using a special kitchen tool, add salt, steam. Then put them into the wok with a little oil, add soup stock to stew well.

Vegetarian: ✗   Muslim: ✗

Xinjiang chicken and potato dish
Xinjiang Da Pan Ji

Ingredients:
Chicken 500 g, potato 500 g, 1 green pepper, 1 red pepper, 1 mushroom, dough

Seasonings:
Green onion, ginger, garlic, Chinese prickly ash, small hot pepper to taste

Preparation:
1. Heat oil in wok and fry Chinese prickly ash.
2. Add chicken, green onion, ginger, garlic and small hot pepper. Stir-fry for several minutes, then add soy sauce, water, white granulated sugar, salt, cooking wine and mushrooms and stew for 15 minutes.
3. Add potatoes and continue braising over low heat.
4. Add green pepper and red pepper for color.
5. Stir-fry and serve.

Vegetarian: ✗   Muslim: ✗

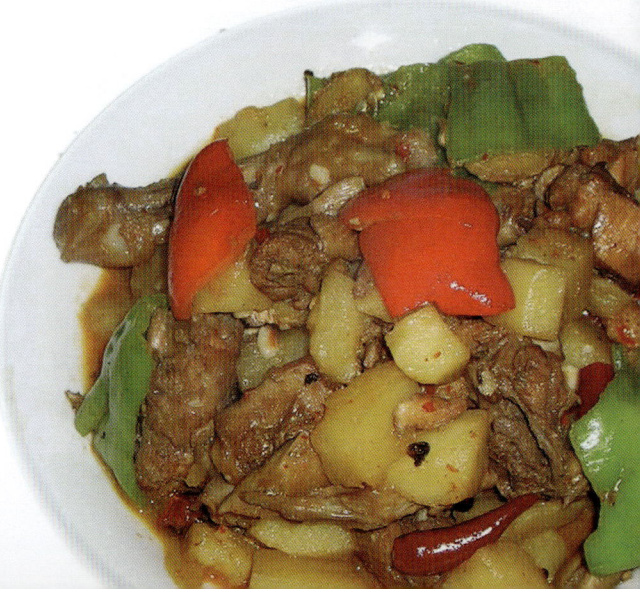

Yulin Three Fresh Delicacies
Yulin Pin Sanxian

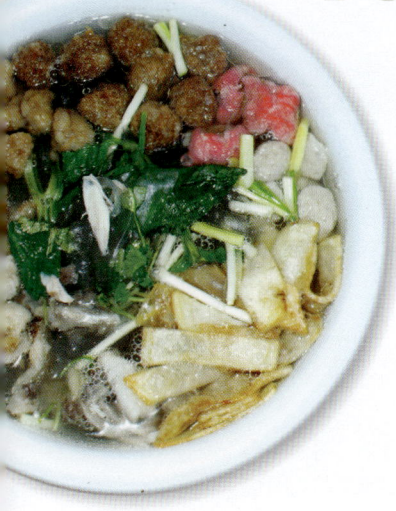

Ingredients:

Potato 500 g, potato starch 150 g, potato noodles 500 g, fried potato chips 200 g, streaky pork 500 g, stewed pork pieces 100 g, pork cooked in soy sauce 200 g, cooked mutton 200 g, cooked chicken 100 g

Seasonings:

Peanut oil 1,000 g, 3 eggs, fennel powder 5 g, minced ginger 5 g, Chinese prickly ash 5 g, table salt 3 g, steeped agaric 200 g, dried daylily flower 100 g, sliced kelp 100 g, ground pepper 3 g, Chinese chives 100 g, chopped green onion 10 g, coriander 10 g, soy sauce 5 g, spinach 10 g, sesame oil 2 g

Preparation:

1. Slice cooked pork and cooked mutton into pieces about 5 cm long and 2 cm thick. Shred cooked chicken by hand.
2. Grind stewed pork and potatoes then mix with potato starch, fennel powder, minced ginger, Chinese prickly ash, table salt, gourmet powder, a little soy sauce and three eggs. Form the mixture into balls and fry in hot oil until golden.
3. Fry potato pieces and stewed pork. Steam balls (refer to methods on how balls are made).
4. Boil the meat soup and add pork, mutton, chicken, stewed pork, meat balls, potato noodles, steeped agaric, steeped dried daylily flower, sliced kelp, minced ginger, ground pepper, Chinese chives, chopped green onion, coriander, table salt, soy sauce, gourmet powder and spinach. Remove, sprinkle with sesame oil and serve.

Vegetarian: ✗   Muslim: ✗

Potato Recipes from Southwest China

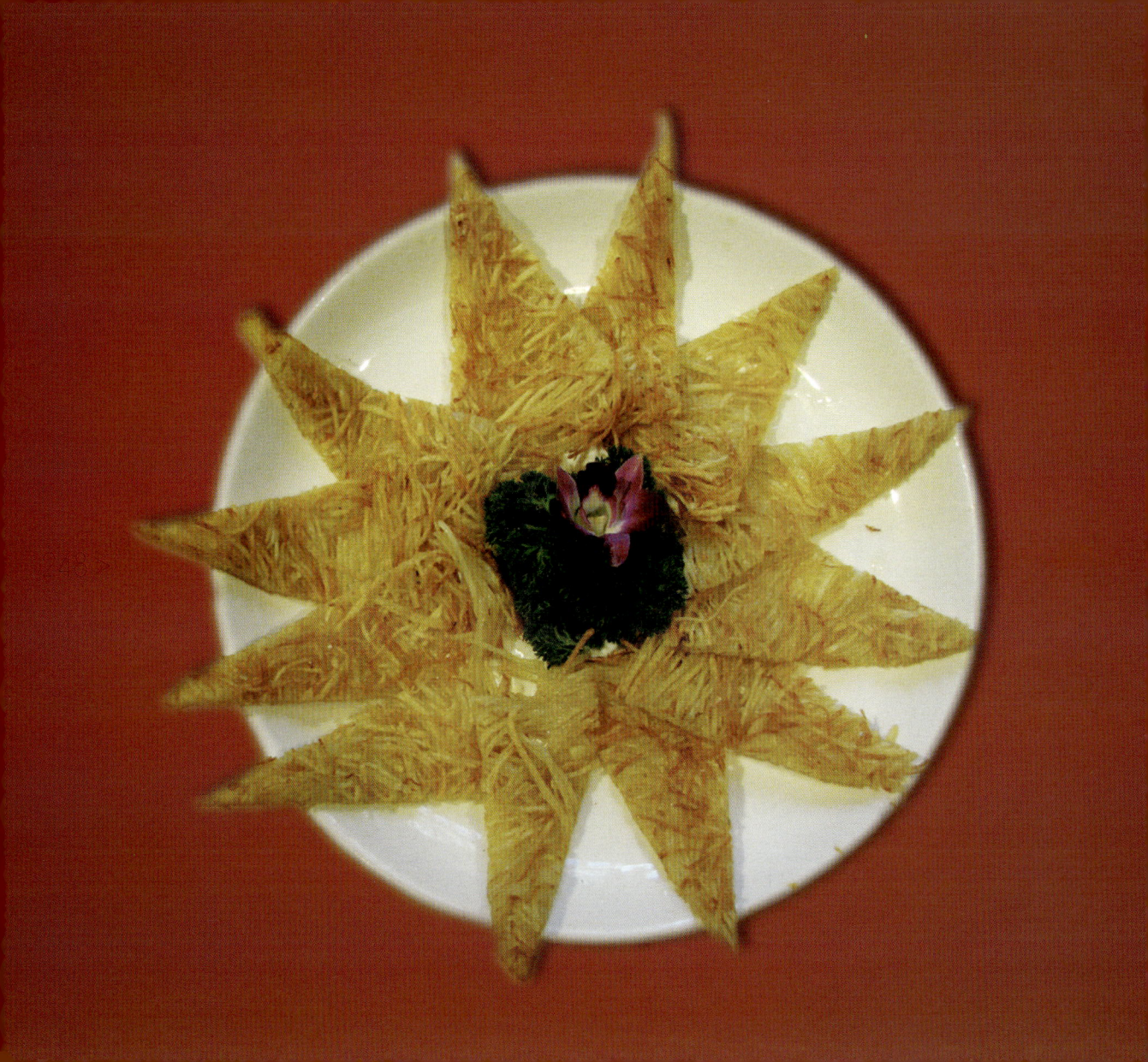

Baked Shredded Potatoes
Gan Bei Yangyu Si

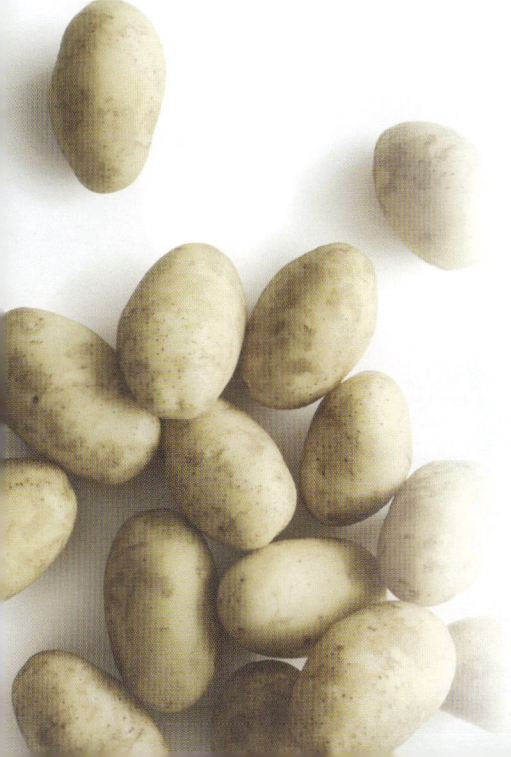

Ingredients:
Potato 500 g, starch 30 g

Seasonings:
Cooking oil 300 g, refined salt 5 g, Chinese prickly ash 2 g

Preparation:
1. Peel and shred potatoes.
2. Mix evenly with starch and press to form paste on a plate.
3. Heat oil over low heat and deep-fry raw potato cake until golden. Sprinkle evenly with salt and Chinese prickly ash.

Note: During frying, press potato cake frequently using pancake ladle.

Vegetarian: ✓   Muslim: ✓

Birds nest-shaped shredded potatoes
Niaochao Shu Si

Ingredients:
Potato 200 g, starch, 2 eggs

Seasonings:
Cooking oil 200 g, refined salt 2 g, fructus tsaoko powder to taste

Preparation:
1. Peel and shred potato. Separate egg yolk and white and whisk yolk in a bowl.
2. Mix the shredded potato, egg yolk, starch, salt and fructus tsaoko powder with water and knead into pan-shaped dough.
3. Heat oil a wok and fry the pancake until both sides are golden

Vegetarian: 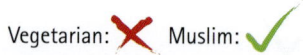 Muslim:

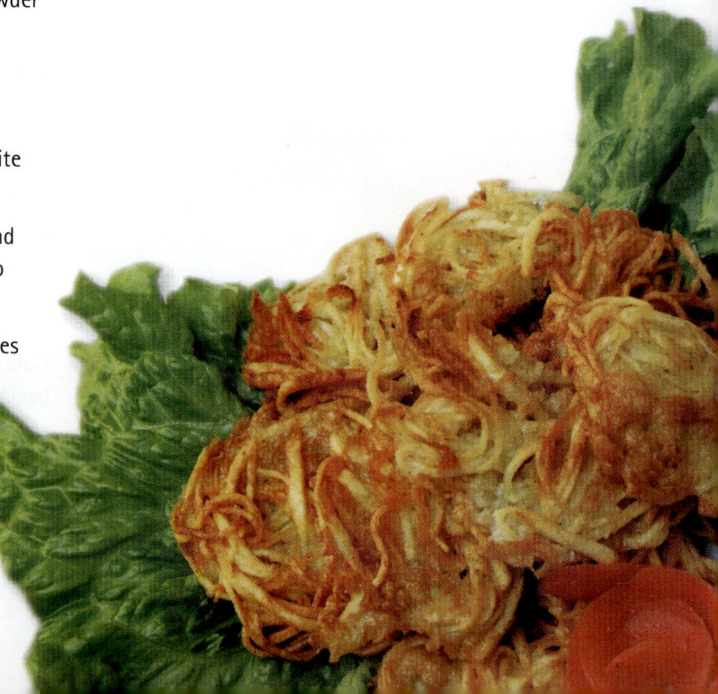

Braised potato balls with black soy sauce
Hongshao Tudouqiu

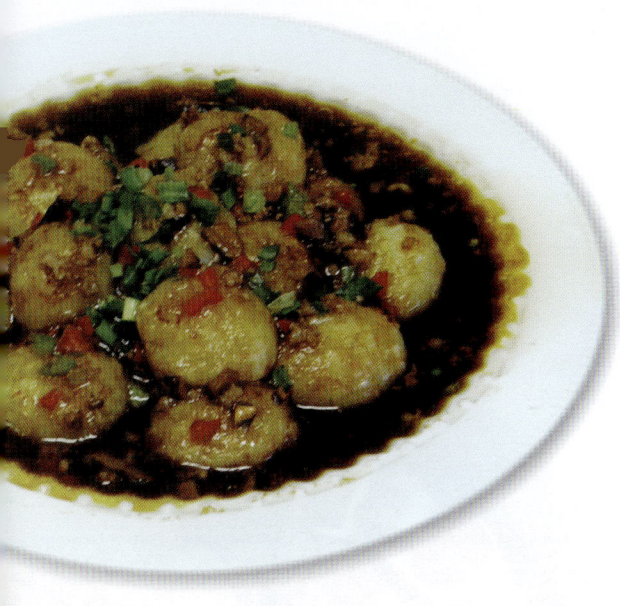

Seasonings:
Salad oil 70 g, salt 2 g, gourmet powder 1 g, white sugar 4 g, ginger 4 g, black soy sauce 7g

Time:
25 minutes

Preparation:
1. Peel cooked potatoes and mash them. Then mix with potato starch, plain flour, salt and gourmet powder. Form mixture into round balls.
2. Dice green and red pepper and ham.
3. Heat salad oil and deep-fry the potato balls until golden brown.
4. Keep some oil in the pan and add the ginger, green and red pepper, ham, soup, potatoes and seasonings. Boil for a while.

Ingredients:
Potato 250 g, potato starch 20 g, plain flour 5 g, green pepper 10 g, red pepper 10 g, ham 5 g

Vegetarian: ✗   Muslim: ✗

Braised potatoes with duck
Tudou Huang Men Ya

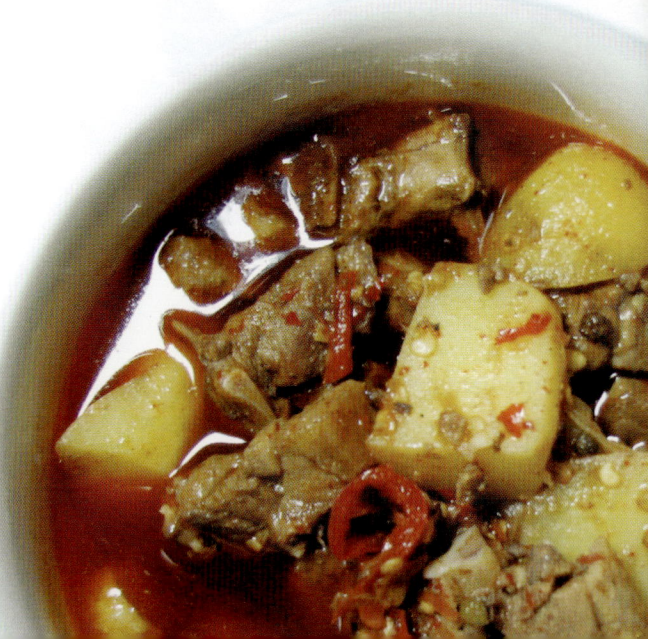

Ingredients:
Duck meat 300 g, potato 300 g, pickled red pepper 3, ginger 1

Seasonings:
Cooking oil 100 g, soy sauce 15 g, cooking wine 20 g, refined salt 5 g, gourmet powder 2 g, starch 20 g, hot pepper oil 10 g

Preparation:
1. Clean and chop duck meat. Clean ginger and slice.
2. Cut pickled red pepper into small sections. Peel potatoes and dice.
3. Put duck meat pieces in hot oil to fry until almost done. Then add potatoes, soy sauce, red pepper, hot pepper oil, ginger, cooking wine, refined salt and water to stew for 30 minutes over low heat until duck meat well-done. Add gourmet powder and use starch to thicken soup, then serve.

Vegetarian: ✗   Muslim: ✓

Braised potatoes with rice
Tudou Men Fan

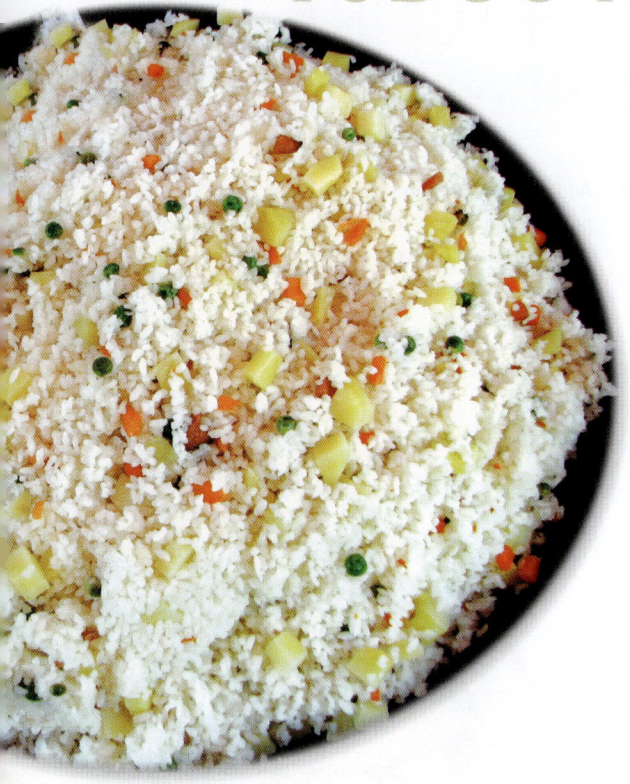

Ingredients:
Rice, potato, peas, carrot, sausage

Seasonings:
Cooking oil, refined salt

Preparation:
1. Peel and dice potatoes and carrots. Clean peas, slice sausage and wash rice.
2. Fry the diced potato for 1–2 minutes, then add other ingredients and seasonings together to the wok. Add water and simmer.

Note: Seasonings should be added to taste.

Vegetarian: ✘   Muslim: ✘

Braised side pork with potatoes in soy sauce
Tudou Hongshao Rou

Ingredients:
Side pork 200 g, potato 300 g, green onion 2, ginger 1

Seasonings:
Oil 50 g, cooking wine 10 g, black soy sauce 20 g, chili powder, Chinese prickly ash to taste, 2 fructus tsaoko

Preparation:
1. Clean side pork and dice into diamonds. Clean and dice potatoes, cut green onion into sections and slice ginger.
2. Heat a little oil and stir-fry the green onion and ginger until it gives off aroma, then add the diced pork and fry. Add soy sauce and cooking wine. Continue stir-frying until meat is brown.
3. Add a little water and boil over high heat. Stew the pork over low heat until nearly cooked, than add potato and white sugar. Continue to cook for 15 minutes until potatoes are flavored, then remove to a bowl and serve.

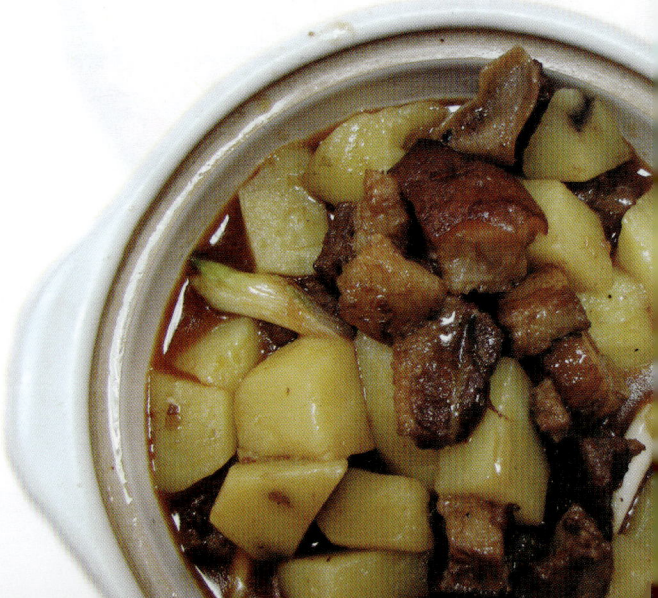

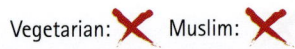

Charcoal-roasted potatoes
Tanhuo Kao Tudou

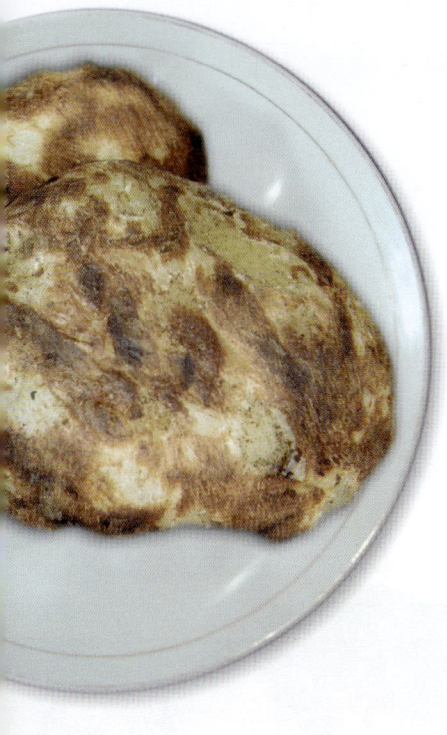

Ingredient:
Potato 200 g

Seasonings:
Salt 2 g, spiced pepper powder 10 g

Time:
25 minutes.

Preparation:
1. Put potatoes on a gentle charcoal fire until they are cooked.
2. Add the spiced pepper powder or other seasonings to taste.

Vegetarian: ✓ Muslim: ✓

Chinese date-filled potato balls with honey
Mizhi Nuoxiang Tudou Zao

Ingredient:

Potato 400 g

Seasonings:

10 Chinese dates, honey 20 g, wheat flour 20 g, white sugar 10 g, vegetable oil 500 g

Preparation:

1. Peel potatoes and steam well. Then mash the potatoes and mix with honey, wheat flour, eggs and white sugar.
2. Add the Chinese dates to the mashed potatoes and form into balls.
3. Fry potato balls well, then set aside in a dish.
4. Put water in wok, add white sugar and honey and boil to make honey sauce. Sprinkle on the potato balls.

Vegetarian: ✗   Muslim: ✓

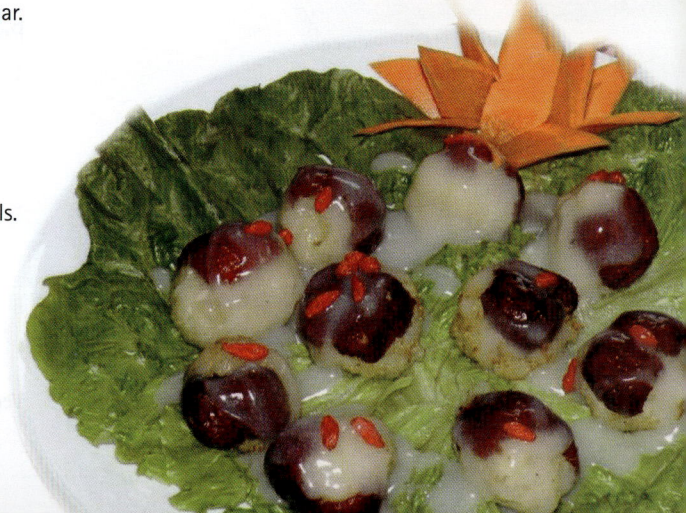

Colorful shredded potatoes
QICAI TUDOU SI

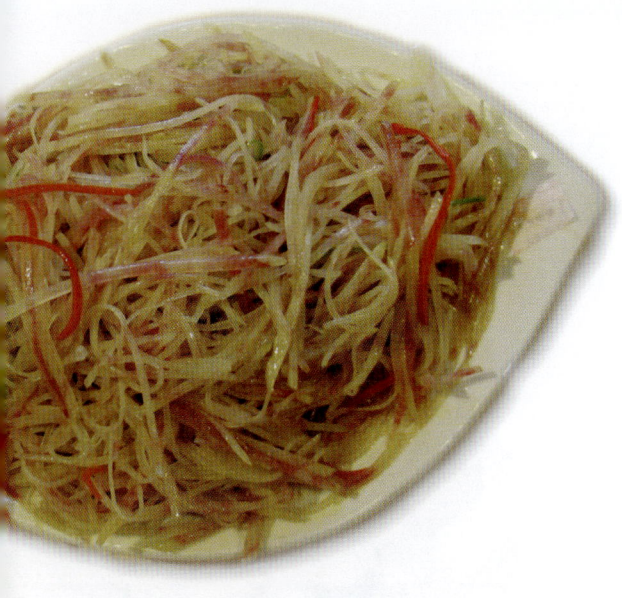

Ingredients:
Colored potato 300 g, 2 green peppers, 2 red peppers

Seasonings:
Cooking oil 70 g, refined salt 3 g, gourmet powder 1.5 g

Preparation:
1. Peel and shred potatoes. Shred the green and red peppers.

2. Heat oil in a wok and fry the shredded potatoes and green and red peppers well. Add salt and gourmet powder, mix evenly.

Vegetarian: ✓   Muslim: ✓

Crisp potato strips I
Xiangsu Shu Tiao I

Ingredient:
Potato 500 g

Seasonings:
Cooking oil 500 g, chili powder 15 g, refined salt 5 g, gourmet powder 2 g, Chinese prickly ash to taste

Preparation:
1. Peel potatoes, and cut into strips 1 cm wide and 10 cm long.
2. Heat oil in a wok and deep-fry the potato strips. Remove once strips are golden and drain the excess oil. Mix gourmet powder, salt, chili powder and Chinese prickly ash in a bowl. Use as dip when serving the potato strips.

Vegetarian: ✓   Muslim: ✓

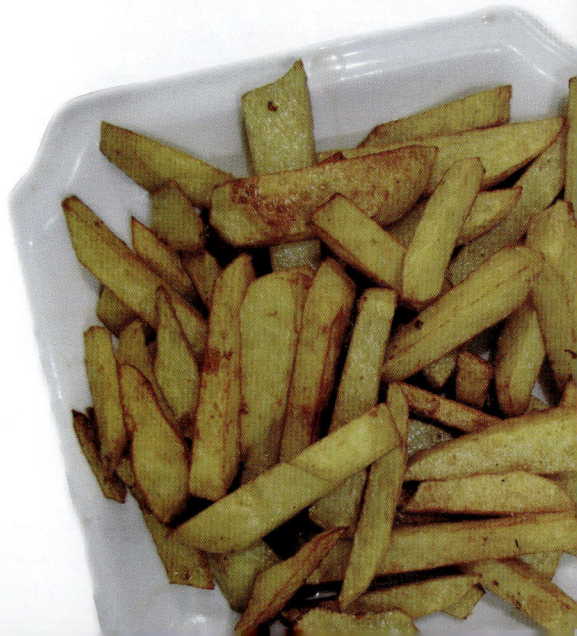

Crisp potato strips II
XIANGSU SHU TIAO II

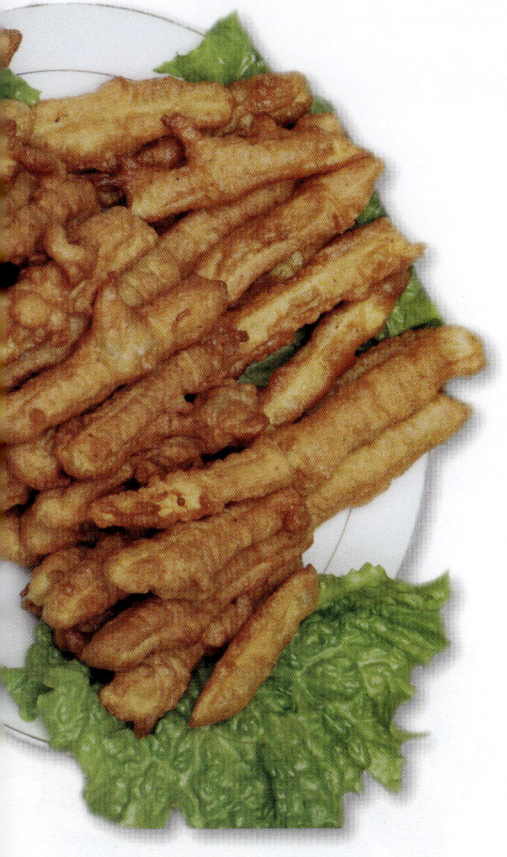

Ingredients:
Big potato 300 g, flour 200 g, 3 eggs

Seasonings:
Cooking oil 400 g, refined salt 5 g, fructus tsaoko powder to taste

Preparation:
1. Peel potatoes and cut into strips. Whisk eggs.
2. Mix egg whites, salt, fructus tsaoko powder, flour and water to form an even paste. Coat the potato strips with the paste.
3. Heat oil and fry the potato strips until golden brown, then serve.

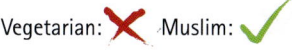

Deep-fried fat pork and diced potatoes
Cuishao Tudou Li

Ingredients:
Potato 500 g, deep-fried fat meat 15 g, green pepper 5 g, red pepper 5 g

Seasonings:
Salad oil 120 g, salt 3 g, gourmet powder 1 g, chicken essence 1 g, pepper oil 15 g, green onion 5 g, ginger 3 g, garlic 3 g

Preparation:
1. Cut the potatoes into small cubes. Heat the oil and deep-fry the diced potatoes until golden brown, then remove to a plate.
2. Keep some oil in the pan and add deep-fried fat meat, green onion, ginger, garlic, green pepper and red pepper together with the diced potatoes and seasonings and stir.

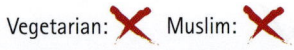

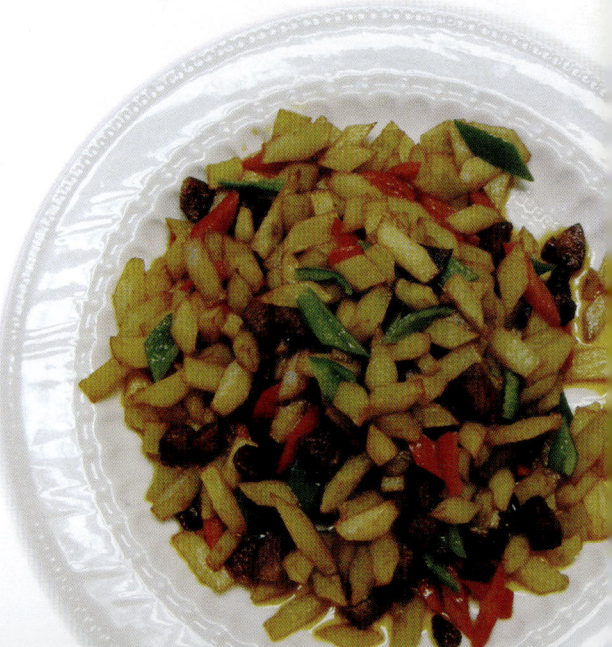

Deep-fried potato chips
Youzha Tudou Pian

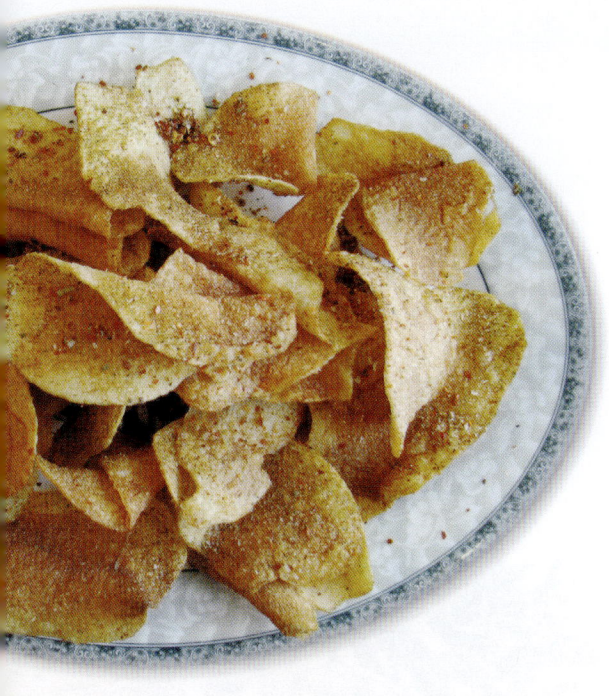

Ingredient:
Potato 300 g

Seasonings:
Cooking oil 500 g, chili powder 20 g, a little Chinese prickly ash, gourmet powder 1 g, refined salt 3 g

Preparation:
1. Clean and peel potatoes. Slice the potatoes, then rinse in cool water and drain.
2. Heat oil in a wok and deep-fry potato chips over low heat. Remove when the chips start to bubble.
3. Mix chili powder, Chinese prickly ash, gourmet powder and salt together, then sprinkle on potato chips and serve.

Vegetarian: ✓   Muslim: ✓

Deep-fried potato chips with peanuts and chili
Youzha San Pin

Ingredients:

Potato chips 150 g, peanuts 150 g, seasoned pepper 50 g

Seasonings:

Cooking oil 300 g, refined salt 3 g, Chinese prickly ash to taste

Preparation:

1. Peel and slice potatoes.
2. Heat oil in wok and deep-fry peanuts, then remove. Deep-fry the potato chips until they give off aroma. Keep a little oil in the wok to fry seasoned hot pepper. Combine all ingredients, sprinkle with salt and Chinese prickly ash, then serve.

Vegetarian: ✓ Muslim: ✓

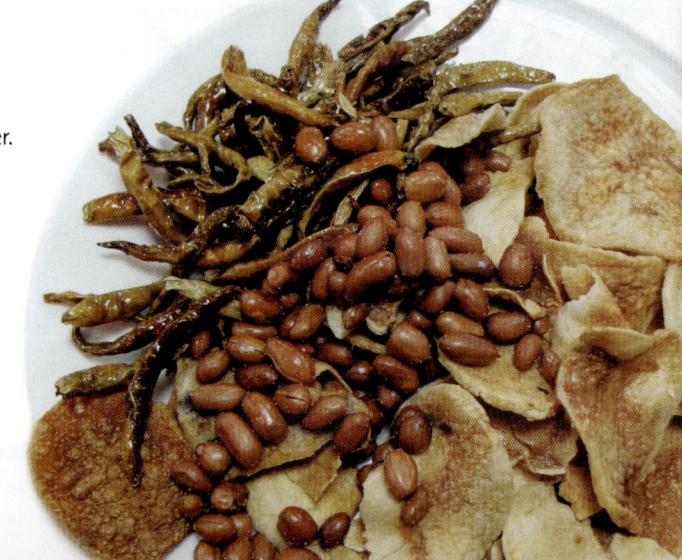

Diced potatoes with salted egg yolk
Yan Danhuang Tudou Li

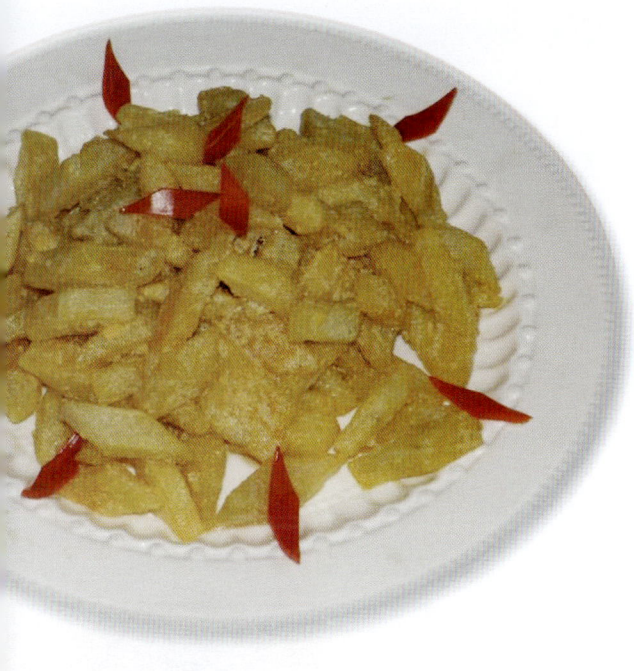

Ingredient:
Potato 500 g

Seasonings:
Custard power 10 g, starch 20 g, chili 20 g, salted egg yolk 20 g, corn kernels 20 g, salt 3 g, gourmet powder 2 g, chicken essence 2 g, vegetable oil 250 g

Preparation:
1. Peel potatoes and cut them into diamond-shaped pieces. Put water and salt in a big bowl and marinate the potato pieces for 15 minutes.
2. Steam salted egg yolk well, then mince.
3. Remove potato pieces and put in another bowl. Add custard powder and starch and mix well.
4. Fry the potato pieces until well-done.
5. Keep a little oil in the wok and fry the salted egg yolk. Then add the potato pieces and fry with seasonings.

Vegetarian: ✗   Muslim: ✓

Finely shredded potatoes with ginger
Jiangwei Longxu Si

Ingredient:
Potato 250 g

Seasonings:
Green pepper 10 g, red pepper 10 g, onion 10 g, salad oil 180 g, green onion 5 g, sesame oil 3 g, salt 2 g, gourmet powder 1 g

Time:
6 minutes.

Preparation:
1. Peel the potatoes and cut into slices. Mince the green peppers, red peppers and onion.
2. Heat 500 g of salad oil and fry the potato slices until golden, then remove to a plate.
3. Keep some oil in the pan, add the green and red pepper, onion, and other seasonings, and stir.

Vegetarian: ✓   Muslim: ✓

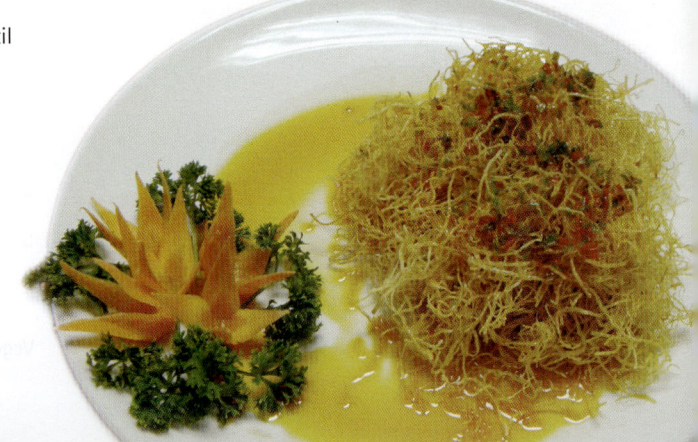

Fried dried potato slices
Zha Gan Yangyupian

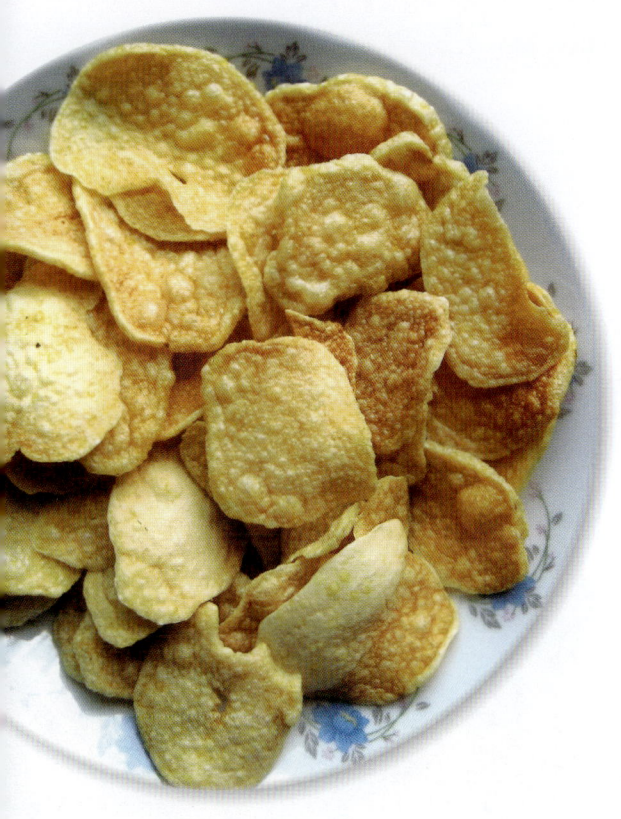

Preparation:

Dried potato pieces:

1. Select potatoes that are about 25 g each. Peel and cut into 2 mm-thick pieces.

2. Quick-boil the potatoes, then remove, drain and cool. Dry the pieces in sunlight and preserve in sealed container.

Fried dried potato pieces:

1. Put 500 ml of vegetable oil in a wok and heat over medium heat. Deep-fry the dried potato pieces until golden brown.

2. Season to taste.

Vegetarian: ✓   Muslim: ✓

Fried Green Pepper and Shredded Potato
Qingjiao Tudou Si

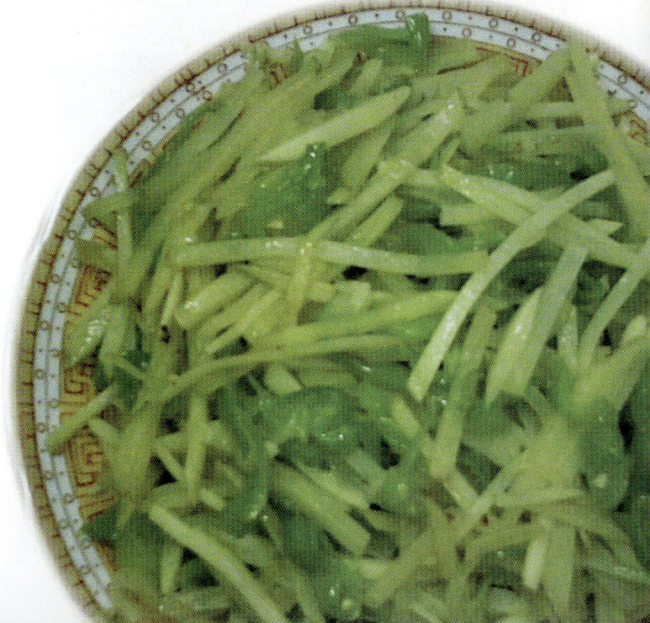

Ingredients:
Potato 300 g, green pepper 50 g

Seasonings:
Cooking oil 60 g, refined salt 3 g, gourmet powder 2 g

Preparation:
1. Peel potatoes and shred into strings. Shred green pepper as well.
2. Heat oil in wok and fry shredded potatoes and green peppers. Add salt and gourmet powder, mix well, and serve.

Vegetarian: ✓   Muslim: ✓

Fried Potato Chips
Su Chao Tudou Pian

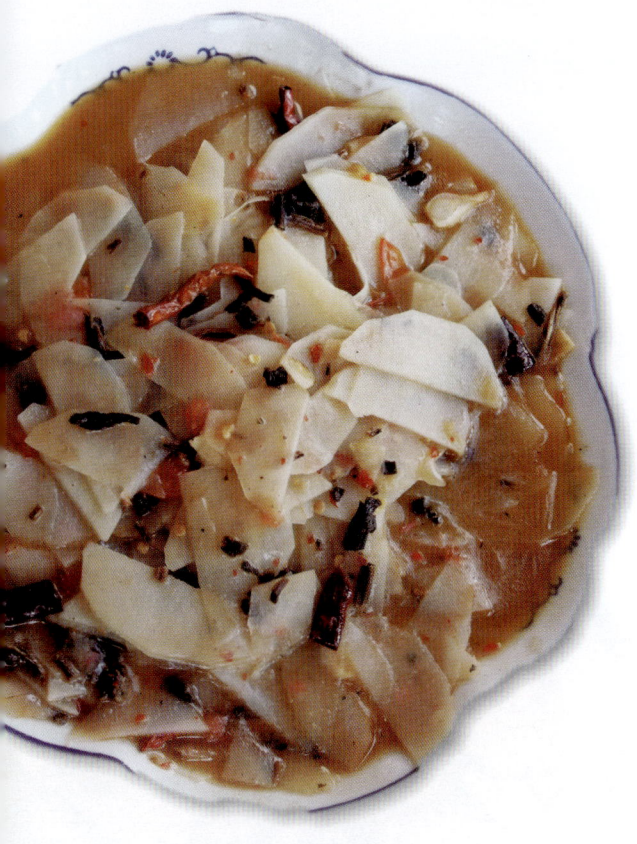

Ingredients:
Potato 300 g, hot pepper 20 g, tomato 50 g

Seasonings:
Cooking oil 30 g, refined salt 5 g, gourmet powder 2 g

Preparation:
1. Peel and slice potatoes into thin pieces. Chop the hot pepper into sections and mince the tomatoes.

2. Heat oil in a wok and stir-fry the tomatoes and hot pepper, then add the potato chips and fry for a while together. Add water and stew until cooked. Mix well with salt and gourmet powder, then serve.

Vegetarian: ✓   Muslim: ✓

Fried potato chips with soy sauce
Jiang Bao Tudou Pian

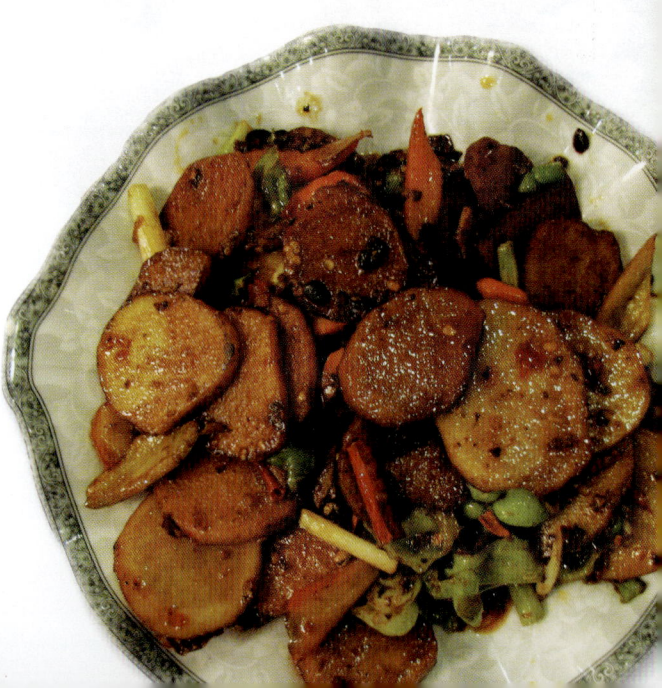

Ingredients:
Potato 200 g, green onion 2, green pepper 30 g, seasoned pepper 10 g, fermented soybean

Seasonings:
Cooking oil 300 g, sweet sauce 40 g, soy sauce 10 g, salt 2 g, gourmet powder 1 g

Preparation:
1. Peel and slice potatoes. Cut green onion and seasoned peppers into section. Slice green pepper.
2. Heat oil in a wok and deep-fry potatoes, stirring at intervals until the chips turn golden yellow.
3. Keep a little oil in the wok and stir-fry green onion, green pepper, seasoned pepper and sweet sauce together until it gives off aroma. Add water, potato pieces, salt, gourmet powder and soy sauce. Stew until boiling, then turn to low heat and stew for flavoring. Remove from heat before the water evaporates.

Vegetarian: ✓ Muslim: ✓

Fried Potato Pancake
Qiaoshou Tuanyuanbing

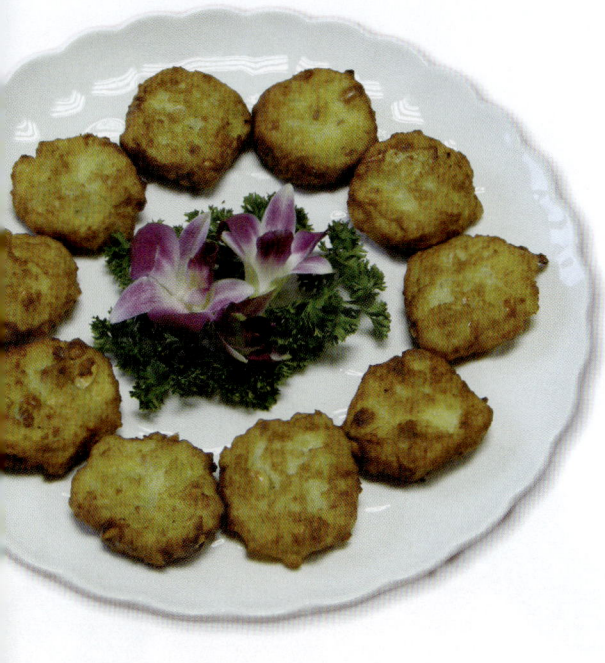

Ingredients:
Potato 250 g, 1 egg, wheat flour 15 g

Seasonings:
Salad oil 200 g, custard powder 1 g, fried peanuts 3 g, salt 3 g, white sugar 6 g

Time:
20 minutes.

Preparation:
1. Peel the cooked potatoes and mash them. Chop the peanuts into pieces.
2. Add the seasonings into the mashed potatoes and mix to make a pancake 5 cm across and 3 cm thick.
3. Heat oil in a saucepan and fry the potato pancakes over low heat until they turn golden brown on both sides.

Vegetarian: ✗   Muslim: ✓

Fried potato pie
Youzha Shu Bing

Ingredient:
Potato 300 g

Seasonings:
Cooking oil 200 g, salt 3 g, fructus tsaoko powder, Chinese prickly ash

Preparation:
1. Peel the steam potatoes, then mash. Mix evenly with fructus tsaoko powder, Chinese prickly ash and salt and knead into a cake.
2. Heat oil in wok and fry potato cake until golden.

Vegetarian: ✓   Muslim: ✓

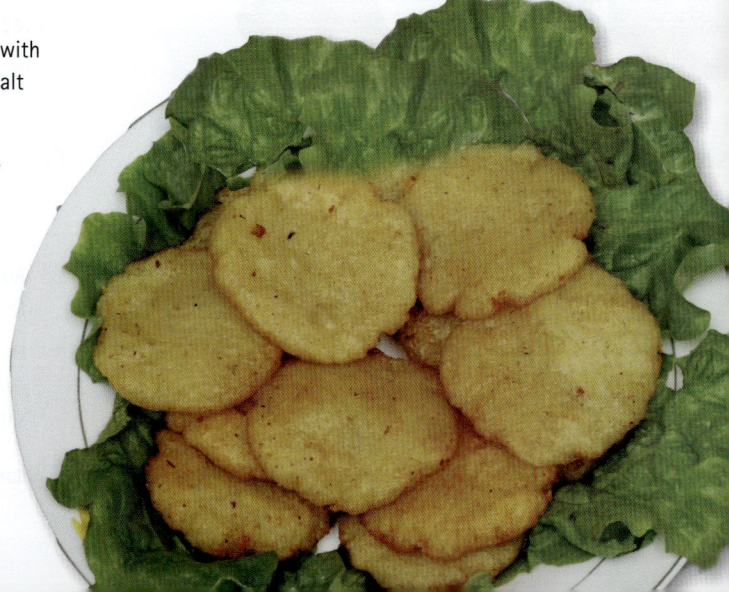

Fried Potato Slices with Dried Pickles
Gan Yancai Chao Shu Pian

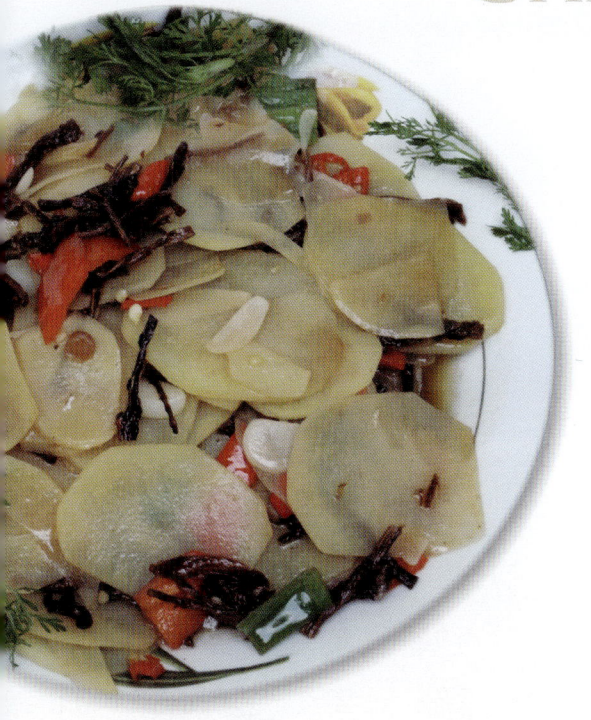

Ingredients:
Potato 300 g, seasoned pickles of ethnic Dai flavor 50 g, 2 red peppers, 2 green peppers, garlic

Seasonings:
Cooking oil 50 g, refined salt 4 g, gourmet powder 2 g

Preparation:
1. Peel and slice potatoes. Cut pickles into sections. Remove stems and seeds from green and red peppers, then dice. Slice garlic.
2. Deep-fry pickles for a while, then add red and green peppers and potato slices and fry together until cooked. Add salt, garlic and gourmet powder before serving.

Vegetarian: ✓ Muslim: ✓

Fried potato slices with sour bamboo shoots
Suan Sun Chao Shupian

Ingredients:
Potato 300 g, sour bamboo shoots of ethnic Dai flavor 50 g, 3 red peppers, garlic to taste

Seasonings:
Cooking oil 50 g, refined salt 4 g, gourmet powder 2 g

Preparation:
1. Peel and slice potatoes. Rinse bamboo shoots and cut them into sections. Remove stems and seeds from red peppers, then dice.
2. Fry the diced red peppers and potato slices well, then add the sour bamboo shoots, salt, garlic and gourmet powder. Fry together, then serve.

Vegetarian: ✓   Muslim: ✓

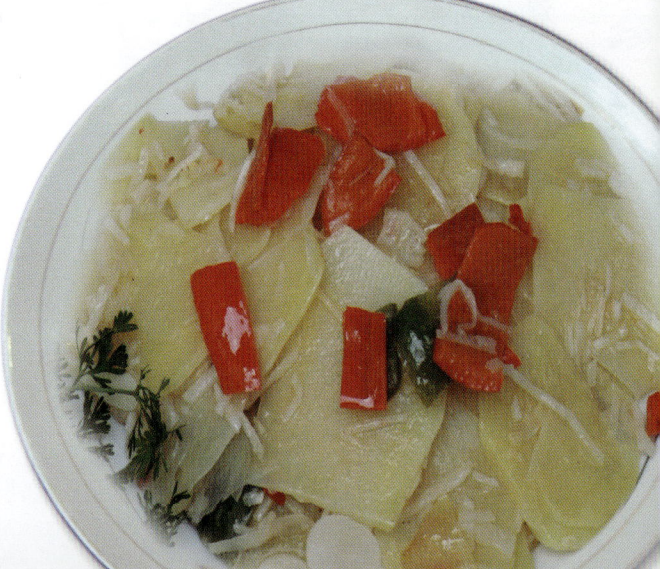

Fried potato strips coated with yolk
Jinsha Tudou Tiao

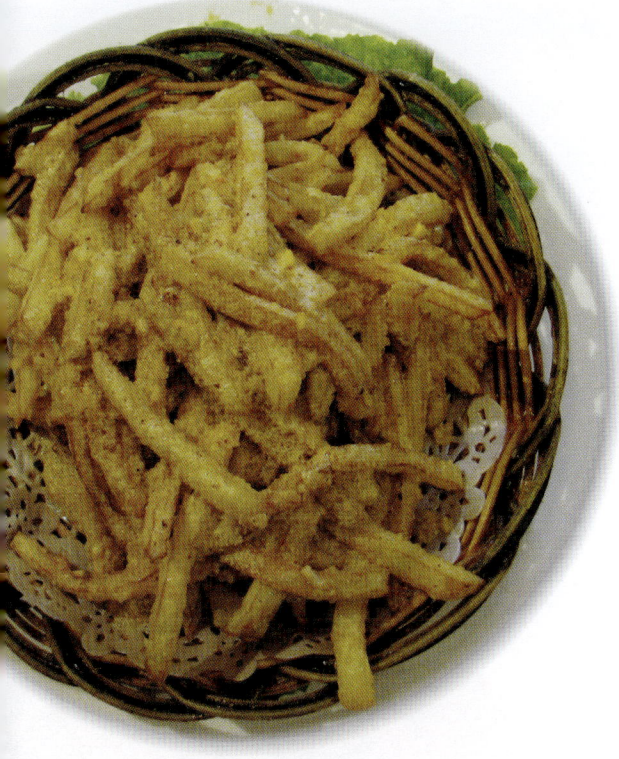

Ingredients:
Potato 300 g, 2 duck eggs, starch

Seasonings:
Cooking oil 500 g, refined salt 5 g, white sugar 10 g

Preparation:
1. Separate duck eggs, discard the egg whites, and whisk the egg yolks.
2. Peel potatoes and cut into 1 cm by 10cm strips, then mix evenly with egg yolk, starch and seasonings.
3. Heat oil over medium heat and deep-fry the potato strips until golden. Remove and drain off oil.
4. Sprinkle gourmet powder and salt on potato strips, mix evenly and place on a plate.

Vegetarian: ✗ Muslim: ✓

Fried potatoes and chicken with pickled pepper
Paojiao Tudou Ji

Ingredients:
Potato 400 g, farmyard chicken 200 g

Seasonings:
Prickled pepper 100 g, celery 15 g, salt 3 g, gourmet powder 3 g, chicken essence 3 g, soy sauce 5 g, pungent sauce 5 g, vegetable oil 500 g (60 g consumed)

Preparation:
1. Dice potatoes and quick-boil in water. Cut celery into sections and chop the chicken into cubes.
2. Heat vegetable oil in a wok and fry the chicken well.
3. Keep a little oil in the wok and fry prickled pepper and celery until it gives off aroma. Add the diced potatoes, chicken, soup stock and seasonings; fry until well-done.

Vegetarian: 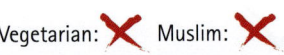 Muslim:

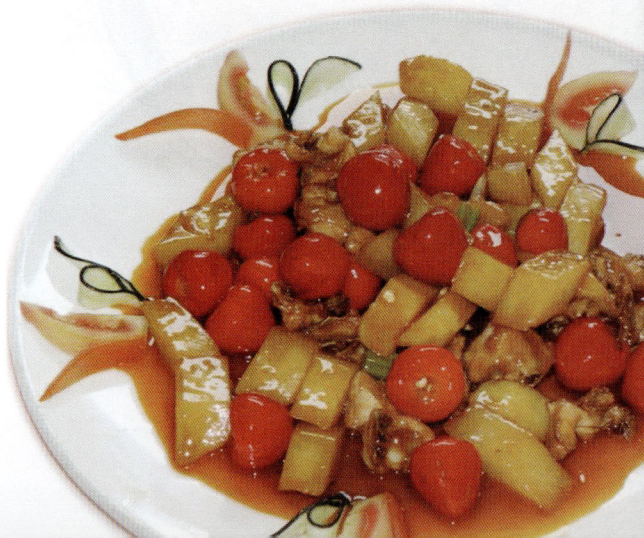

Fried Potatoes and Pork with Pickled Pepper
Jiang Rou Tudou Ding

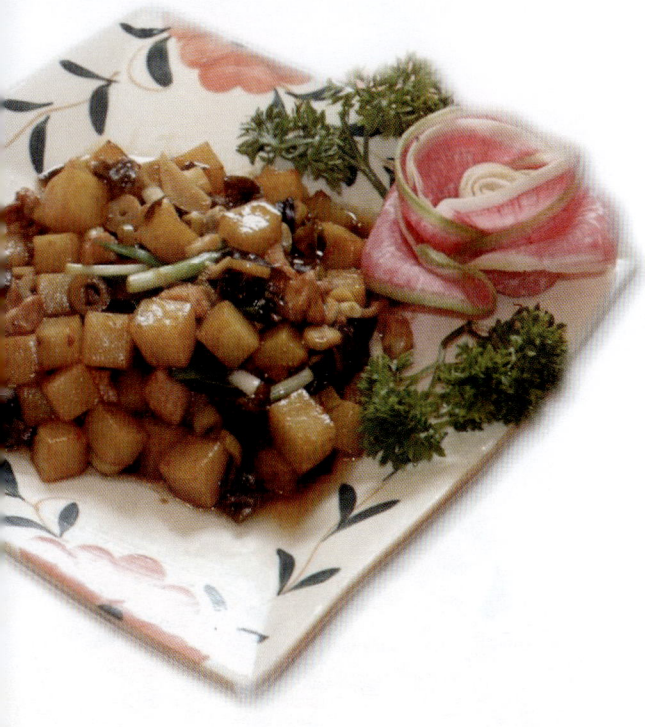

Ingredients:
Potato 300 g, pork 100 g

Seasonings:
Black agarics 3 g, green onion 3 g, garlic 2 g, starch 5 g, bamboo shoots 5 g, salt 2 g, salted and fermented soy paste 5 g, white sugar 3 g, vegetable oil 60 g

Preparation:
1. Peel potatoes and dice them into 2 cm cubes. Mince black agarics and bamboo shoots and cut green onion into 2 cm sections. Cut the pork into cubes, the same size as the potatoes.
2. Heat oil and fry the pork.
3. Keep oil in the wok and fry garlic. Then add salted and fermented soy paste and fry until the color changes. Add in the remaining ingredients and seasonings, stir-fry and then serve.

Vegetarian: ✗ Muslim: ✗

Fried potatoes with four treasures
Jin Shu Hui Sibao

Ingredient:
Potato 250 g

Seasonings:
Shiitake mushroom 10 g, carrot 10 g, slippery Jack mushroom 10 g, green beans 20 g, corn kernels 20 g, salt 3 g, gourmet powder 2 g, chicken essence 2 g, sesame oil 5 g, vegetable oil 30 g

Preparation:
1. Peel potatoes and dice them. Mince shiitake mushroom, carrot and slippery Jack mushroom.
2. Quick-boil mushrooms, carrot and green beans in water.
3. Put vegetable oil in a wok; add all ingredients, seasonings and a little soup stock, then fry for 1 minute.

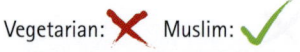
Vegetarian: ✗ Muslim: ✓

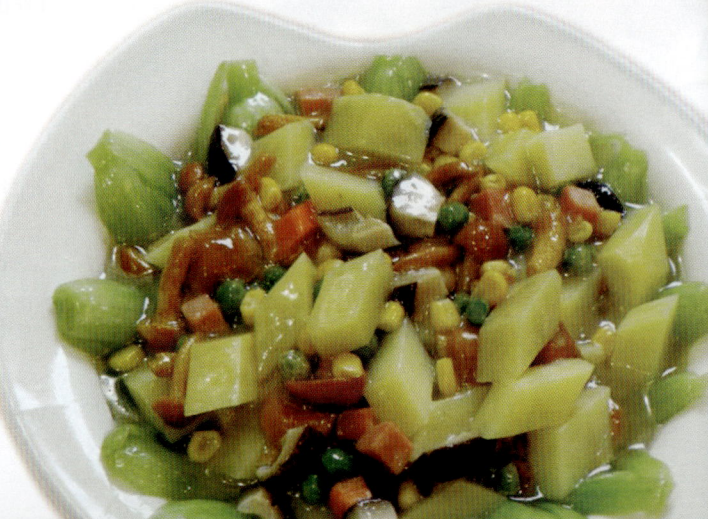

Fried Prawn Coated with Fine Potato Strings
Jinsi Fengwei Xia

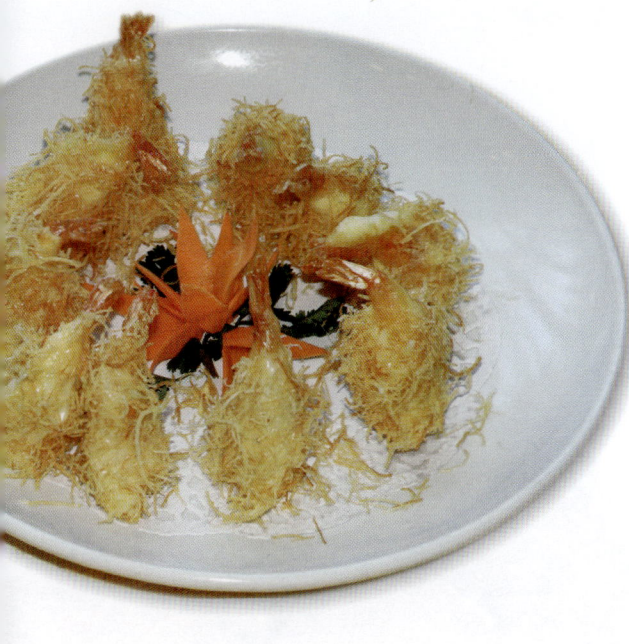

Ingredients:
Potato 400 g, prawns 100 g

Seasonings:
Ginger 8 g, 2 eggs, salad dressing 100 g, salt 5 g, starch 6 g, vegetable oil 500 g

Preparation:
1. Peel and clean potatoes, then shred them and soak in water.
2. Remove prawn shells but keep the tails. Marinate with a little salt and ginger.
3. Mix starch, egg and salt until it turns into paste.
4. Fry the shredded potatoes until golden brown.
5. Coat the prawns with the starch paste and fry until crisp. Dip in salad dressing and coat with shredded potato, then serve.

Vegetarian: ✗   Muslim: ✗

Golden potato string cake
Jinhuang Dousi Bing

Ingredients:
Potato 300 g, flour, 2 eggs

Seasonings:
Cooking oil 100 g, refined salt 3 g, gourmet powder 2 g

Preparation:
1. Peel potatoes and cut into strings.
2. Beat eggs and mix evenly with potato strings, refined salt and flour to make paste.
3. Heat oil in a wok over medium heat, then fry both sides of the potato string cake over low heat until golden.

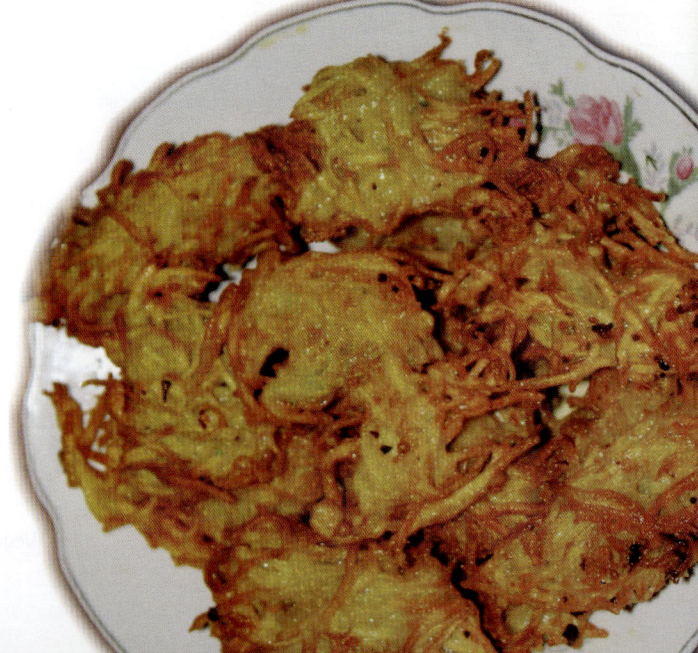

Vegetarian: ✗   Muslim: ✓

Green onion-flavored potato chips
Conghua Shu Pian

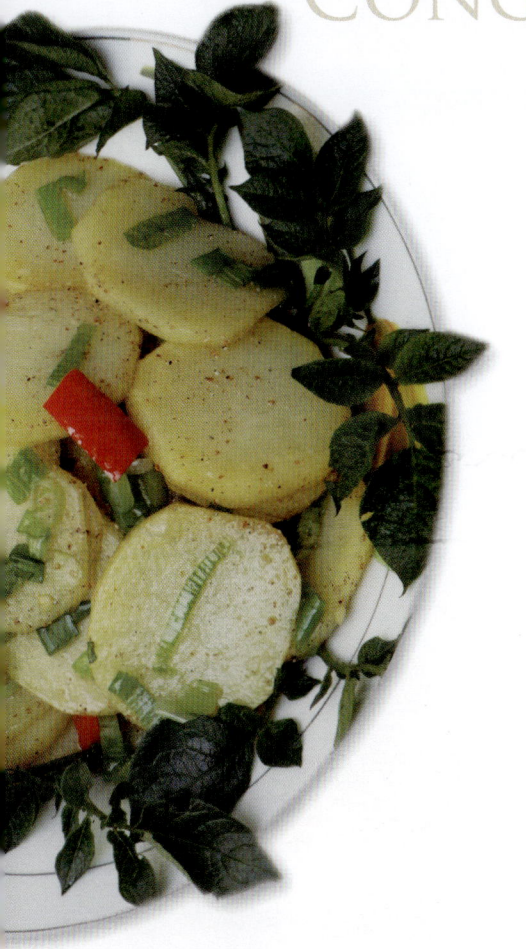

Ingredients:
Potato 300 g, 2 red peppers, green onion 3

Seasonings:
Cooking oil 70 g, salt 3 g, fructus tsaoko powder

Preparation:
1. Peel and slice potatoes. Mince the green onion. Remove the stem and seeds of the red pepper, then dice.
2. Heat oil in a wok and deep-fry the potato chips. Drain excess oil, then combine with red pepper, minced green onion, fructus tsaoko powder and salt and mix well, then serve.

Vegetarian: ✓   Muslim: ✓

Ham-flavored potato strings
Huotui Fengwei Tudou Si

Ingredients:
Ham juice 100 g, potato 300 g, 3 seasoned hot peppers, 2 green peppers, 2 red peppers

Seasonings:
Cooking oil 60 g, refined salt 3 g

Preparation:
1. Peel and shred potatoes. Cut the dried hot pepper into sections and shred the red and green peppers into strings. Stew ham to get the juices, then set aside.
2. Put shredded potatoes in hot water and quickly remove. Heat oil in a wok and quickly fry the shredded potatoes and seasoned hot pepper. Add the ham cooking juice and covers the wok to stew for 3 minutes. Then add red and green peppers and salt and quickly stir-fry, then serve.

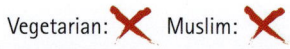
Vegetarian: ✗   Muslim: ✗

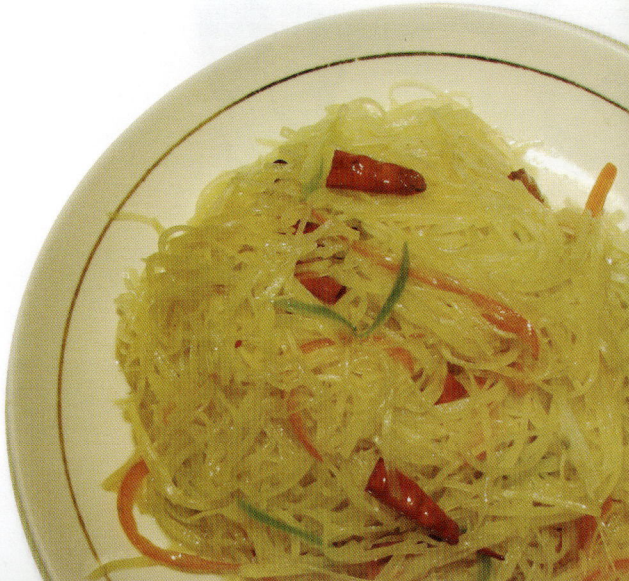

Honeycomb-shaped Potatoes
Fengwo Tudou

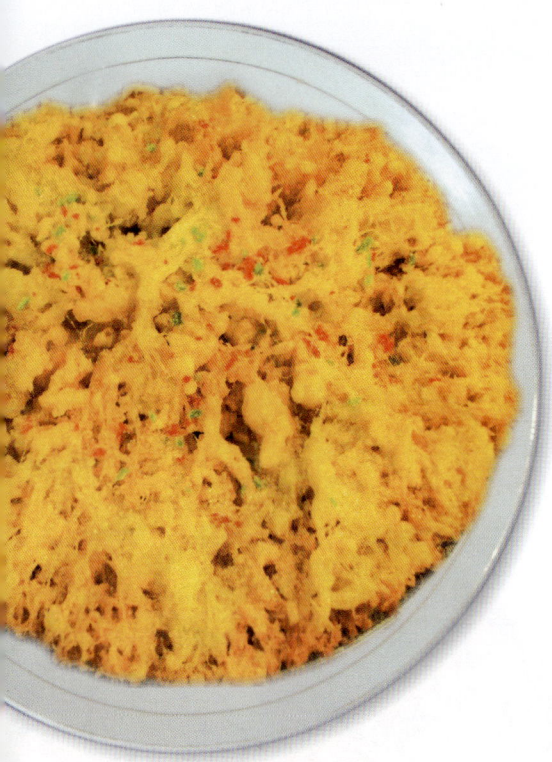

Seasonings:
White sugar 50 g, refined salt 3 g, cooking oil 500 g, candied fruit 20 g

Preparation:
1. Peel potatoes and finely chop. Rinse in water and set aside. Shred candied fruit.
2. Mix egg, flour, peanut meal and refined salt in a bowl. Add water to form a paste, then add the potatoes.
3. Add soy sauce into wok and heat until half cooked. Remove the potato pieces from the paste by hand and sprinkle slowly into the wok to form a mesh skeleton. Continue sprinkling potatoes, building up the honeycomb structure until all the potato and paste is used up.
4. When the honeycomb becomes crisp, remove from the wok and drain the oil. A few minutes later, place the honeycomb on a dish, sprinkle with white sugar and candied fruit, then serve.

Ingredients:
Potato 200 g, 1 egg, wheat flour 40 g, starch 10 g

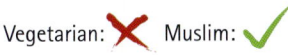

Hot and spicy diced potatoes I
Mala Tudou Ding

Ingredients:
Potato 500 g, green onion 50 g

Seasonings:
Cooking oil 500 g, chili powder 20 g, Chinese prickly ash 3 g, chili sauce 30 g, refined salt 5 g, gourmet powder 2 g

Preparation:
1. Peel and dice the potatoes, then soak in water. Remove and drain.
2. Heat oil and deep-fry the diced potatoes, then remove and mix with chili powder, Chinese prickly ash, refined salt, gourmet powder and starch. Fry the flavored potatoes in a little oil, then serve.

Vegetarian: ✓   Muslim: ✓

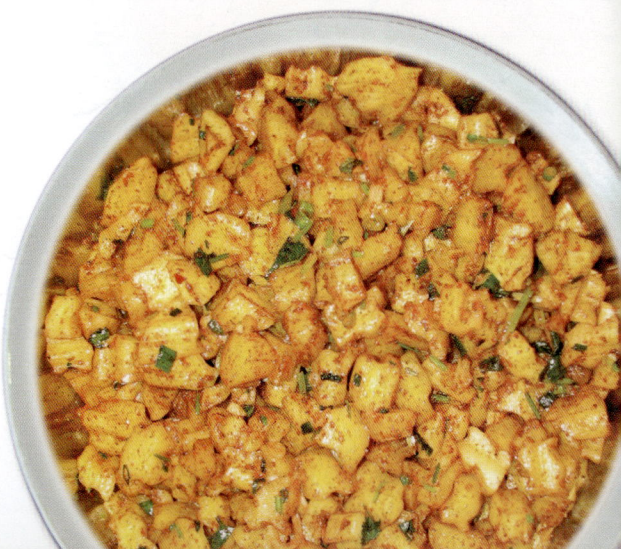

Hot and spicy diced potatoes II
Xiangma Tudou Ding

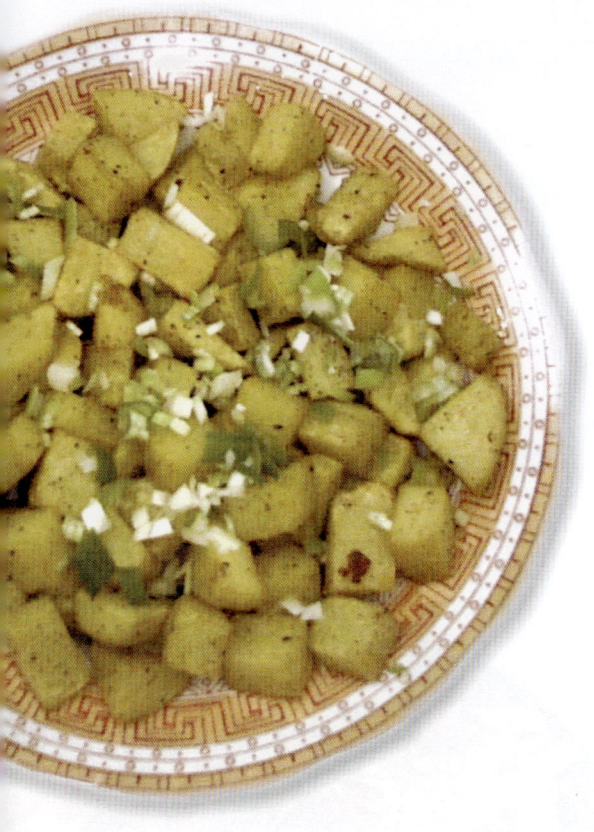

Ingredients:
Potato 500 g, green onion

Seasonings:
Cooking oil 100 g, refined salt 3 g, Chinese prickly ash to taste

Preparation:
1. Peel and dice the potatoes, mince the green onion.
2. Heat oil in a wok and deep-fry diced potatoes. When almost cooked, add salt and Chinese prickly ash and mix well. Sprinkle with minced green onion before serving.

Vegetarian: ✓   Muslim: ✓

Hotpot potatoes with preserved ham and radish
Yi Guo Hui

Ingredients:
Potato 600 g, preserved ham 200 g, radish 300 g

Seasonings:
Cilantro 20 g, garlic sprout 30 g, horse beans 20 g, ginger 10 g, dried pepper 100 g, Chinese prickly ash 40 g, salt 4 g, gourmet powder 3 g, soy sauce 10 g, vegetable oil 50 g

Preparation:
1. Cut potatoes, preserved ham and radish into 6 cm-long strips.
2. Fry ginger, garlic and horse beans, then add potatoes and preserved ham strips. Stir-fry together and add a little water to stew with seasonings. When well cooked, add radish, garlic sprouts, fried dried pepper and Chinese prickly ash.
3. Sprinkle with cilantro before serving.

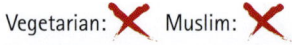
Vegetarian: ✗ Muslim: ✗

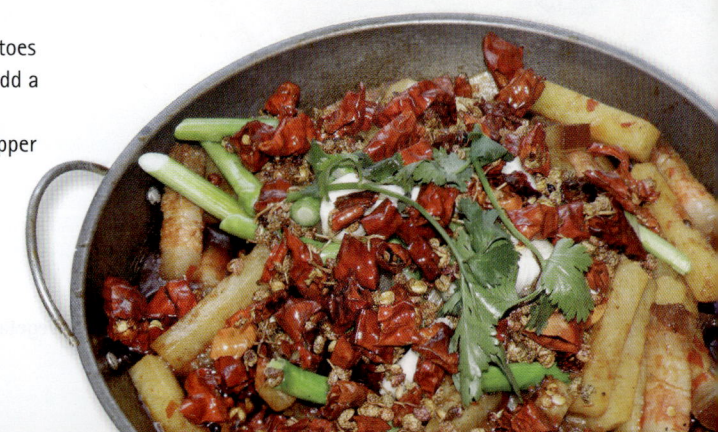

Long life shredded potatoes
Changshou Tudou Si

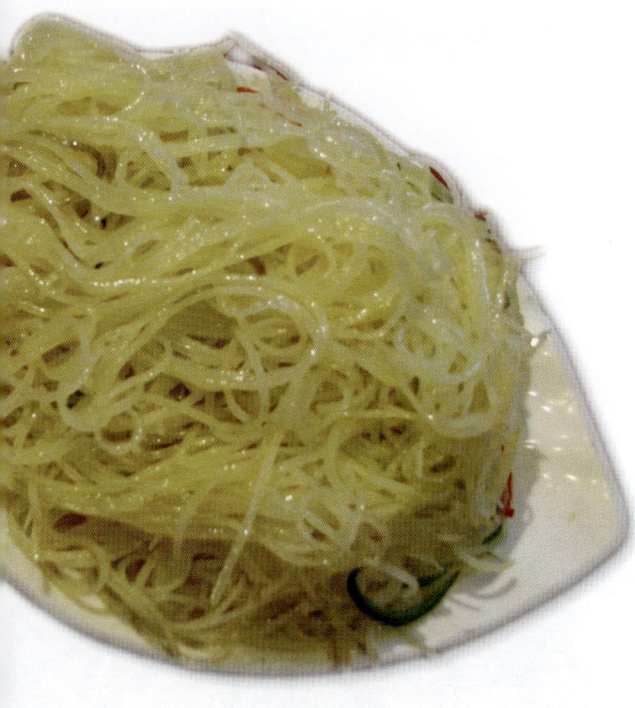

Ingredients:
Several big potatoes, 1 red pepper, 1 green pepper

Seasonings:
Cooking oil 100 g, aromatic vinegar 3–6 g, salt 3 g, chicken essence 1 g

Preparation:
1. Clean potatoes and shred into long strings. Quick-boil the potato strings. Shred the peppers.
2. Heat oil in a wok and fry the shredded potatoes together with hot pepper strings until done. Add salt, vinegar and chicken essence and mix well.

Vegetarian: ✗   Muslim: ✓

Mashed potatoes fried with fennel
Huixiang Tudou Ni

Ingredients:
Fennel 25 g, potato 300 g, starch to taste

Seasonings:
Cooking oil 70 g, refined salt 3 g, gourmet powder 2 g

Preparation:
1. Steam potatoes, then peel. Mash the potatoes in a bowl. Mince the fennel.
2. Combine some water with starch to make a thic liquid.
3. Heat oil in a wok and fry the mashed potatoes, then add starch liquid, fennel, refined salt and gourmet powder. Stir-fry and serve.

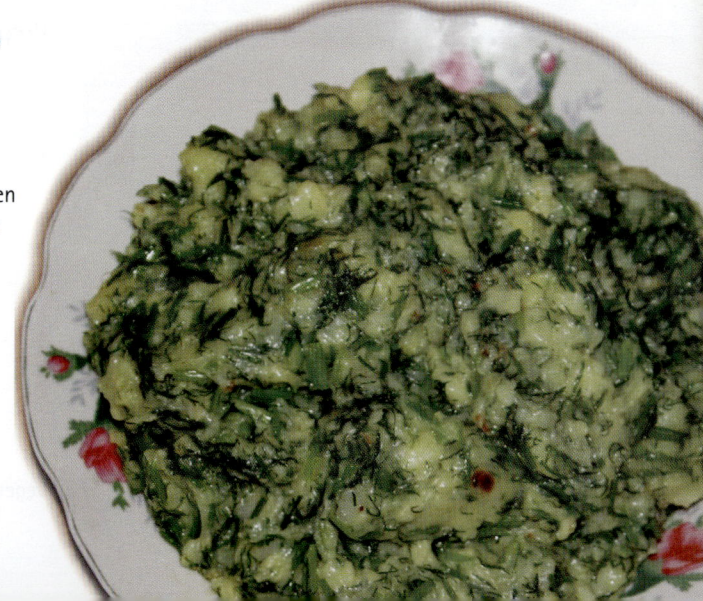

Vegetarian: ✓   Muslim: ✓

Mashed potatoes in lotus leaf
Heye Tudou Ni

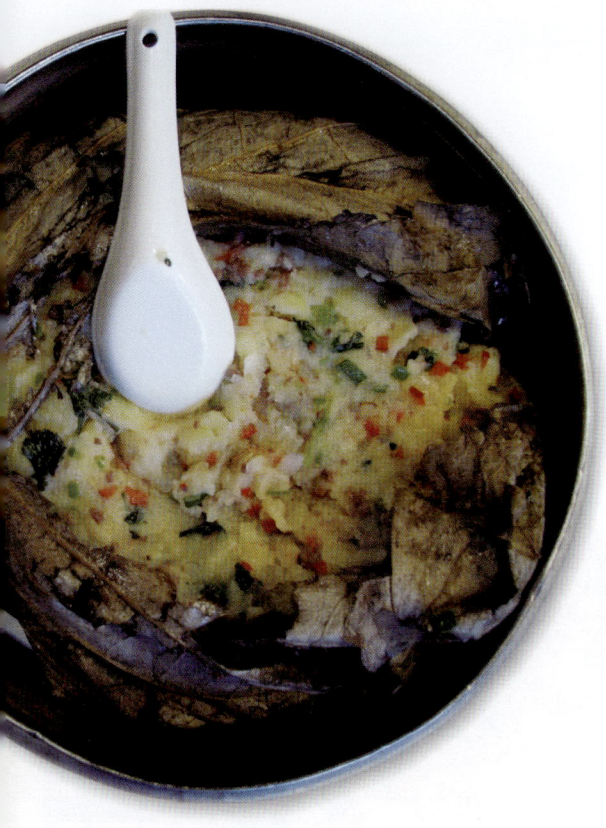

Ingredients:
Potato 300 g, 2 red peppers, green onion 20 g, starch

Seasonings:
Cooking oil 50 g, refined salt 3 g, gourmet powder 2 g

Preparation:
1. Steam potatoes, then peel. Mash potatoes in a bowl. Scald lotus leaf to soften for use (fresh lotus leaf is better).
2. Remove the stem and seeds from the red pepper. Mince the green onion.
3. Add some oil to the mashed potatoes, mix together with refined salt, starch, a little water, red pepper and green onion, stirring evenly. Then wrap the mixture with the lotus leaf and steam for 30 minutes in a steamer.

Vegetarian: ✓   Muslim: ✓

Mashed potatoes with pine nuts
Songren Tudou Ni

Ingredients:
Potato 300 g, pine nuts 50 g, 2 eggs, starch

Seasonings:
Cooking oil 400 g, refined salt 5 g, white sugar 6 g, gourmet powder 3 g, 3 green onion

Preparation:
1. Peel and steam potatoes, then mash in a bowl.
2. Whisk egg in a bowl then combine with refined salt, white sugar and gourmet powder and mix well, making a paste. Form into a cake and sprinkle with pine nuts.
3. Mince green onion.
4. Heat oil in a wok and fry both sides of the mashed potato cake until golden. Remove and sprinkle with minced green onion, then serve.

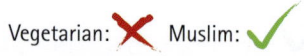

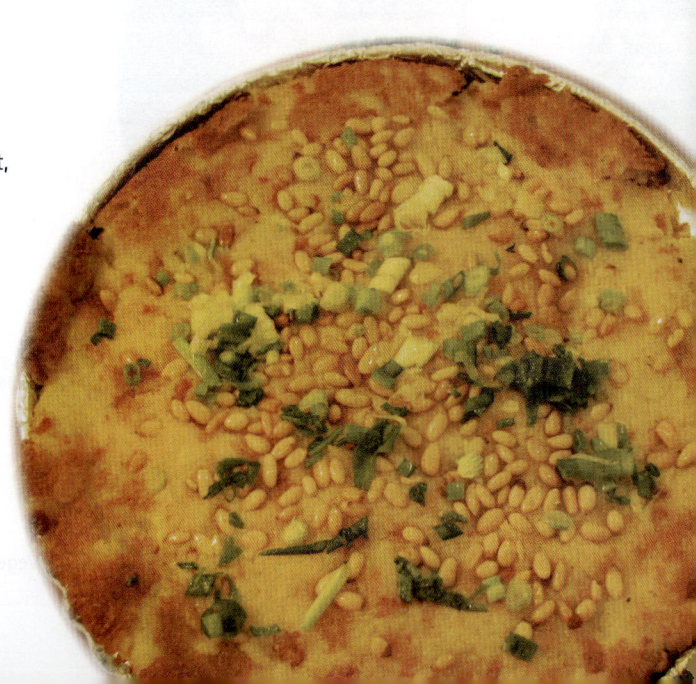

Mashed Potatoes Wrapped in Sticky Rice Pancakes
Zhibao Tudou Ni

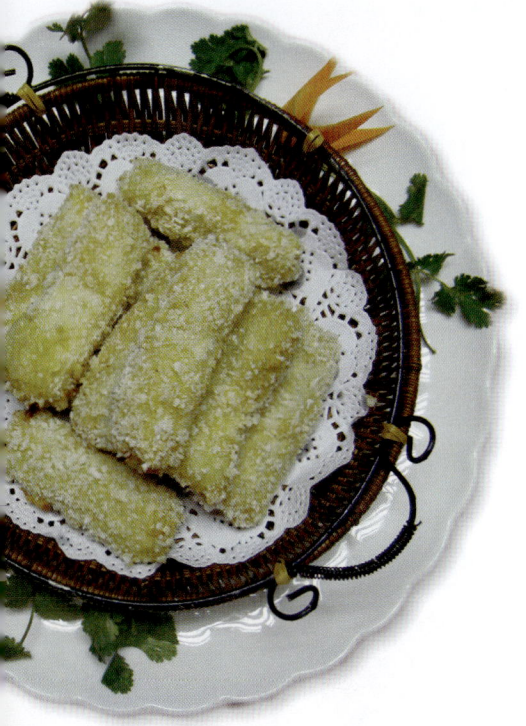

Seasonings:
White sugar 30 g, fried peanut 10 g, 2 eggs, condensed milk 20 g, salt 2 g, crust 25 g, thickening 5 g

Time:
25 minutes

Preparation:
1. Peel the cooked potatoes and mash them. Finely chop the fried peanuts.
2. Heat a frying pan and add in the mashed potatoes, 1 egg, salt, condensed milk, fried peanuts and white sugar. Stir the contents of the pan, letting them dry.
3. Make the potato paste into the rice pancake at the size of 8 cm in length and 3 cm in width.
4. Put the mashed potatoes into the prepared egg mixture and sprinkle the crust.
5. Heat the salad oil and fry the mashed potatoes until golden brown.

Ingredients:
Potato 50 g, 10 sticky rice pancakes

Vegetarian: ✗   Muslim: ✓

Megranate-shaped Fried Chicken
Fugui Shiliu Ji

Ingredients:
Potato 400 g, chicken breast 100 g, sticky rice 80 g

Seasonings:
20 thin sticky rice wrappers, 2 eggs, bread crumbs 500 g, salt 5 g, chicken essence 3 g, dark soy sauce 5 g, oyster oil 5 g, vegetable oil 1,500 g

Preparation:
1. Peel the potatoes and mince them. Mince the chicken breast. Steam the soaked sticky rice.
2. Fry the minced potatoes and chicken breast well, then add the steamed sticky rice, salt, chicken essence, dark soy sauce and oyster oil and fry together. Use this mixture as filling.
3. Whisk the eggs. Wrap the fried fillings in the thin sticky rice wrappers, dip in the eggs and then coat with bread crumbs. Fry until golden brown, then serve.

Vegetarian: ✗   Muslim: ✓

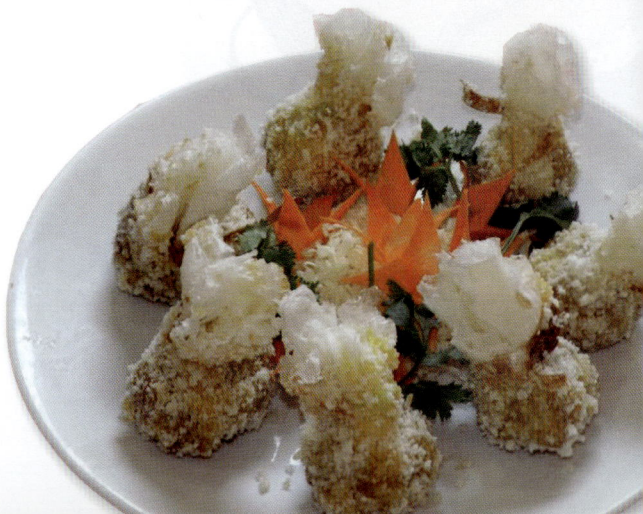

Minced beef in potato bowls
Yi Wan Chi

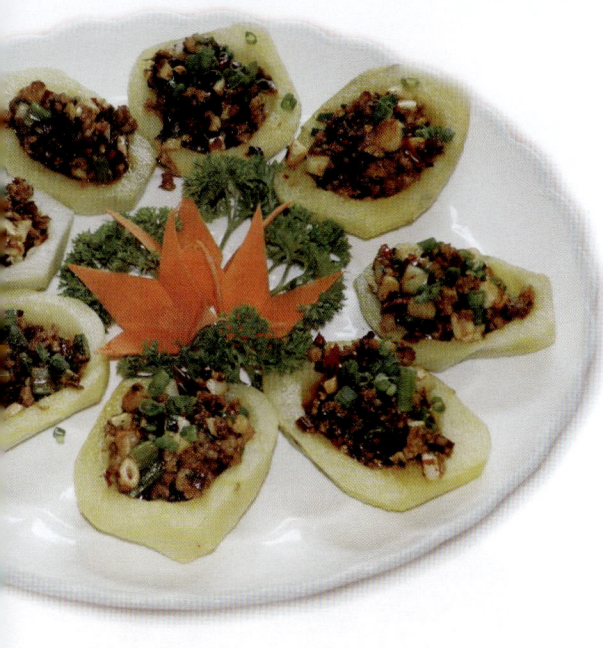

Ingredient:
Potato 800 g

Seasonings:
Bamboo shoots 300 g, spicy sauce 200 g, dried lily flower 20 g, minced beef 50 g, salt 3 g, gourmet powder 3 g, vegetable oil 80 g

Preparation:
1. Peel potatoes and carve them into bowl shapes. Steam the bamboo shoot well and cut into columns.

2. Heat wok and add vegetable oil, then quick-fry the bamboo shoots and remove. Put the spicy sauce, dried lily flower and minced beef in the wok, then add the fried bamboo shoots, salt, gourmet powder, and minced green onion and stir-fry. Serve in the potato bowls.

Vegetarian: ✗   Muslim: ✓

Pan-fried potato pastry
Xiangjian Tudou Bing II

Ingredients:
Potato 300 g, pork 50 g

Seasonings:
Table salt 5 g, gourmet powder 2 g

Preparation:
1. Boil two potatoes, then peel and mash into paste.
2. Combine the cooked minced pork, table salt and gourmet powder with the potato paste and form into a pastry.
3. Pan-fry over low heat until brown, then serve.

Vegetarian: ✗ Muslim: ✗

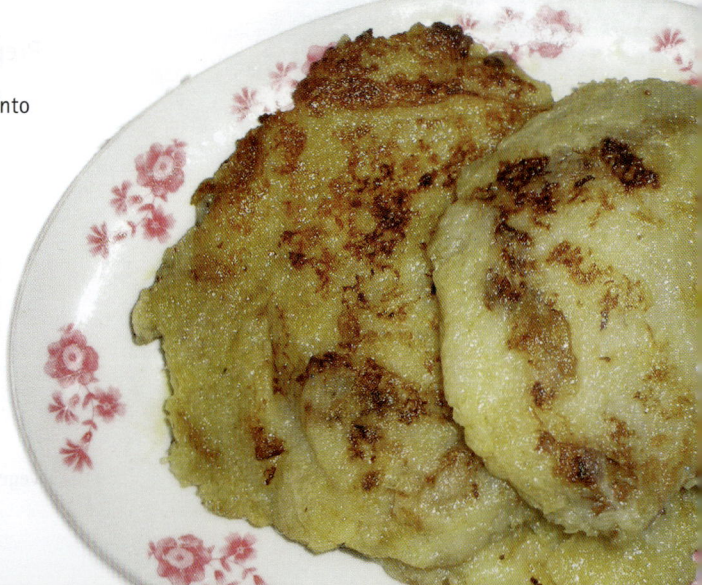

Potato and chicken with chili powder
Yangyu Lazi Ji

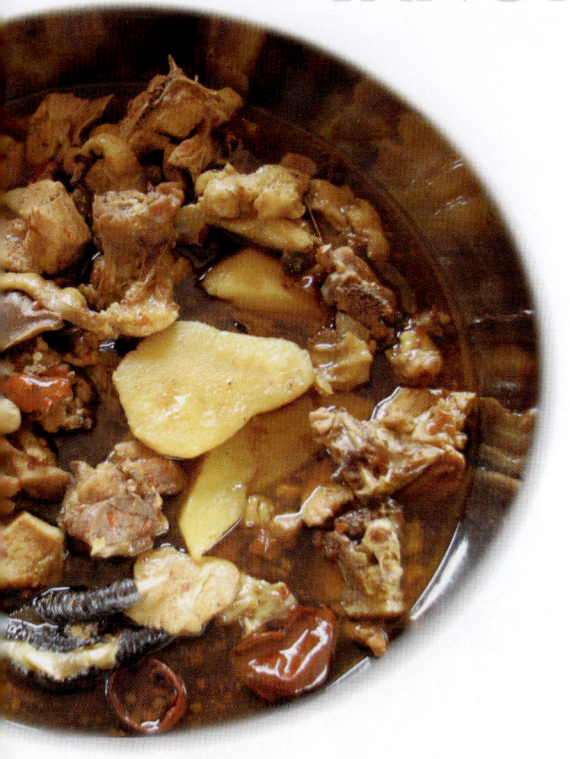

Ingredients:
Potato 200 g, chicken 600 g, ginger 1, starch to taste

Seasonings:
Cooking oil 50 g, soy sauce 20 g, cooking wine 15 g, refined salt 10 g, dried hot pepper to taste, chili powder to taste, 1 star anise

Preparation:
1. Clean and dice chicken. Peel and dice potatoes. Peel and mince ginger.
2. Put diced chicken in a bowl and mix well with salt, water and cooking wine.
3. Heat oil in a wok and fry diced chicken until almost cooked, then add potato, soy sauce, dried hot pepper, chili powder, ginger, water and refined salt to stew for an hour over low heat. Add starch to thicken the soup, then serve.

Vegetarian: ✗   Muslim: ✗

Potato chips served with Yunnan ham
Yuntui Tudou Pian

Ingredients:
Xuanwei-brand ham 100 g, potato 200 g

Seasoning:
Green onion to taste

Preparation:
1. Slice the ham, peel and slice cleaned potatoes and mince the green onion.
2. Lay out the sliced potatoes and sliced ham by turns in a steamer. Steam until well-done, remove to a plate and sprinkle with minced green onion, then serve.

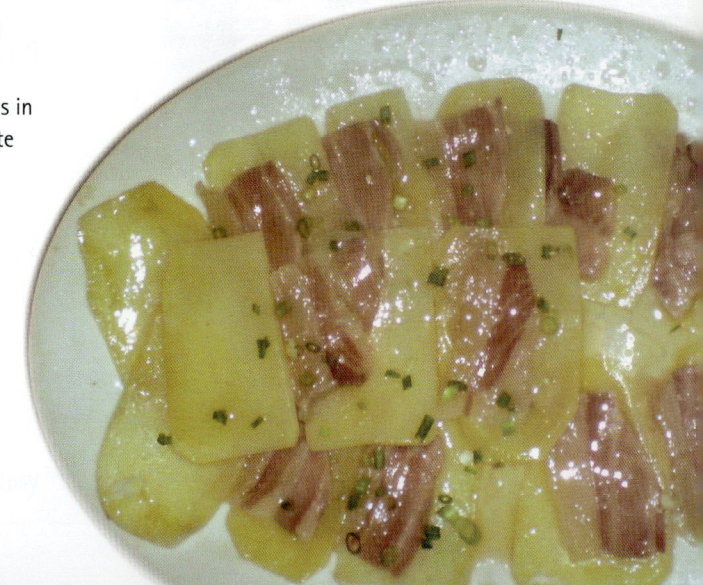

Vegetarian: ✘ Muslim: ✘

Potato pancake with salted vegetables
Xuecai Tudou Bing

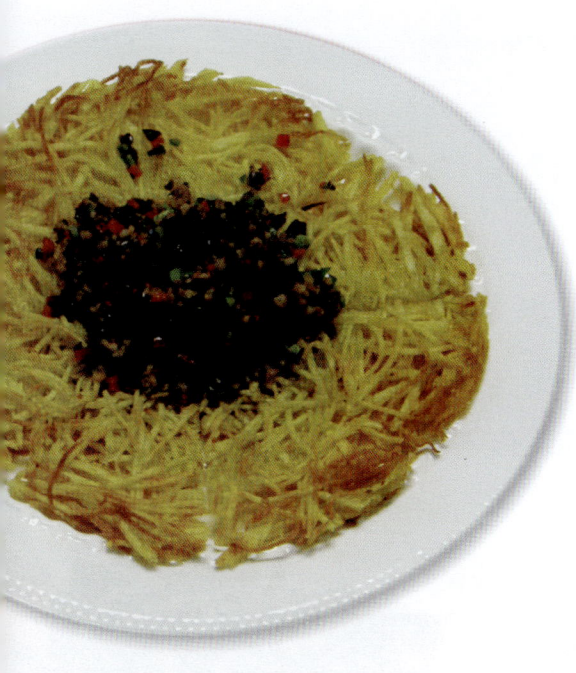

Seasonings:
Salad oil 200 g, gourmet powder 2 g, chicken essence 1 g, potato starch 10 g, salt 3 g

Time:
5 minutes.

Preparation:
1. Slice the potatoes and mix with some salt and a little potato starch.
2. Heat the salad oil and stir-fry the potato slices until golden brown, then remove to a plate.
3. Keep some oil in the pan and add some minced meat, green pepper, red pepper and salted vegetable and stir them until they are dry.
4. Transfer the fried potato pancake and the prepared salted vegetable onto one plate and serve.

Ingredients:
Potato 500 g, salted vegetable 10 g, green pepper 10 g, red pepper 10 g, minced pork 10 g

Vegetarian: ✗   Muslim: ✗

Potato shoot salad in vinegar
Liangban Shumiao

Ingredients:
Potato shoots 200 g, tomato 70 g, 2 hot peppers

Seasonings:
Refined salt 2 g, gourmet powder, vinegar and garlic

Preparation:
1. Clean the potato shoots and put in boiling water to stew well. Remove and set aside to cool, then cut into sections. Slice some of the tomatoes and mince the rest. Mince the hot pepper and mash the garlic.
2. Remove the cooked potato shoots to a dish and mix evenly with salt, gourmet powder, vinegar, tomato, hot pepper and garlic mash.

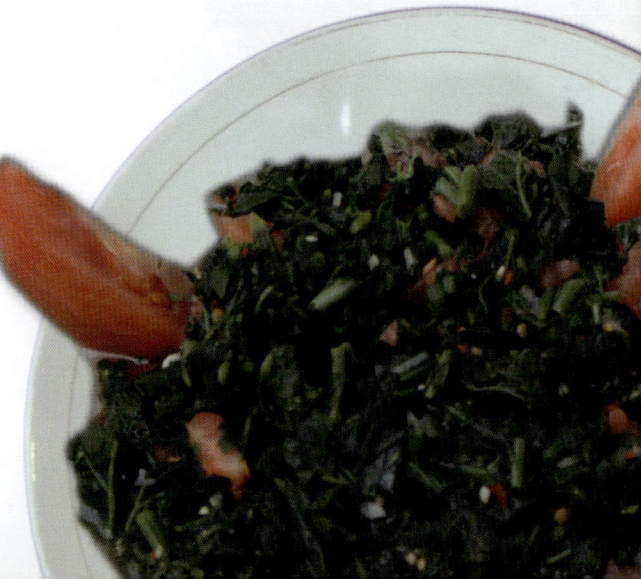

Vegetarian: ✓   Muslim: ✓

Potato shoot soup with sour bamboo shoots
Suan Sun Shumiao Tang

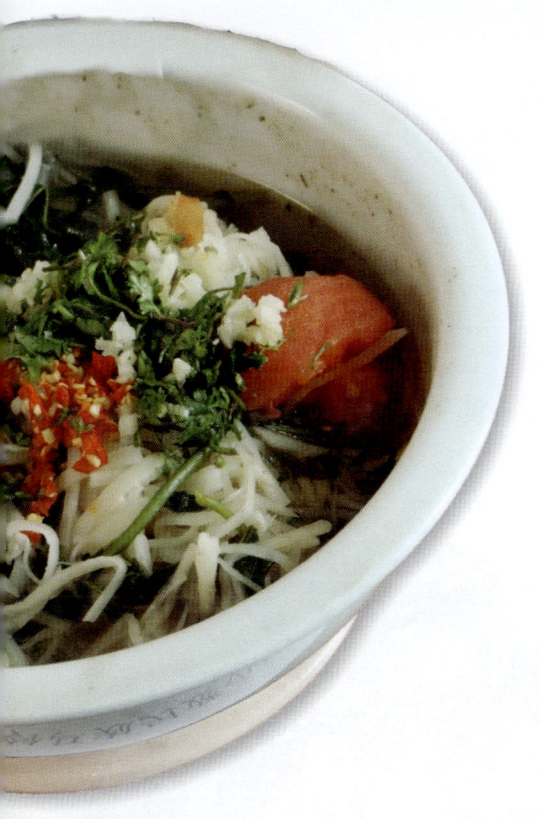

Ingredients:
Potato shoots 200 g, Dai-made sour bamboo shoots 200 g, tomato 100 g, coriander 5 g, small hot pepper 10 g, garlic

Seasonings:
Peanut oil 50 g, green onion 3 g, red pepper 2 g, soy sauce 2 g, ginger powder 2 g, Chinese prickly ash 2 g, table salt 1 g, gourmet powder 1 g

Preparation:
1. Rinse the bamboo shoots and stew for a moment, then add the potato shoots, tomato and salt to stew well.
2. Mix in coriander, garlic mash, small hot pepper, salt and gourmet powder, then serve.

Vegetarian: ✓   Muslim: ✓

Potato soup with pickled cabbage
Suancai Tudoupian Tang

Ingredients:
Potato 200 g, pickled cabbage 30 g

Seasonings:
Salad oil 15 g, salt 2 g, gourmet powder 1 g, pepper powder 0.5 g, small green onion 7 g, ginger pieces 3 g

Time:
6 minutes.

Preparation:
1. Peel potatoes and cut them into pieces. Cut the pickled cabbage into small sections.
2. Heat the salad oil and fry ginger together with pickled cabbage. Add some water and bring to a boil, then add the potatoes into the soup and cook them for a while. Add salt and gourmet powder, and sprinkle minced green onion before remove.

Vegetarian: ✓   Muslim: ✓

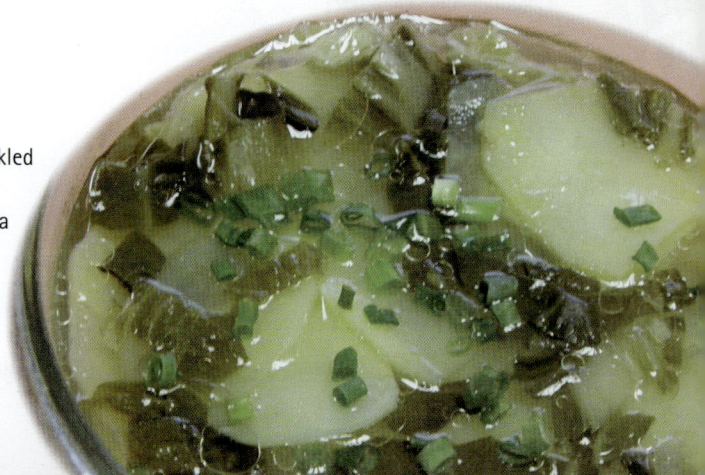

Potato string cake with five spices
Wuxiang Tudou Si Bing

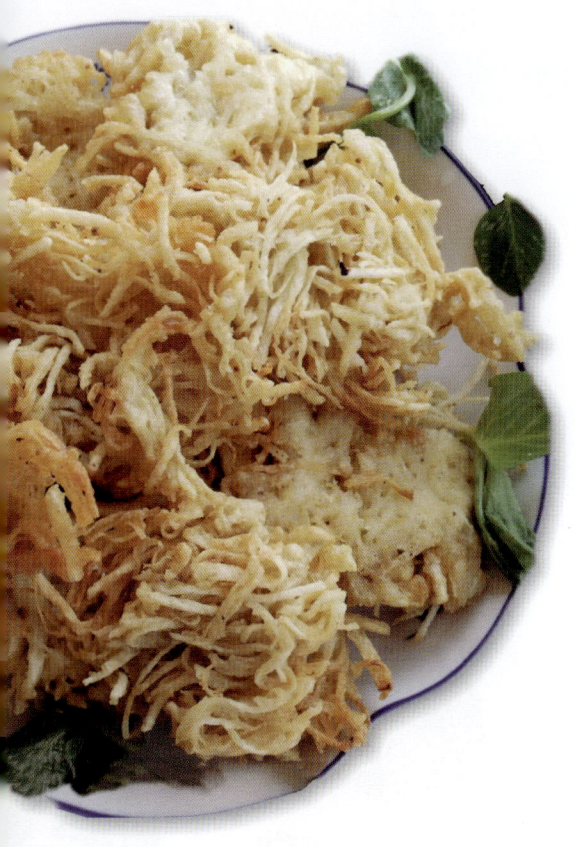

Ingredients:
Potato 300 g, flour 100 g

Seasonings:
Cooking oil 300 g, refined salt 3 g, five spices

Preparation:
1. Peel and shred potatoes. Combine water and flour to make a paste and mix into the shredded potatoes. Stir until sticky.
2. Heat the oil over medium heat and deep-fry the raw potato cake. When it is done, remove excess oil and turn off heat. Sprinkle with salt and flavored spices while stirring, then serve.

Vegetarian: ✓   Muslim: ✓

Potato with Laver
Zi Cai Tudou Bing

Ingredient:
Potato 500 g

Seasonings:
Dried laver 10 g, starch 100 g, minced pork 200 g, carrot 50 g, onion 20 g, salt 3 g, gourmet powder 2 g, sugar 20 g, chili pepper 2 g

Preparation:
1. Peel and steam potatoes, then mash them. Add starch and porphyra capensi to make the wrapper.
2. Dice the carrots and onion.
3. Fry the minced pork well, add diced carrot and onion and fry together to make the filling.
4. Wrap the fillings and make into a cake. Steam the cake and serve.

Vegetarian: ✗   Muslim: ✗

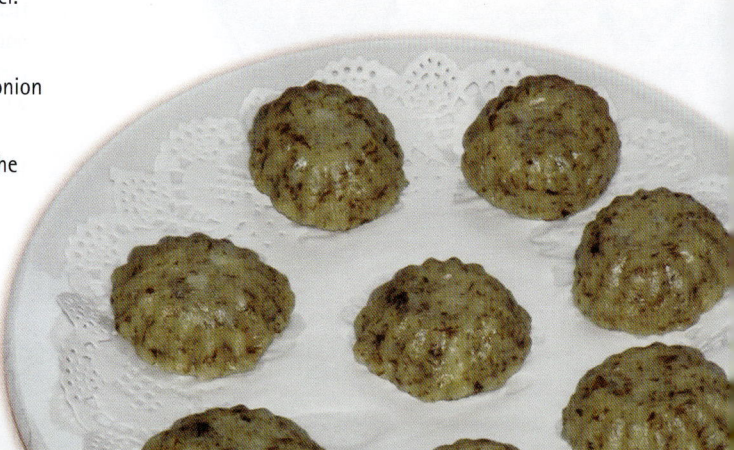

Potato with Twice-Cooked Pork
Tudou Huiguo Rou

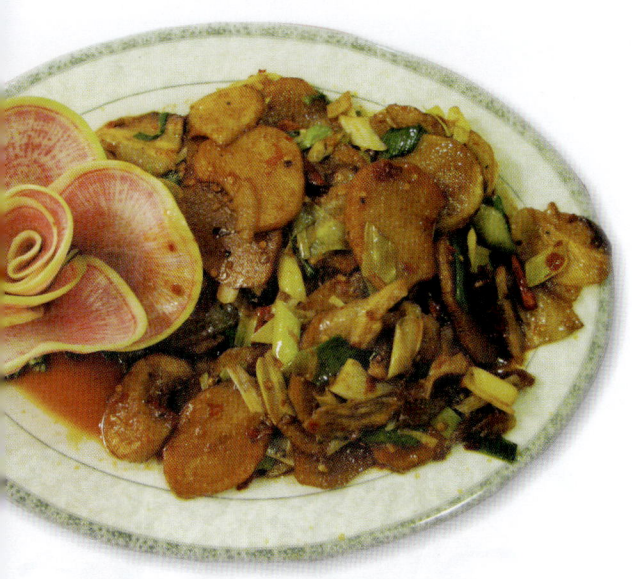

Preparation:

1. Clean the meat and stew it for about 20 minutes. Poke meat with chopsticks; remove and slice if no bloody liquid seeps out.
2. Clean and peel red peppers, removing the stems and seeds, then dice them. Clean tender garlic shoots and cut into sections. Peel cleaned potatoes and slice.
3. Put oil in a wok and quick-fry the sliced meat, then add potato chips to fry together. Once the fatty part of the meat starts to reduce, add red pepper and stir-fry, then remove.
4. Leave some oil in the wok and fry sweet sauce and fermented soybean until it gives off aroma. Add the cooking wine and gourmet powder and fry evenly, then add the fried meat and potato chips and stir-fry. Before turning off the heat, add tender garlic shoots to fry together, then remove and serve.

Ingredients:

Potato 200 g, side pork 300 g, 1 red pepper, tender garlic shoots 50 g

Seasonings:

Garlic to taste, cooking oil 50 g, cooking wine 20 g, fermented soybean 30 g, sweet sauce 20 g, refined salt 3 g, soy sauce 10 g, gourmet powder 2 g

Vegetarian: ✗   Muslim: ✗

Potatoes cooked in tin foil
Xizhi Tudou

Ingredients:
Potato 500 g; about 50 g per piece

Seasoning:
Chaotung-brand hot sauce

Time:
25 minutes

Preparation:
Clean potatoes, wrap with tin foil, then steam in food steamer. Cut the steamed potatoes into four pieces each and cover with hot sauce before serving. Garnish with cherries for appearance, if desired.

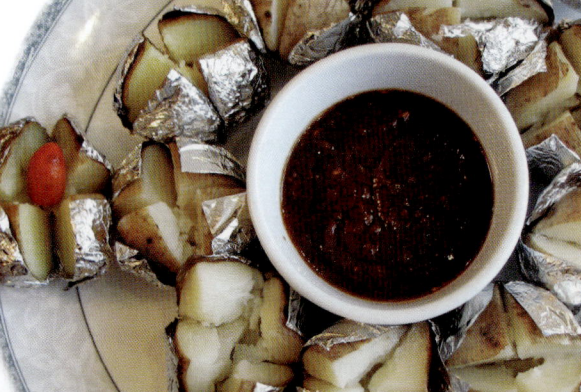

Vegetarian: ✓   Muslim: ✓

Potatoes in Soy Sauce
Jiang Xiang Tudou

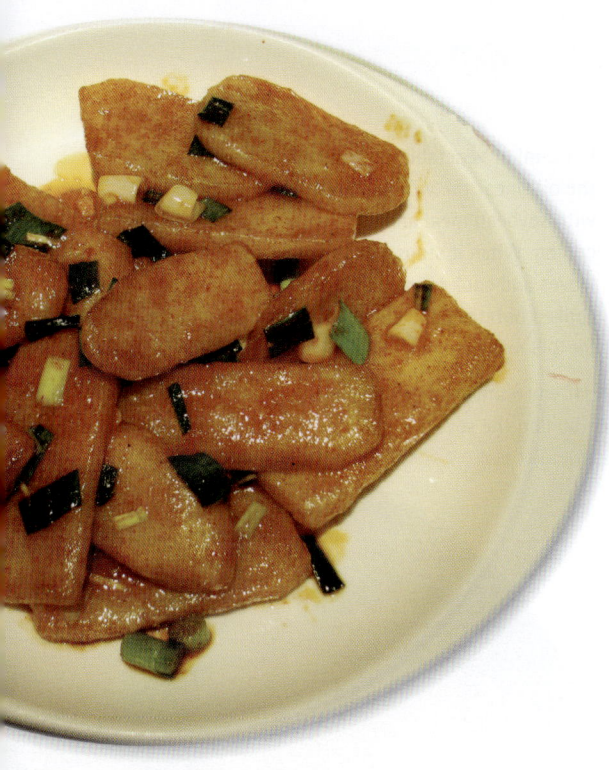

Ingredients:
Potato 300 g, green onions 3

Seasonings:
Cooking oil 50 g, hot sauce 30 g, refined salt 2 g, gourmet powder 1 g

Preparation:
1. Peel potatoes and slice them into 3 mm-thick chips. Cut green onion into sections.
2. Put a little water in a wok and stew potato chips for 2 minutes, then remove and drain.
3. Heat oil in the wok and fry the hot sauce, then add in the potato chips and green onion to quick-fry. Mix in other seasonings evenly and serve.

Vegetarian: ✓   Muslim: ✓

Potatoes in soybean milk
Hezha Yangyu

Ingredients:
Fresh potato 250 g, dry soybean 200 g

Seasonings:
Tender radish leaves 10 g, vegetable oil 5 ml, salt 2 g

Preparation:
1. Peel potatoes and cut into halves, then boil them in water.
2. Soak soybean in warm water until it becomes soft, then put in a blender to make about 1 liter of soybean milk. Keep the soybean meal in the soybean milk. Mince radish leaves.
3. Put 5 ml of vegetable oil in a wok and turn it to let the oil smear the whole wok. Add the soybean milk with soybean meal and stir over medium heat until boiling. When it stops foaming, add the minced radish leaves and cook together for 2 minutes, then add cooked potatoes and salt to taste. Continue to cook for 3-5 minutes.

Note: If you want to make porridge, just add some rice when boiling the soybean milk.

Vegetarian: ✓   Muslim: ✓

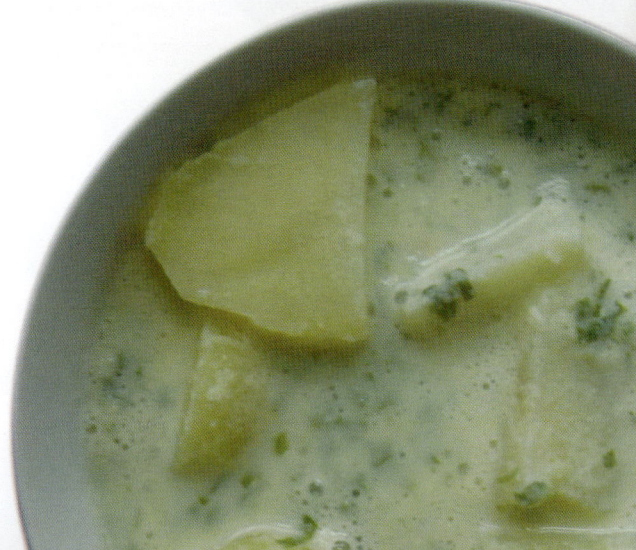

Roasted potatoes
Kang Yangyu

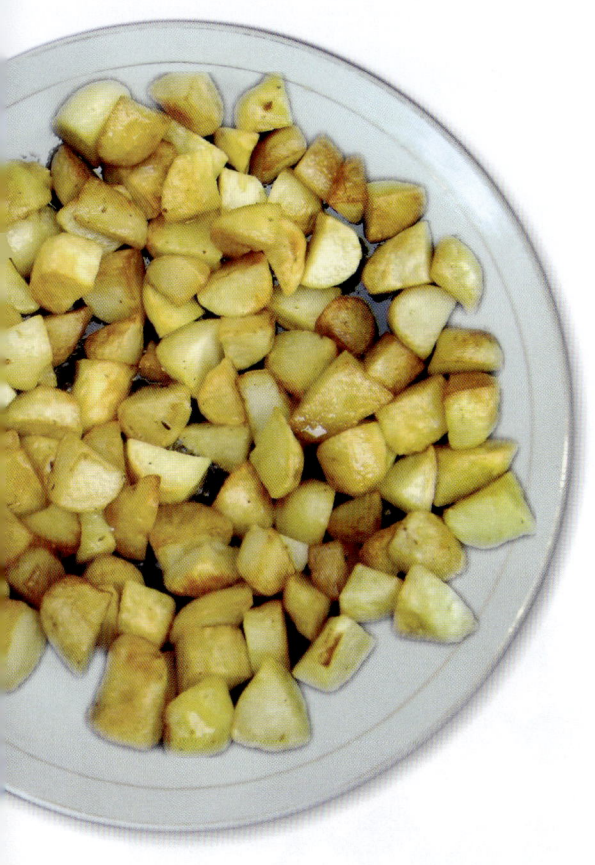

Ingredients:
Fresh potato 1,000 g; 25 g per piece

Seasonings:
Vegetable oil 30 ml, salt 3 g

Preparation:

1. Peel potatoes and rinse in cool water, then drain.

2. Put vegetable oil in heated wok and fry potatoes for 5 minutes. Then add salt and stir-fry until potatoes become transparent. Add 300 ml of water and cover. Stew to a boil over high heat, then turn to low heat to stew until the soup is almost dry. Stir potatoes to make sure they are evenly roasted until golden brown.

Vegetarian: ✓   Muslim: ✓

Salted meat with colored potatoes
Yanrou Caiyangyu

Ingredients:

Colored potato 500 g, salted meat 50 g, 5 dried hot peppers, green onion 2

Seasonings:

Cooking oil 50 g, refined salt 3 g

Preparation:

1. Cut dried hot pepper and green onion into sections. Slice salt meat and peel and slice potatoes.

2. Heat oil in a wok and quick-fry the sliced meat together with the dried hot pepper. Then add the potato chips and water to fry together until the fatty parts of the meat start to reduce. Add green onion and stir-fry, then serve.

Vegetarian: ✘ Muslim: ✘

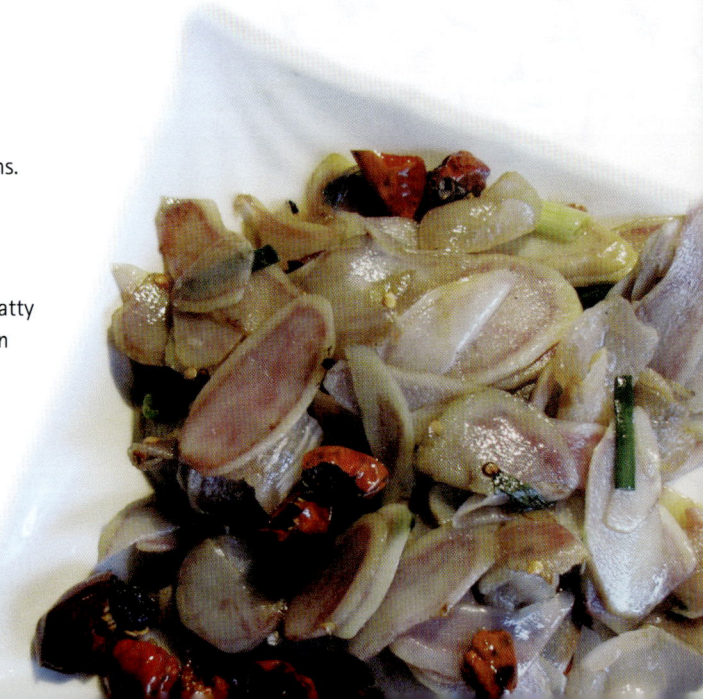

Shredded potato salad in vinegar
Liangban Shu Si

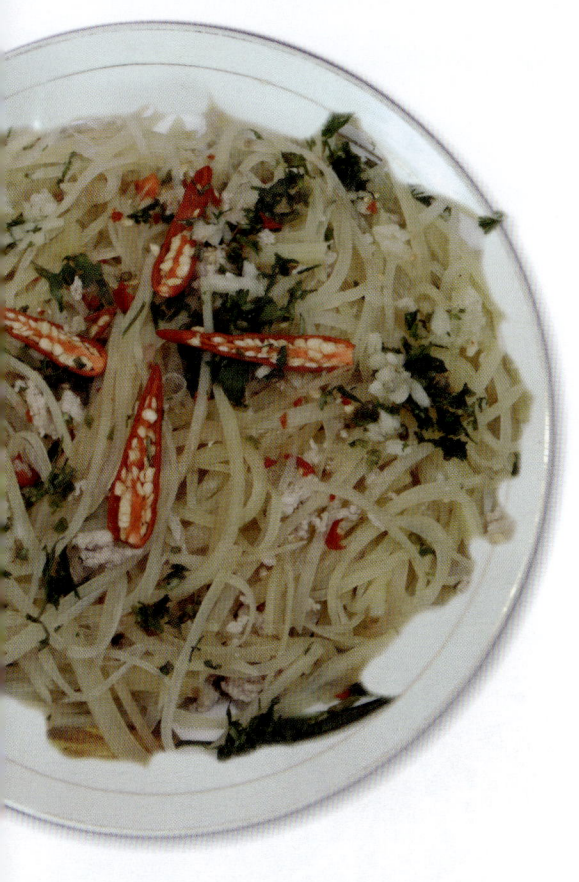

Ingredients:
Potato 300 g, garlic, coriander, small hot pepper

Seasonings:
Refined salt 3 g, vinegar, gourmet powder 1 g

Preparation:
1. Peel potatoes and shred them into strings. Mince small hot pepper and coriander. Mash the garlic.
2. Put the shredded potatoes into boiling water and stew until almost cooked, then remove and set aside to cool. Mix cooled potatoes with vinegar, coriander, garlic mash, salt and gourmet powder, then serve.

Vegetarian: ✓   Muslim: ✓

Shredded potatoes with beef jerky
Ganba Yanyu Si

Ingredients:
Beef jerky 50 g, potato 300 g, 10 dried hot peppers, green onion 5 g

Seasonings:
Cooking oil 400 g (65 g in use), refined salt 3 g

Time:
25 minutes

Preparation:
1. Peel and shred potatoes. Shred beef jerky and cut hot pepper and green onion into pieces.
2. Heat oil in a wok and fry shredded potatoes, then remove. Keep a little oil in the wok and fry dried hot pepper until it gives off aroma. Then fry beef jerky. Once it is cooked, add shredded potatoes and fry together. Mix in green onion and salt and stir-fry quickly, then serve.

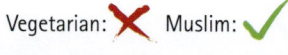

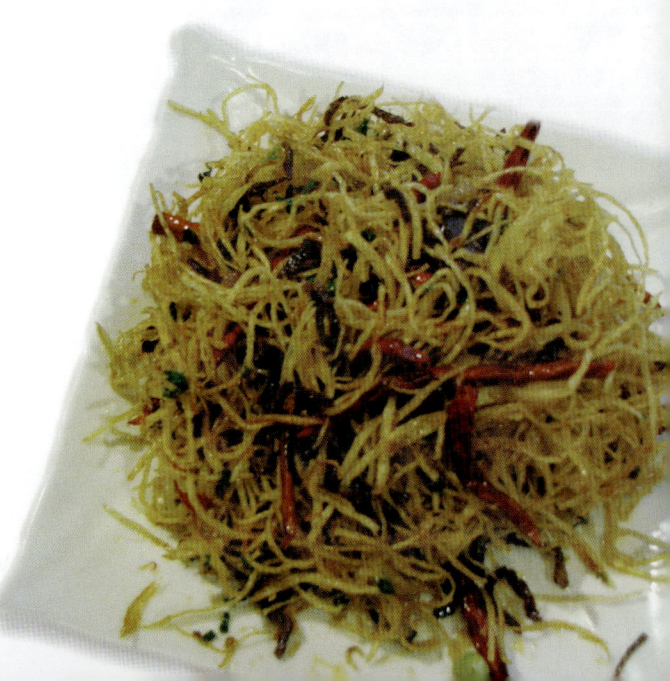

Shredded Potatoes with Pickles
Yangyu Si Xiancai

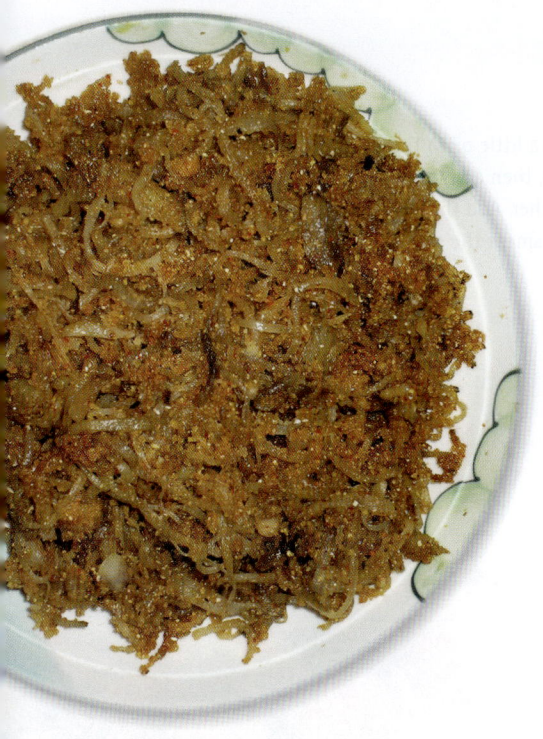

Ingredients:
Potato 500 g, corn meal 150 g

Seasonings:
Oil 150 g, sesame oil 10 g, pepper powder 20 g, salt 15 g

Preparation:
1. Shred the potatoes and marinate in lightly salted water for 30 minutes.
2. Heat sesame oil. When it smokes, add the shredded potatoes and bake over gentle heat, then remove and cool. Mix the potato strings with corn meal and pepper powder.
3. Heat oil and stew the mixed shredded potatoes and pickles over low heat.

Note: This is a typical dish in east Chongqing municipality.

Vegetarian: ✓   Muslim: ✓

Silver thread noodles and potato strings
Yinsi Tudou Chuan

Ingredients:
Silver thread noodles 50 g, a dozen potatoes (20 g each), minced meat 20 g, 2 red peppers, 2 green peppers, starch to taste

Seasonings:
Cooking oil 400 g, soy sauce 5 g, refined salt 5 g, fermented soybean 15 g, chili powder 10 g, gourmet powder 2 g

Preparation:
1. Soak silver thread noodles for 20 minutes in boiling water, then drain.
2. Peel cooked potatoes, string with the bamboo slip.
3. Heat oil in a wok and deep-fry silver thread noodles until they give off aroma, then remove to a dish.
4. Deep-fry the potato string until golden, then remove and put on the dish with the silver thread noodles.
5. Keep a little oil in the wok and quickly fry the minced meat, then add the seasonings and peppers and fry together. Add the wet starch and fry until it thickens, then smear the sauce on the potato strings and serve.

Vegetarian: ✗ Muslim: ✗

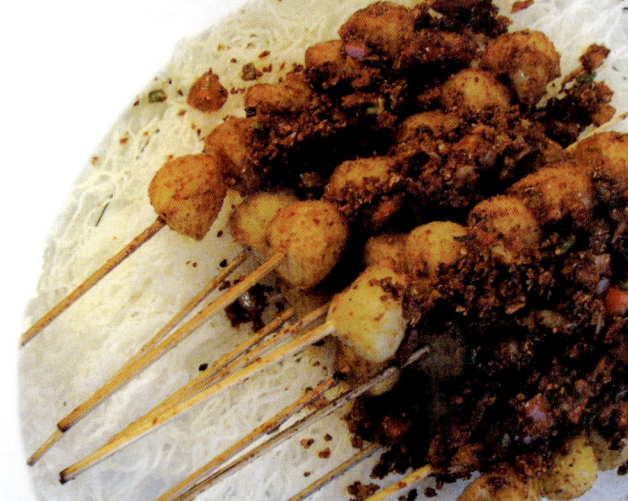

Sizzling Potato
Tieban Tudou

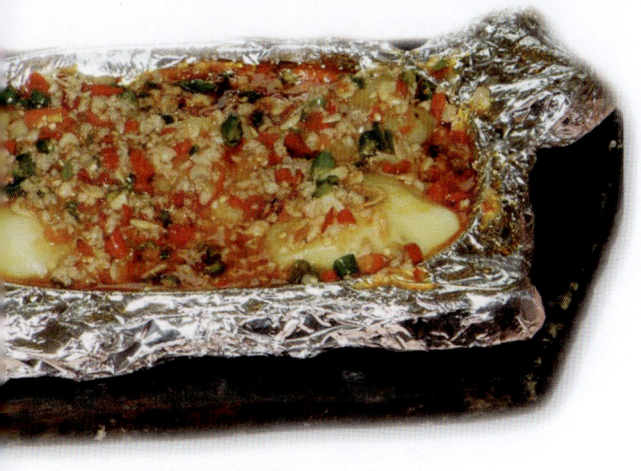

Ingredient:
Potato 400 g

Seasonings:
Small hot pepper 20 g, minced pork 20 g, water starch 5 g, dried small shrimp 10 g, garlic mash 2 g, ginger mash 2 g, salt 3 g, gourmet powder 3 g, hot pepper sauce 5 g, vegetable oil 100 g

Preparation:
1. Peel potatoes and cut them into big pieces, then steam well.
2. Fry small hot pepper, minced pork, hot pepper sauce and dried small shrimp, then add a little water, salt, gourmet powder and water starch.
3. Heat an iron platter and place the steamed potatoes with sauce on it.

Vegetarian: ✘   Muslim: ✘

Soft-fried sliced potatoes
Ruanzha Tudoupian

Ingredient:
Potato 250 g

Seasonings:
Salad oil 100 g, salt 2 g, pepper salt 2 g

Time:
15 minutes.

Preparation:
1. Slice the potatoes into 8 cm x 5 cm x 0.5 cm chips. Marinate them in salt water for 10 minutes.
2. Heat the salad oil and deep-fry the chips until they are crisp. Then place on a plate and sprinkle with some pepper salt.

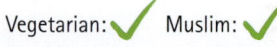
Vegetarian: ✓   Muslim: ✓

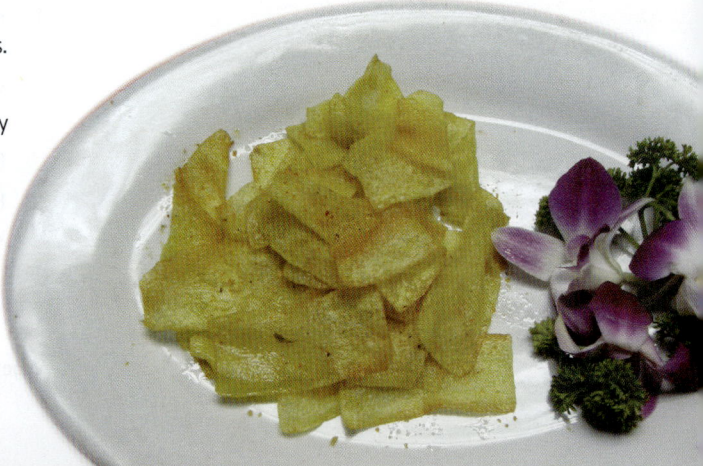

Sour and Spicy Potato Chips
Suanla Tudou Pian

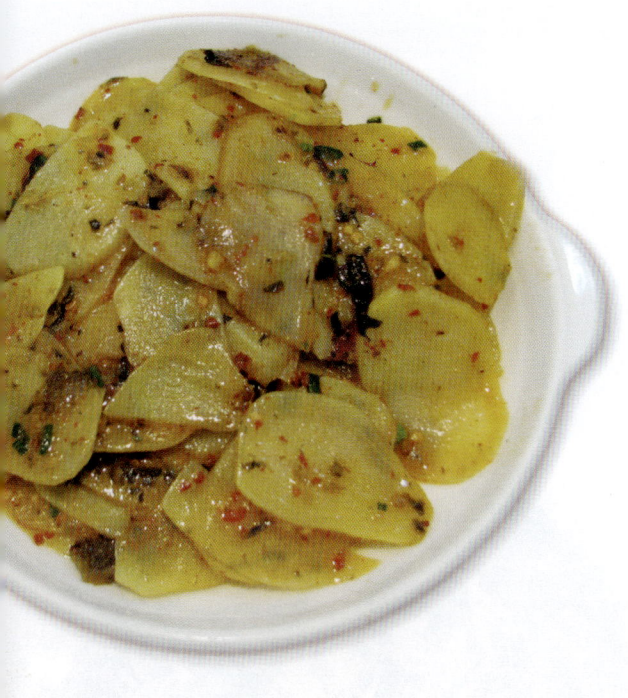

Ingredients:
Sour pickles 15 g, potato 300 g, pickled hot pepper sauce to taste, onion and starch to taste

Seasonings:
Cooking oil 70 g, refined salt 10 g, gourmet powder 2 g, chili powder

Preparation:
1. Peel and slice potatoes. Combine water and starch to make a thick liquid.
2. Heat oil in a wok and fry potato chips. Mix in the starch thick liquid and stew until potato chips are cooked. Then add sour pickles, salt, pickled hot pepper sauce, green onion, chili powder, refined salt and gourmet powder and serve.

Vegetarian: ✓   Muslim: ✓

Sour and spicy shredded potato soup
Suanla Tudou Si Tang

Ingredients:
Potato 500 g, sour pickles 50 g, 10 pickled hot peppers, green onion 10 g

Seasonings:
Cooking oil 20 g, refined salt 10 g, gourmet powder 2 g

Preparation:
1. Peel potatoes and shred into strings together with the sour pickles. Mince the pickled hot pepper and green onion.
2. Put water in a wok and add shredded potatoes, sour pickles and pickled hot pepper to stew together. When potatoes are done, add green onion, refined salt and gourmet powder. Mix well, then serve.

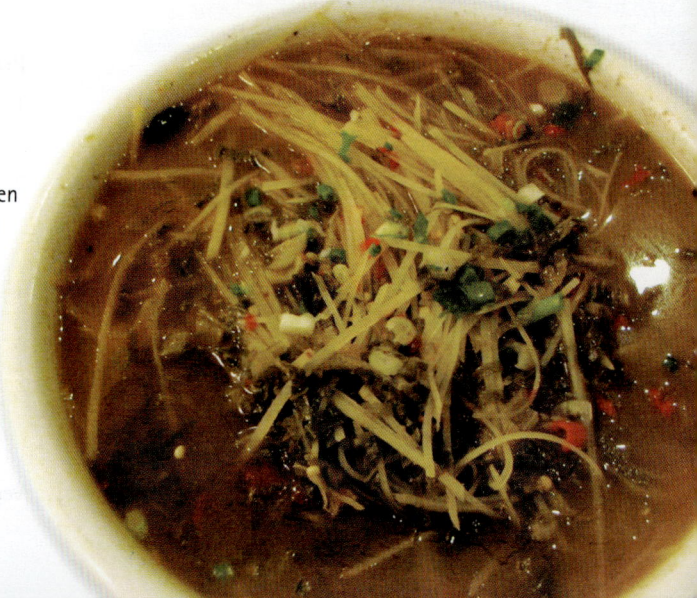

Vegetarian: ✓   Muslim: ✓

Sour diced potato soup
Shu Kuai Suan Tang

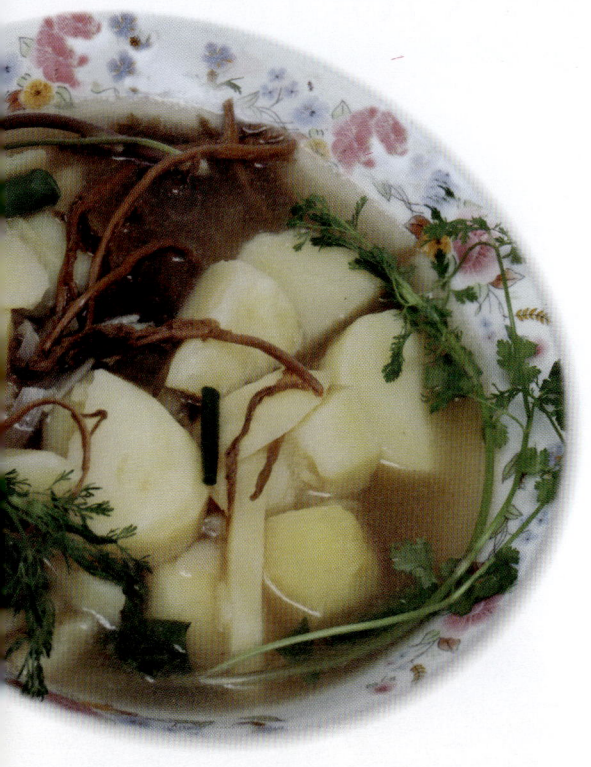

Ingredients:
Potato 300 g, pickles of ethnicl Dai flavor 50 g, 1 ginger, 2 green onion, 2 Coriander, garlic

Seasonings:
Cooking oil 20 g, refined salt 5 g, gourmet powder 2 g

Preparation:
1. Fry the diced potatoes for a few minutes, then add some water and stew.
2. Add pickles, ginger, green onion, garlic and coriander, and continue stewing for 5 minutes. Then season with salt and gourmet powder.

Vegetarian: ✓   Muslim: ✓

Sour pickle and chive flower potato soup
Suanyancai Tudou Tang

Ingredients:
Potato 500 g, sour pickles 50 g, sour salt chive flower 20 g

Seasonings:
Cooking oil 15 g, refined salt 10 g, gourmet powder

Preparation:
1. Clean potatoes and boil well. Mince sour pickles.
2. Boil sour pickles and sour salt chives in water. Add potatoes and boil for 5 minutes, then add refined salt and gourmet powder and serve.

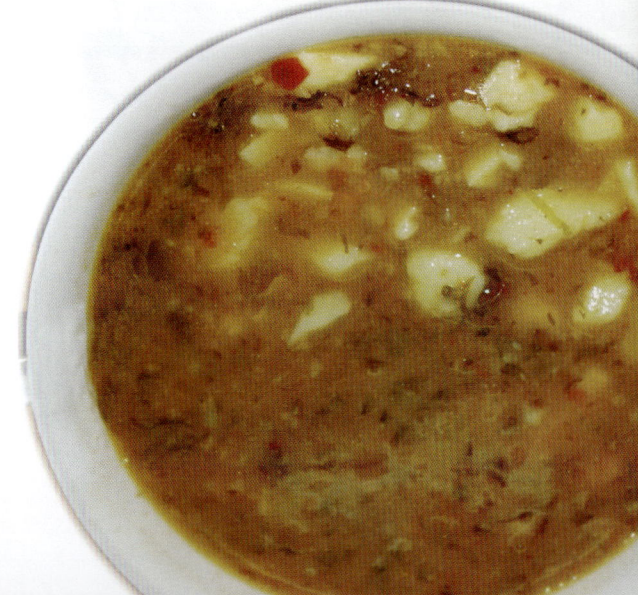

Vegetarian: ✓   Muslim: ✓

Sour Pickle and Potato Chip Soup
Suanyancai Tudou Pian Tang

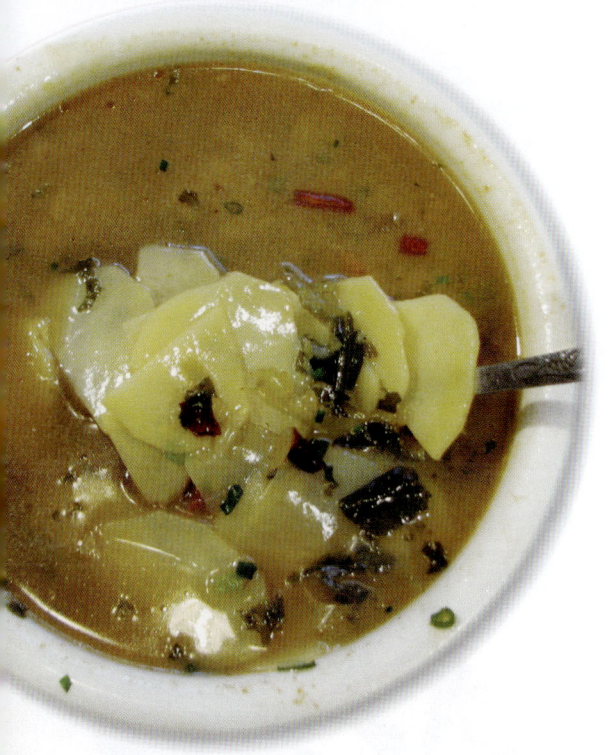

Ingredients:
Potato 500 g, sour pickles 50 g, seasoned hot pepper, green onion 5 g

Seasonings:
Cooking oil 15 g, refined salt 8 g, gourmet powder to taste

Preparation:
1. Peel and slice potatoes. Shred sour pickles. Cut dried hot pepper into sections and mince green onion.
2. Put water in wok and stew potato chips, sour pickles, dried hot pepper and green onion together until potatoes are well-cooked. Add refined salt and gourmet powder for flavor.

Vegetarian: ✓   Muslim: ✓

Spicy and hot potatoes
Xiangla Tudou

Ingredients:
Potato 300 g, fermented soybean 50 g, 3 green peppers, 3 red peppers, 2 green onion

Seasonings:
Cooking oil 50 g, soy sauce 3 g, refined salt 3 g, spicy sauce 15 g, sesame seeds

Preparation:
1. Clean the potatoes. Dice green and red peppers and cut green onion into sections.
2. Steam potatoes, then peel and dice. Heat oil in a wok and fry green and red peppers, green onion, fermented soybean and spicy sauce. Once it gives off aroma, add the potatoes and mix well together with soy sauce and salt. Then sprinkle with sesame seeds and serve.

Vegetarian: ✓ Muslim: ✓

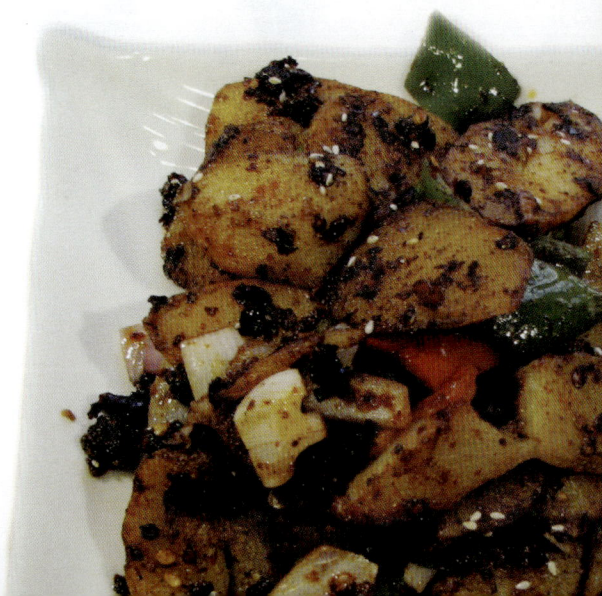

Spicy Diced Potatoes II
Xiangla Shu Kuai

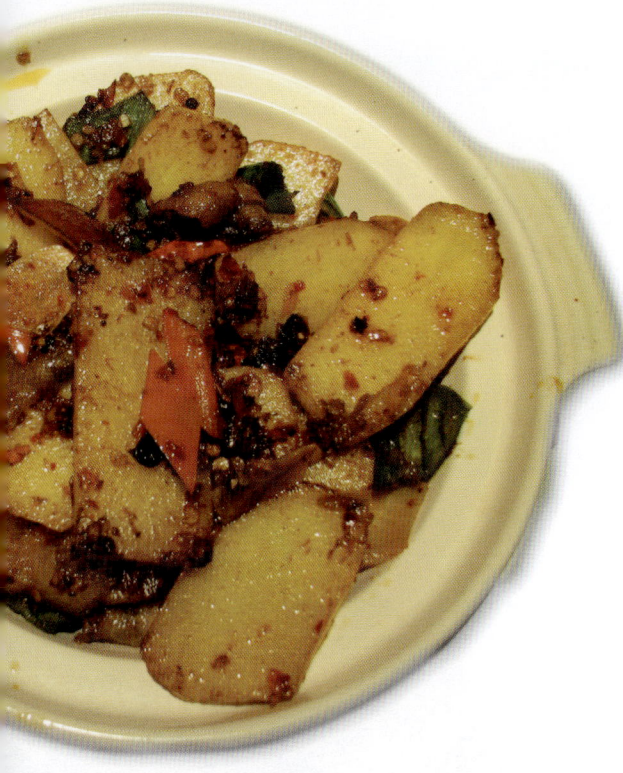

Ingredients:
Potato 300 g, 2 green peppers, 2 red peppers

Seasonings:
Cooking oil 200 g, hot pepper sauce 20 g, refined salt 3 g, fermented soybean 10 g

Preparation:
1. Peel potatoes and dice to 2 cm-thick pieces. Dice green and red peppers.
2. Heat cooking oil and fry the potatoes. Remove excess oil.
3. Add green and red pepper and seasonings, then fry together and mix well.

Vegetarian: ✓   Muslim: ✓

Spicy potato chips
Xiangla Tudou Pian II

Ingredients:
Potato 300 g, pickled hot pepper sauce to taste, a little green onion, a little starch

Seasonings:
Cooking oil 70 g, refined salt 10 g, gourmet powder 2 g, chili powder

Time:
25 minutes

Preparation:
1. Peel and slice cleaned potatoes. Add water into starch to form a thick starch soup.
2. Heat oil in a wok and fry sliced potatoes, then add the thick soup and stew until the potato chips are well cooked. Add green onion, chili powder, refined salt and gourmet powder. Mix and fry.

Vegetarian: ✓   Muslim: ✓

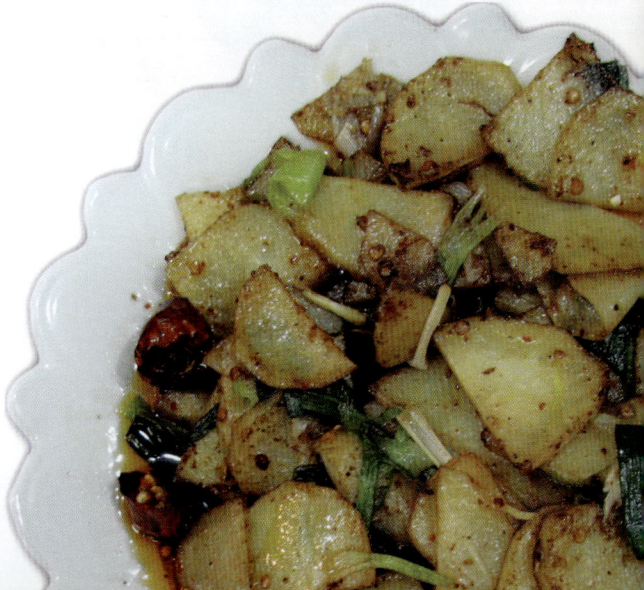

Spicy Potato Slices
Xiangla Tudou Pian I

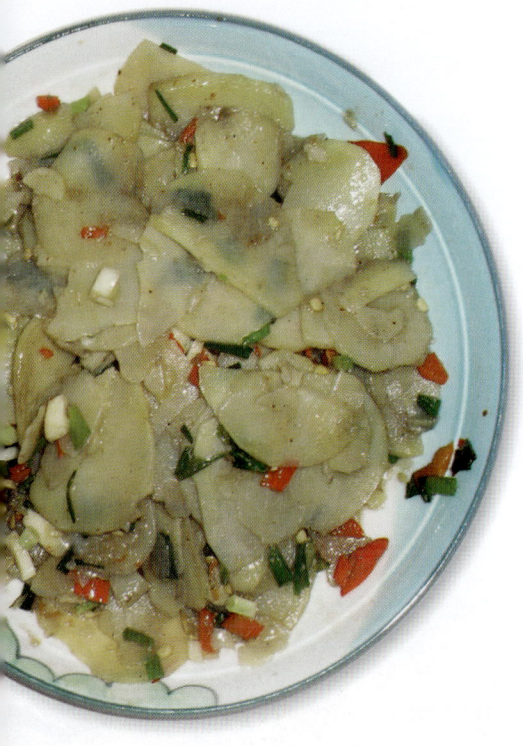

Ingredients:
Potato 500 g, minced garlic, chili powder to taste

Seasonings:
Vegetable oil 100 g, a little Chinese prickly ash, salt to taste, gourmet powder, chili pepper, white vinegar, cilantro and sesame oil

Preparation:
1. Slice potatoes.
2. Heat vegetable oil and pepper oil until they smoke, then add potato slices and stir-fry for 6–7 minutes. Add 150 ml of water, cover the wok and stew.
3. Add a little salt, gourmet powder, chili powder, white vinegar, and caraway or sesame oil and braise until cooked.

Vegetarian: ✓   Muslim: ✓

Spicy Sichuan-style potato strings
Ganbian Tudou Si

Ingredient:
Potato 250 g

Seasonings:
2 chilis, green onion 20 g, table salt 3 g, gourmet powder 2 g, oil 50 g

Preparation:
1. Shred potatoes and cut green onion into pieces.
2. Wash potato strings to remove excess starch, then drain.
3. Heat the oil and red pepper, then add the potato strings and stir-fry over high heat.
4. After 2 minutes, add the onion and stir-fry over medium heat.
5. Add some table salt and gourmet powder, then serve.

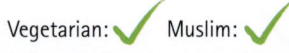
Vegetarian: ✓   Muslim: ✓

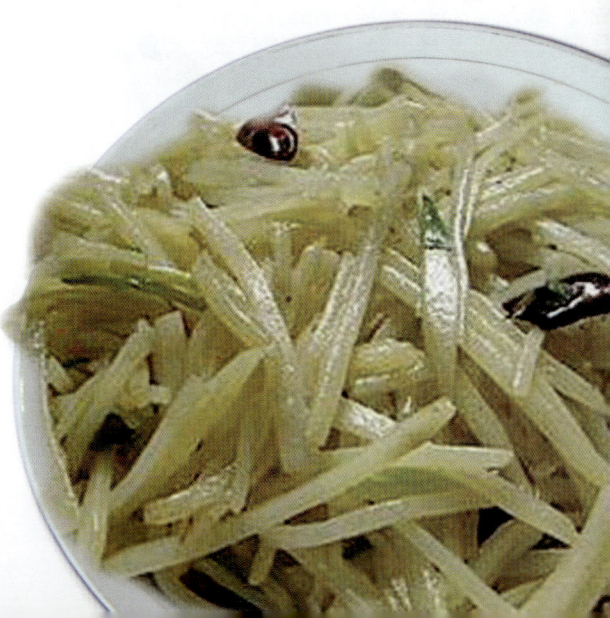

Steamed potatoes and spareribs
Fen Zheng Tudou Paigu

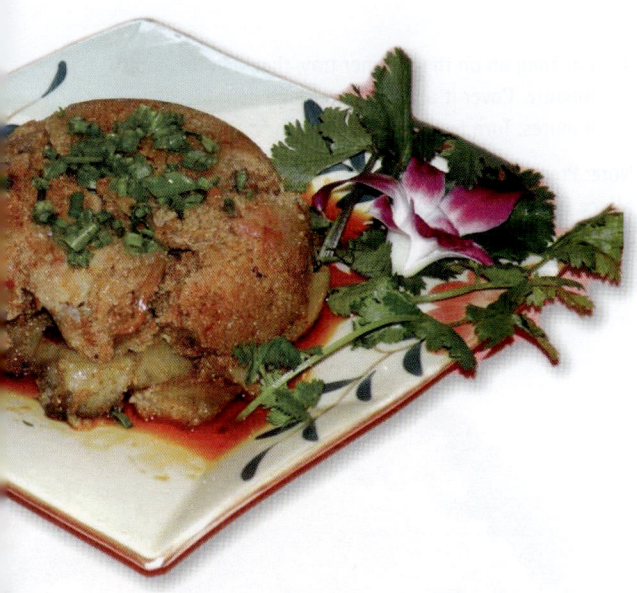

Seasonings:
Shredded ginger 5 g, minced green onion 5 g, sliced green onion 5 g, garlic 5 g, salt 5 g, gourmet powder 5 g, red oil 5 g.

Time:
25 minutes

Preparation:
1. Cut potatoes into cubes. Chop spareribs into sections.
2. Stew spareribs with green onion, shredded ginger and mashed garlic for 30 minutes. Put the steamed pork with rice on the spareribs, mix well.
3. Put the spareribs in a small bowl with potato cubes and steam for 10 minutes over high heat. Then steam for 50 minutes over low heat. Remove and place on a plate and sprinkle with minced green onion.

Ingredients:
Potato 400 g, pork spareribs 500g

Vegetarian: ✘   Muslim: ✘

Steamed potatoes with pickled chili
Culajiao Zheng Tudou

Ingredients:
Fresh potato 500 g, pickled chili 50 g

Seasonings:
Smoked sausage 100 g, ginger 2–3 g, Chinese prickly ash 2 g, Tong oh 200 g

Preparation:
1. Peel potatoes and cut them into cubes of about 25 g each. Rinse in cool water and drain.
2. Cut smoked sausage into 0.5 cm cubes. Mince ginger. Clean Tong oh and drain water.
3. Mix the potatoes, pickled chili, smoked sausage, minced ginger and Chinese prickly ash in a soup bowl and marinate for 5 minutes.
4. Put Tong oh on the steamer tray, then add the potato mixture. Cover it and heat over high heat for 30 minutes. Turn to low heat to steam for 15 minutes.

Note: Preparation of pickled chili
Mince fresh chili and combine with corn flour and salt in a special pot. Let stand to pickle for 1 month.

Vegetarian: ✗   Muslim: ✗

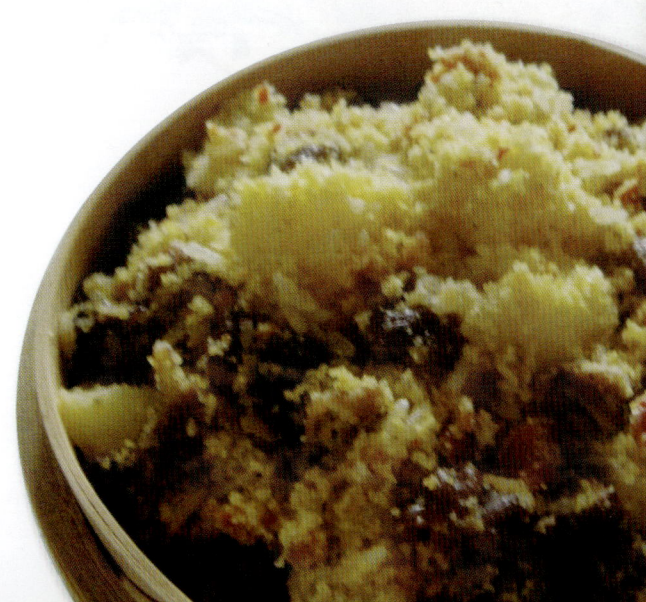

Stewed potatoes and pork ribs with spices
Xiangla Paigu Men Tudou

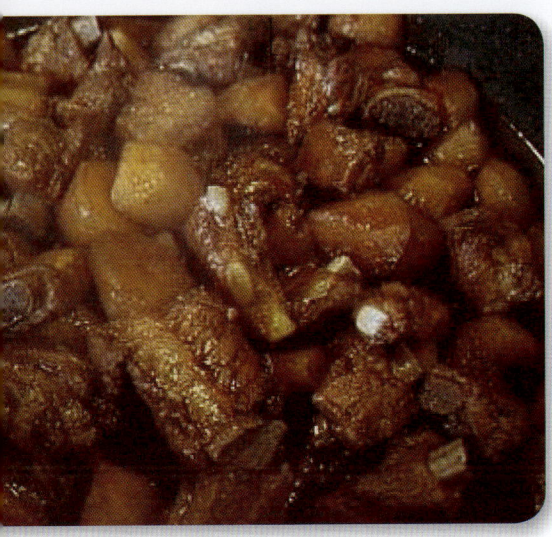

Preparation:

1. Cut the pork ribs into small pieces and dice potatoes to the same size as the pork ribs.
2. Heat oil in a pan and stir-fry the ginger pieces over high heat.
3. Add the pork ribs and continue stir-frying over high heat until they are dry.
4. Add the light soy sauce, dark soy sauce, white sugar and wine and stir for a few seconds, then add some water.
5. Add in potatoes and cover the pan. Stew for a while.
6. Mix in some spicy sauce and water and simmer for 20–25 minutes.

Ingredients:

Pork ribs 500 g, potato 500 g

Seasonings:

Dark soy sauce 5 g, light soy sauce 15 g, oil 20 g, sugar 5 g, ginger 5 g, cooking wine 15 ml, broad bean paste 10g

Vegetarian: ✗   Muslim: ✗

Stewed potatoes served in wok
Ganguo Tudou

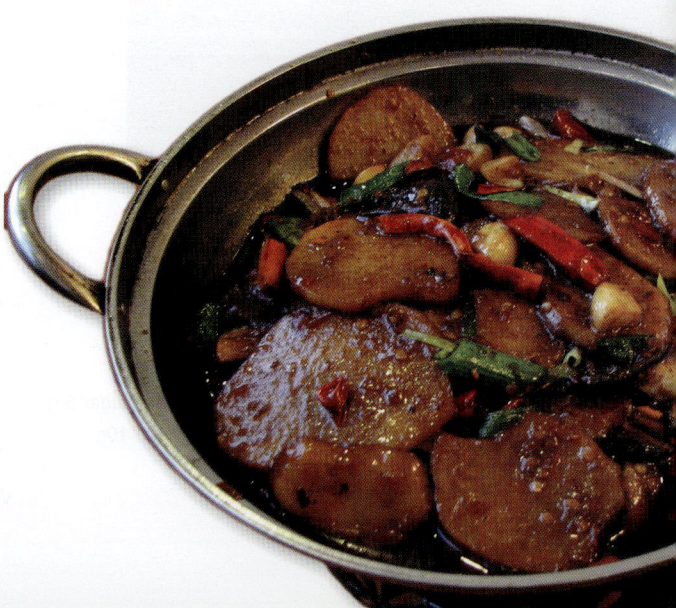

Ingredients:
Potato 500 g, 2 red peppers, 5–8 baked hot peppers, green onion 5

Seasonings:
Cooking oil 100 g, soy sauce 15 g, Chaotung sauce 30 g, refined salt 6 g, gourmet powder 2 g

Preparation:
1. Peel potatoes and slice into pieces about 2 mm thick. Dice green onion, red pepper and hot pepper.
2. Heat oil in a wok and fry green onion, red pepper and hot pepper with Chaotung sauce until it gives off aroma, then add potato slices and fry together. When it is almost done, add some water, salt, soy sauce and gourmet powder and simmer until the sauce thickens.

Note: Use solidified alcohol to heat the wok on the table when serving.

Vegetarian: ✓ Muslim: ✓

Stewed potatoes with cucurbit
Xiao Gua Men Yangyu

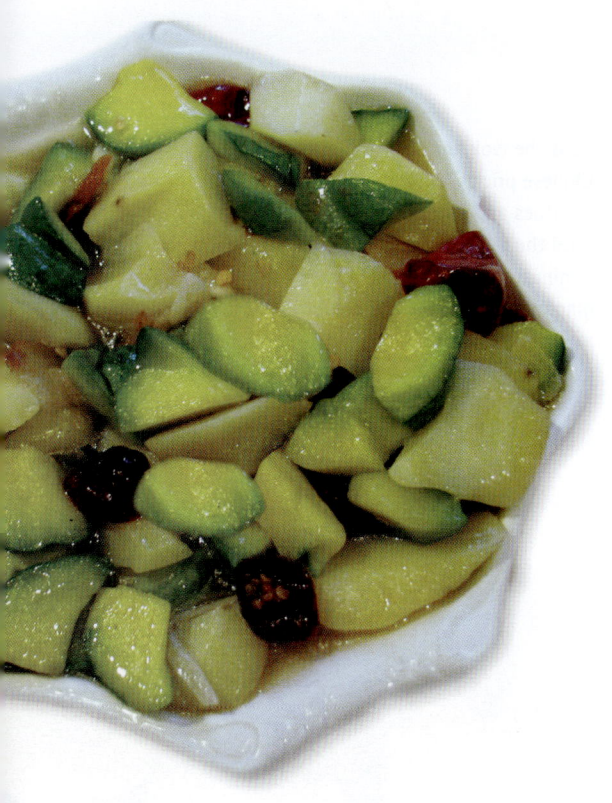

Ingredients:
Potato 200 g, cucurbit 200 g, 3 dried hot peppers

Seasonings:
Cooking oil 30 g, refined salt 3 g, gourmet powder 2 g

Preparation:
1. Peel and dice potatoes. Cut dried hot pepper into sections and dice cucurbit.
2. Add all seasonings in cooking pot to stew for 15 minutes, then serve.

Vegetarian: ✓   Muslim: ✓

Stewed potatoes with pumpkin II
Nangua Dun Tudou

Ingredients:
Fresh potato 500 g (about 50 g per piece), pumpkin 500 g

Seasonings:
Vegetable oil 15 ml, garlic 1, ginger 1, Chinese prickly ash 2 g, salt 1.5 g

Time:
25 minutes

Preparation:
1. Peel potatoes and cut in halves. Rinse in cool water, then drain.
2. Clean pumpkin and remove stem and seeds, then cut into cubes. Mash garlic and ginger.
3. Heat the wok and then add vegetable oil. Fry the Chinese prickly ash until it gives off aroma, then add potatoes and pumpkin and stir-fry over high heat until the pumpkin juice come out. Add salt and fry for 2 minutes. Add 500 ml of water, mashed garlic and ginger, then cover and boil over high heat. Turn to medium heat and simmer for 8–10 minutes.

Vegetarian: ✓   Muslim: ✓

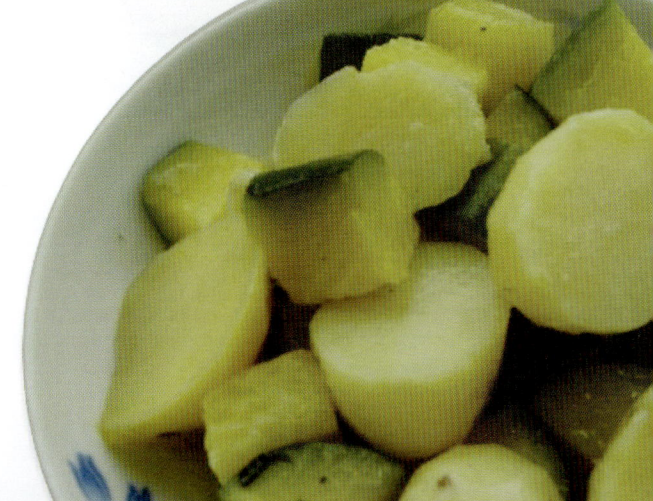

Stewed potatoes with rice
Yangyu Kongganfan

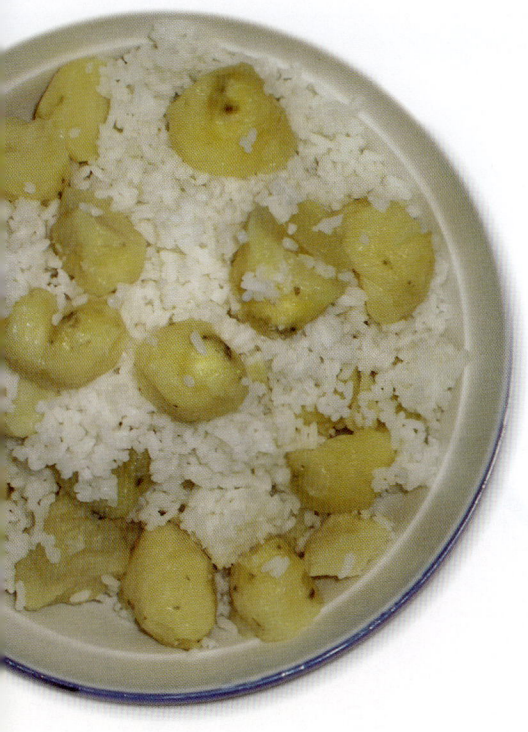

Ingredients:
Rice 500 g, potato 500 g

Seasoning:
Oil 100 g

Preparation:
1. Boil the rice until half-cooked then set aside for later use. Heat vegetable oil and stir-fry the potatoes for 5 minutes.
2. Put the half-cooked rice on top of the potatoes and add water to cover the potatoes. Simmer over low heat.

Note: This is the main staple dish in northeast Sichuan Province.

Vegetarian: ✓   Muslim: ✓

Stewed silver carp soup
Guiyu Zahui Tang

Ingredients:
Silver carp 300 g, potato 100 g, tofu 100 g, shiitake mushroom 30 g, celery 30 g, red pepper 20 g, green onion 2, ginger 1, garlic

Seasonings:
Refined salt 10 g, yellow wine, bean hot sauce 20 g, vegetable oil 20 g, gourmet powder 2 g

Preparation:
1. Clean silver carp and chop in pieces. Slice tofu and potatoes into thick pieces. Rip shiitake mushroom into large pieces. Cut celery into 5 cm-long pieces. Mince ginger, garlic, green onion and red pepper.

2. Heat oil and quick-fry minced green onion, ginger, garlic and bean hot sauce, then add water, shiitake mushroom, fish, bean curd, potatoes, celery, yellow wine, refined salt and heat to a boil. Turn to low heat and cook for 15 minutes. Add gourmet powder and serve.

Vegetarian: ✗   Muslim: ✓

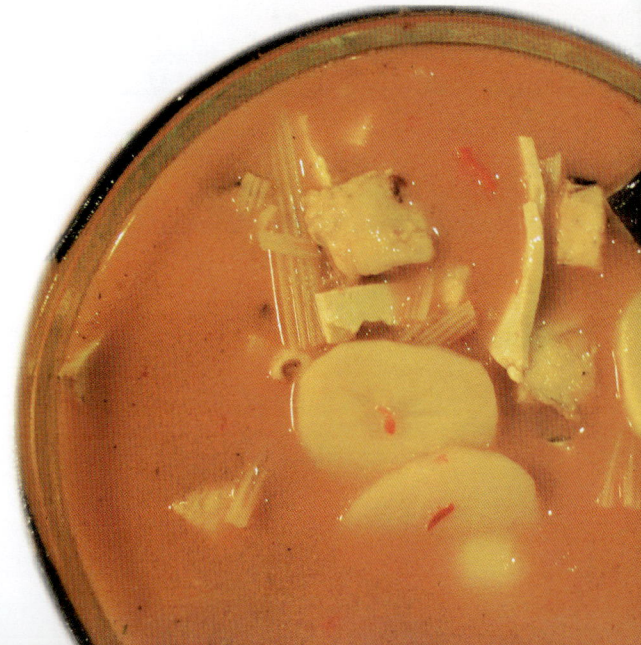

Stewed small potatoes
Youmen Xiao Tudou II

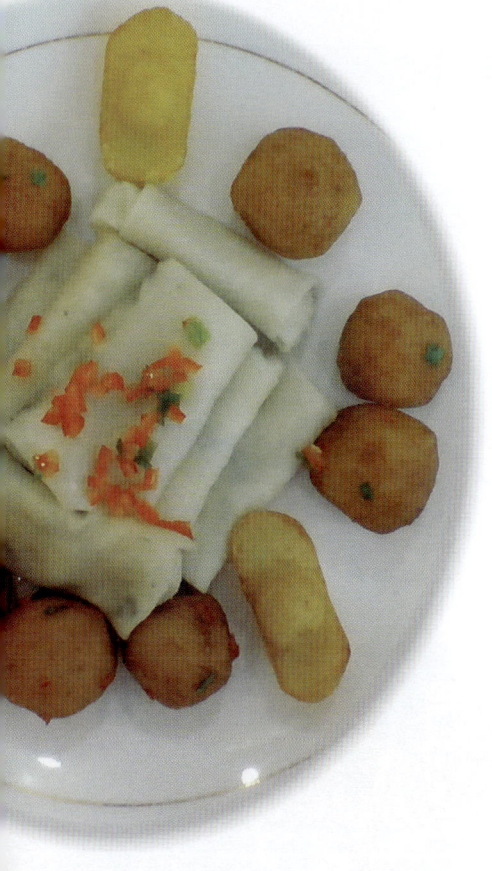

Ingredients:
Potatoes 500 g, several round small potatoes, several spring rolls, candied fruit

Seasonings:
Cooking oil 100 g, refined salt to taste

Preparation:
1. Steam and then peel the potatoes. Carve the longer potatoes into the shape of Yuanbao and put into wok together with the smaller, round potatoes. Fry until golden, then remove.
2. Put steamed spring rolls in a dish, then add the fried potatoes. Sprinkle with diced candied fruit and serve.

Vegetarian: ✓   Muslim: ✓

Stir-fried potato shoots
Su Chao Shumiao

Ingredients:
Fresh potato seedling bud 200 g, tomato 50 g, 3 red peppers, 3 dried peppers

Seasonings:
Cooking oil 30 g, fermented soybean 20 g, refined salt 3 g, gourmet powder 1 g

Preparation:
1. Select a fresh bud from potato shoots. Clean it and cut into sections. Dice tomato and red peppers.
2. Heat oil and stir-fry potato seedling bud, tomato, red peppers and fermented soybean.
3. Add salt and gourmet powder, mix well and serve.

Vegetarian: ✓   Muslim: ✓

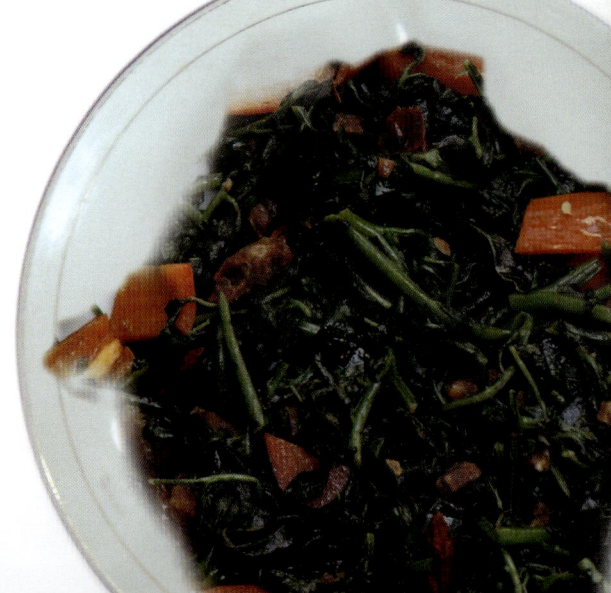

Stir-fried Shredded Vegetables
Chao San Si

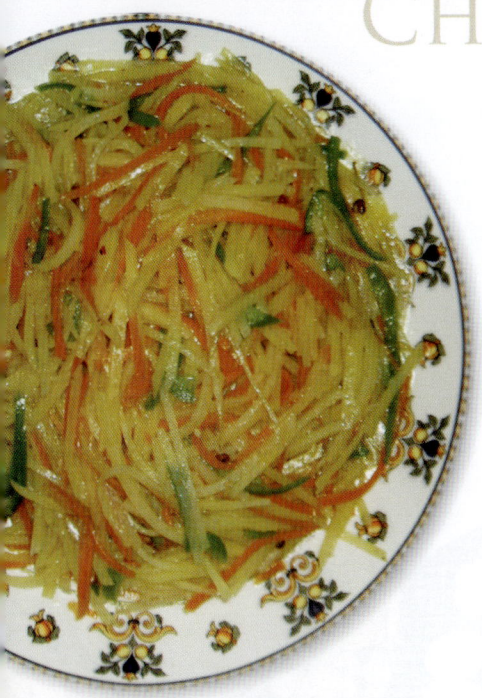

Preparation:

1. Peel and finely shred potatoes. Marinate in water for later use. Shred the green pepper, carrot, garlic and ginger.

2. Heat oil in a frying pan and fry Chinese prickly ash. When it gives off aroma, add the potato strings and fry. Sprinkle frequently with water while frying potatoes, to avoid stickiness.

3. Add green pepper and carrot when potato strings become translucent. Then add ginger and garlic. Fry for about 2 minutes. Season with salt and pickled chili paste. Use light soy sauce to thicken the juice, then serve.

Note: The dish has a pleasant color. Crispy taste and the light hot is good to eat with rice as a popular local dish in E xi, Hubei Province.

Ingredients:
Potato 100 g, green pepper 50 g, carrot 50 g

Seasonings:
Oil 10 ml, 2 cloves of garlic, ginger 2 g, Chinese prickly ash 0.5 g, salt 1 g, pickled chili paste 1 tsp, light soy sauce 1 tsp

Vegetarian: ✓   Muslim: ✓

Street potato snacks from Yunnan
Jie Bian Xiao Chi

Note: These recipes are popular potato snacks along streets in Yunnan. Frying and baking are the two most popular ways to cook them.

334 >

Vegetarian: ✗   Muslim: ✗

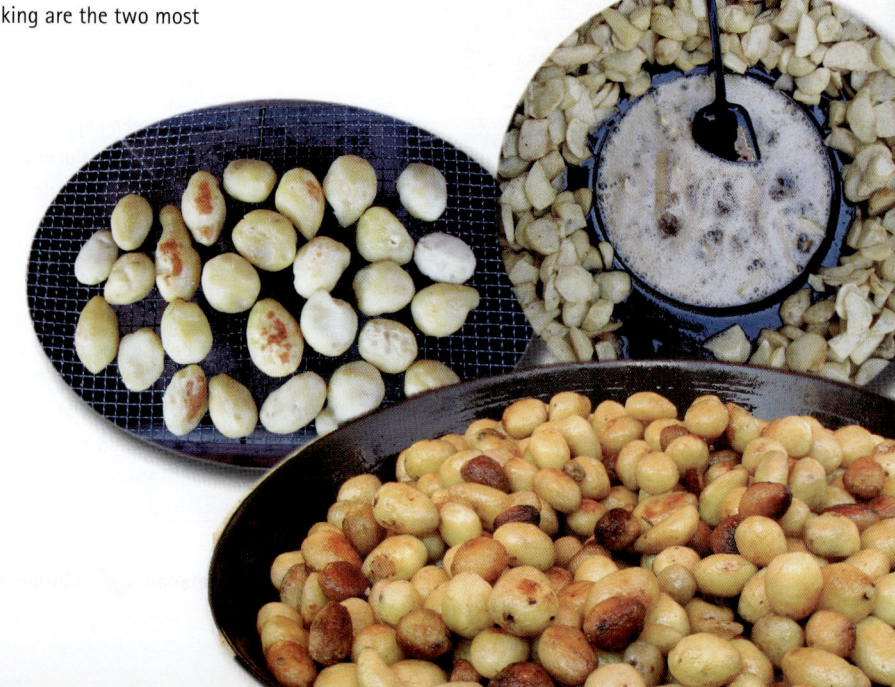

Sweet and sour potato sandwiches
Tangcu Tudou Jia

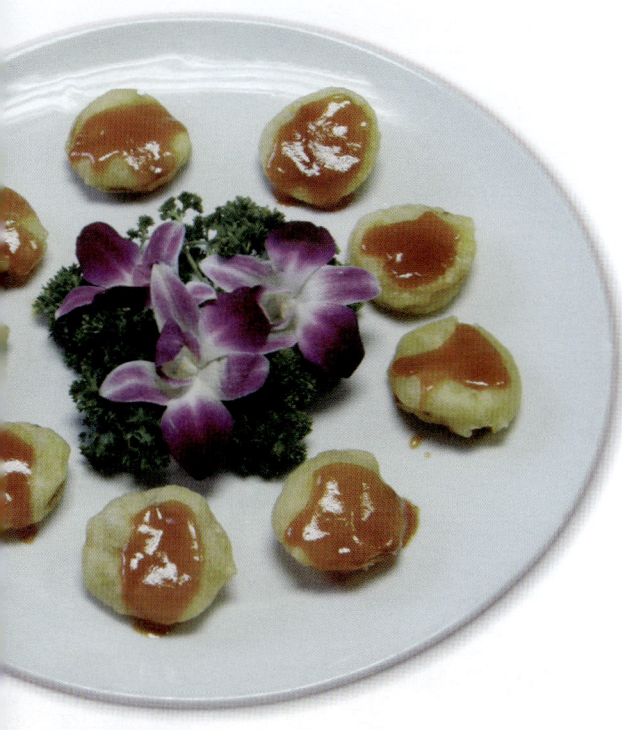

Seasonings:
Salad oil 150 g, vinegar 5 g, white sugar 20 g, salt 2 g, gourmet powder 1 g

Time:
10 minutes.

Preparation:
1. Peel the potatoes and cut them into round pieces with two lips. Put the seasoned minced beef between the lips.

2. Pour the potato starch into a bowl and mix into a paste with the egg, salt, gourmet powder. Then coat the potato sandwiches with the paste and fry them until golden brown.

3. Heat salad oil and add white sugar, tomato sauce, vinegar and starchy sauce and spread the mixture onto the potato sandwiches.

Ingredients:
Potato 200 g, minced beef 20 g, 1 egg, tomatoes sauce 30 g, starchy sauce 70 g

Vegetarian: ✗   Muslim: ✓

Toothpick potato diamonds
Yaqian Tudoukuai

Ingredient:
Potato 250 g

Seasonings:
Salad oil 70 g, spiced pepper powder 20 g

Time:
25 minutes

Preparation:
1. Peel the potatoes and dice into diamond-shaped pieces.
2. Cook the potato pieces in boiling water with a little salt. Remove after boiling and drain.
3. Heat oil in a pan and fry the potato pieces until golden brown. Skewer the potato pieces with toothpicks and sprinkle with spiced pepper powder.

Vegetarian: ✓   Muslim: ✓

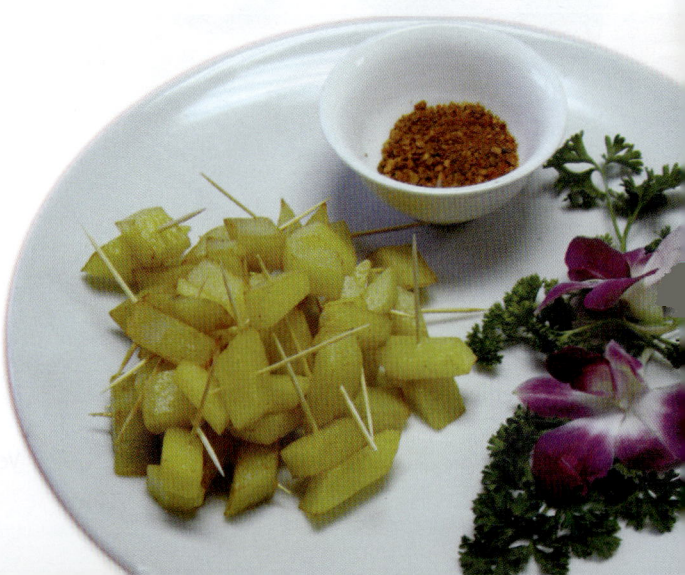

Tree tomato-flavored potatoes
Shu Fanqie Fenwei Tudou Si

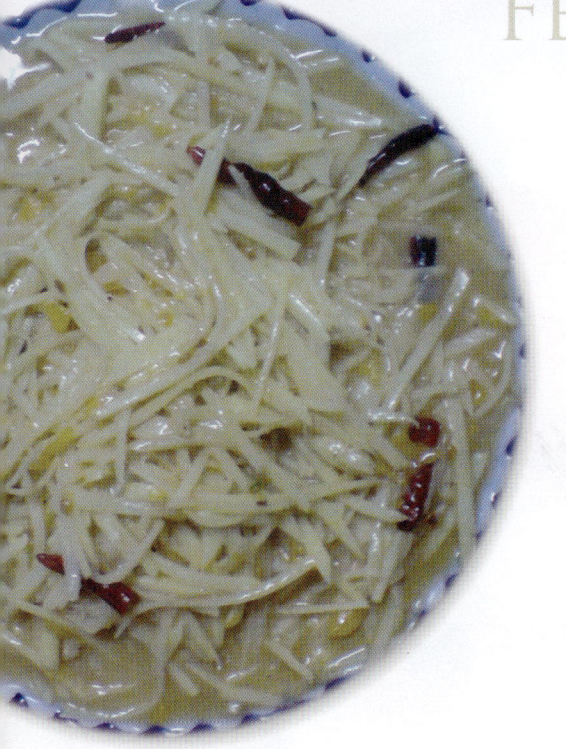

Ingredients:
Potato 300 g, baked hot pepper 20 g

Seasoning:
Cooking oil 30 g, refined salt 5 g, gourmet powder 1 g, tree tomato 50 g

Preparation:
1. Shred the peeled potatoes, cut the hot pepper into sections and the mince tree tomato.
2. Heat oil in a pot and fry the tree tomato and minced hot pepper until it gives off aroma. Add the shredded potato and stir-fry for a while. Then add water and cook well. Add salt and gourmet powder and mix evenly.

Vegetarian: ✓   Muslim: ✓

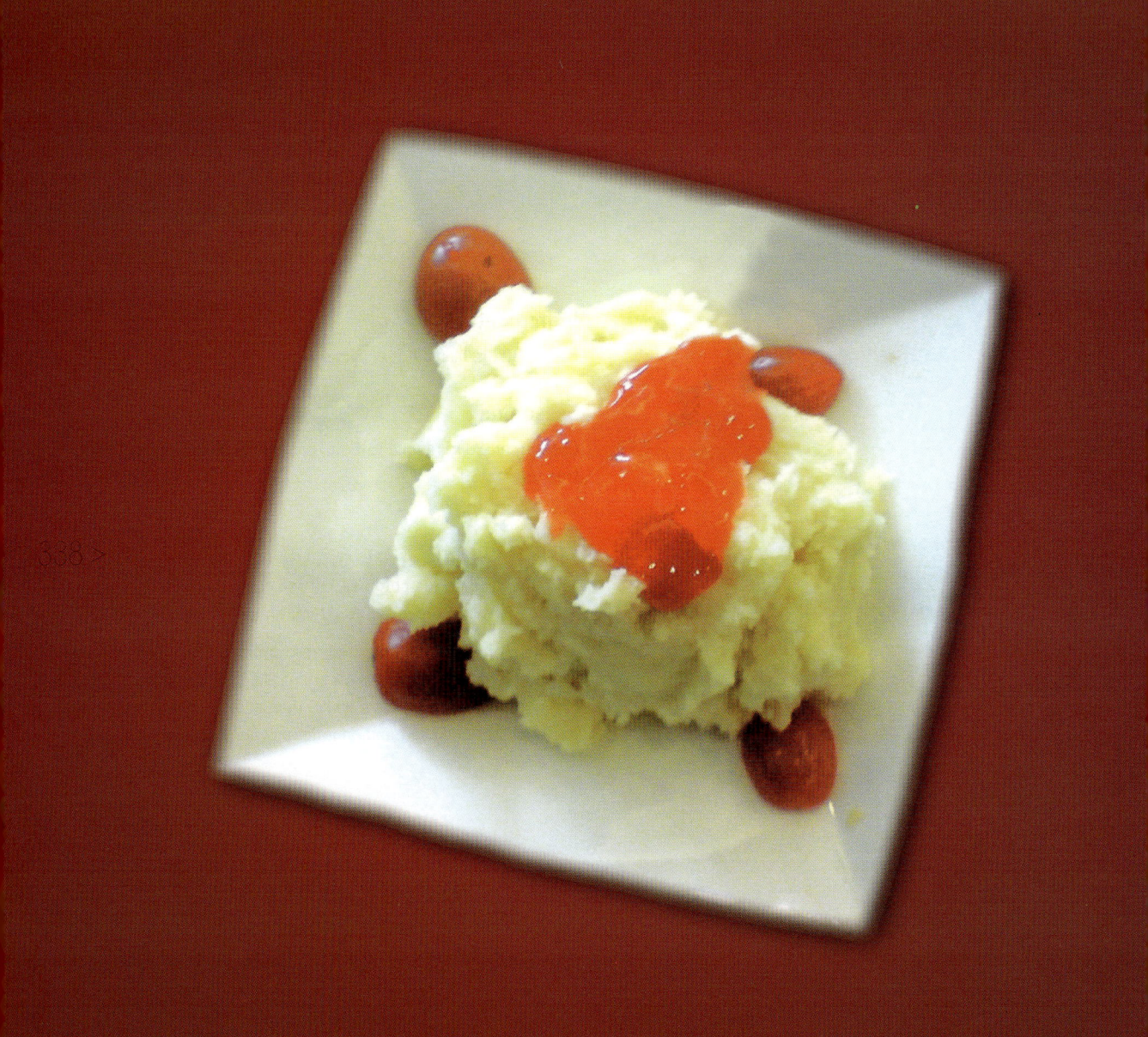

Western-style Mashed Potatoes
Xi Shi Tudou Ni

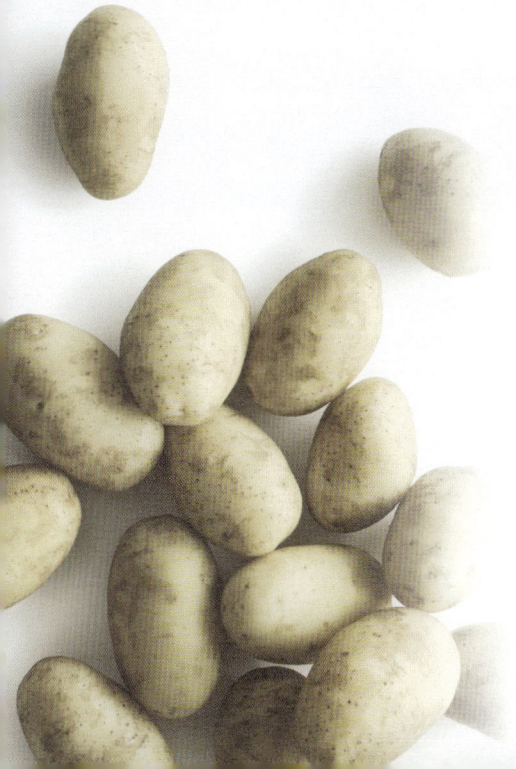

Ingredients:
Potato 150 g, 2 fruit tomatoes

Seasoning:
Ketchup to taste

Preparation:
1. Steam potatoes, then peel and mash them. Cut fruit tomatoes into halves.
2. Remove the mashed potatoes to a dish, with the tomato halves. Spread ketchup on the mashed potatoes and serve.

Vegetarian: ✓   Muslim: ✓

Western-style potato dishes and those from OTHER REGIONS

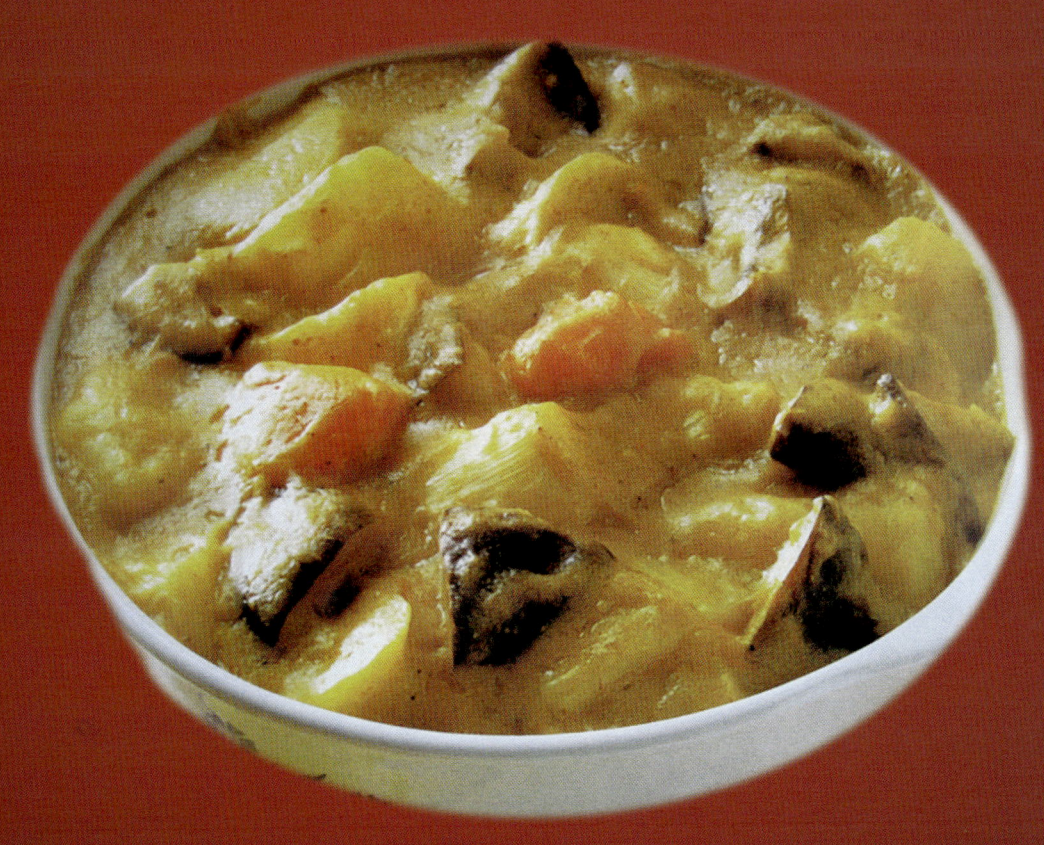

Curry potatoes
Gali Malingshu

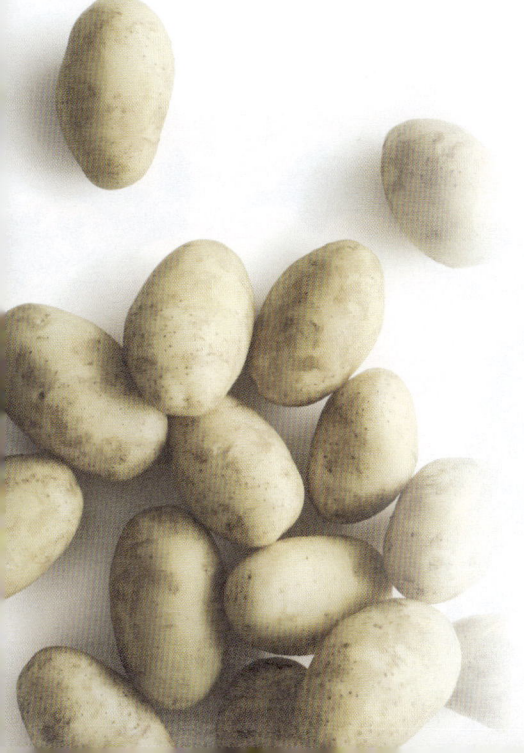

Ingredients:
Potato 400 g, small carrot 100 g, onion 75 g, shiitake mushroom 50 g

Seasonings:
Vegetable oil 75 g, curry 10 g, salt 5 g, sugar 5 g, milk 125 g, a little wheat flour

Preparation:
1. Peel the potatoes and carrots and cut them into irregular pieces. Dice the onions and shiitake mushroom.

2. Heat 45 g of vegetable oil in a wok and fry the diced onion. Then add garlic powder and fry until it gives off aroma. Add the potatoes, carrots and shiitake mushroom, salt, sugar and water, then boil. Change to low heat, stew well, then remove.

3. Heat oil and fry the wheat flour, then slowly add milk, salt and a little water. Fry until thick, then put in the boiled ingredients and fry together. When the cooking liquid thickens, remove to a baking dish.

4. Bake in the oven for 10 minutes at 250°C until brown.

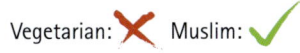

Deep-fried potato balls
Cuizha Tudou Qiu

Ingredients:
Potato 500 g, starch, yeast powder

Seasonings:
A little salt, gourmet powder and sugar

Preparation:
Mash potatoes, then add some table salt and gourmet powder. Form the mashed potatoes into small round balls, coat them with starch and deep-fry.

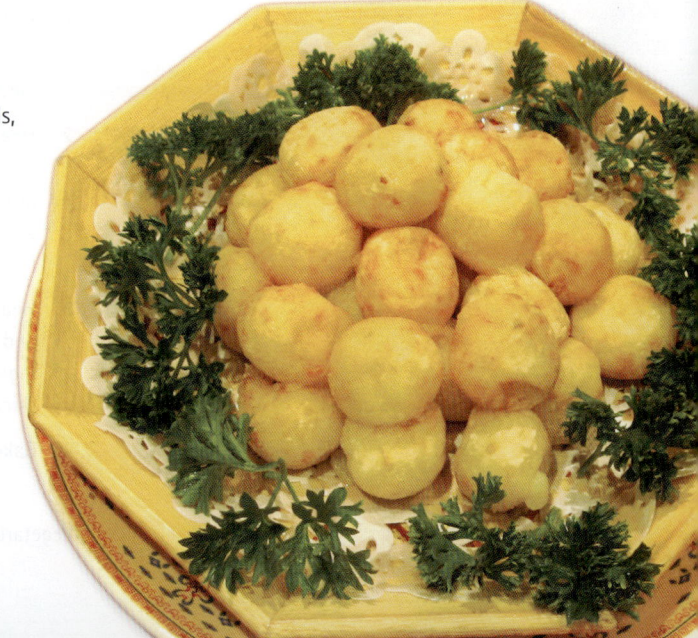

Vegetarian: ✓ Muslim: ✓

French-style Mushroom and Potato Salad
Fashi Xianggu Malingshu Shalazi

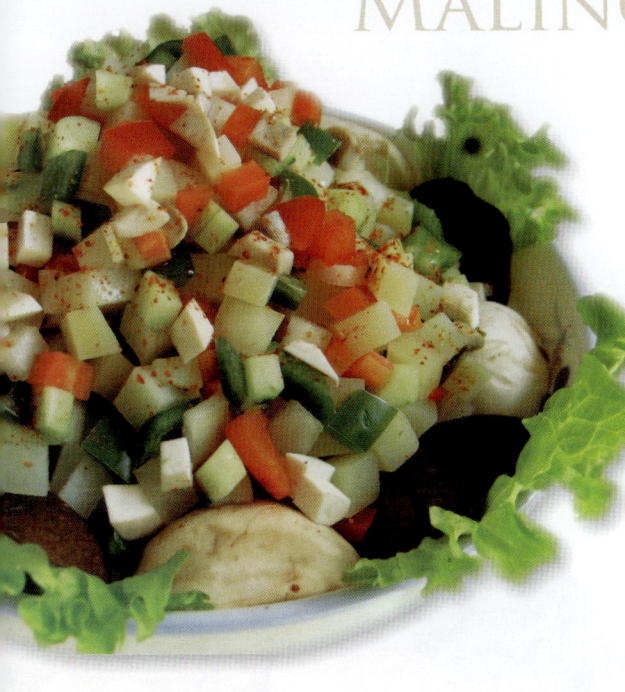

Ingredients:
Potato 750 g, fresh mushrooms 500 g, cucumber 150 g, carrot 150 g, onion 100 g, green pepper 50 g, red pepper 50 g, a little greengrocery

Seasonings:
Vegetable oil 50 g, mustard 2.5 g, salt 15 g, a little vinegar, chili pepper, hot pepper powder, fresh mushroom soup

Preparation:
1. Steam potatoes and carrots well, then peel and dice. Dice onion and one third of the mushrooms. Peel and dice the cucumber. Remove seeds from the pepper and dice.

2. Put all the diced ingredients in a bowl, add vegetable oil, mustard, salt, vinegar, chili pepper, hot pepper powder and fresh mushroom soup and mix well Pile everything in a bowl and use fresh mushrooms and greengrocery to surround the pile, then serve.

Vegetarian: ✓   Muslim: ✓

Fried country-style potato balls
Shancun Zha Malingshu Wanzi

Ingredients:
Potato 1,000 g, lettuce 50 g

Seasonings:
Salt 2 g, white sugar 2 g, wheat flour 3 g, vegetable oil 800 g, a little chili pepper, black sesame seeds

Preparation:
1. Peel potatoes and steam well, then mash them. Mix with salt, white sugar and wheat flour. Knead the potato dough into rolls.
2. Heat vegetable oil over medium heat and deep-fry the kneaded potato rolls until golden yellow. Remove and drain off excess oil.
3. Keep a little oil in the wok and stir-fry the fried potato rolls with chili pepper and black sesame seeds. Place on lettuce leaves on a plate and serve.

Vegetarian: ✓   Muslim: ✓

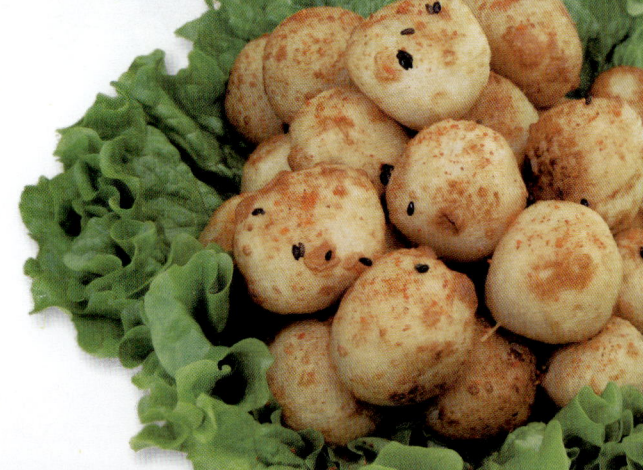

Fried diced potatoes and lettuce stems
Chao Malingshu Wosunding

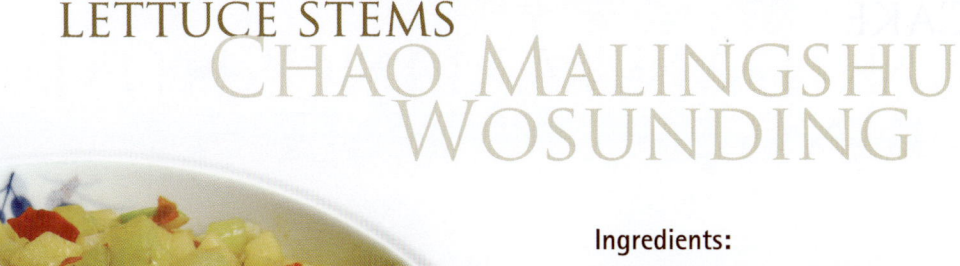

Ingredients:
Potato 500 g, lettuce stems 250 g

Seasonings:
Water starch, ginger, garlic, soy sauce to taste

Preparation:
1. Dice peeled potatoes and lettuce, then set aside.
2. Heat oil in a wok and stir-fry the diced potatoes well.
3. Heat a little oil in the wok and fry the ginger and garlic until it give off aroma, then stir-fry the diced potatoes and lettuce in the wok. Add salt or soy sauce and use water starch to thicken the cooking liquid, then serve.

Vegetarian: ✓   Muslim: ✓

Fried egg and potato string cake
Jianjidan Malingshusi Bing

Ingredients:
Potato 750 g, 3 eggs, wheat flour 25 g

Seasonings:
Vegetable oil 100 g, refined salt 5 g, a little chili pepper

Preparation:
1. Peel and shred potatoes, then wash in water, drain and put in a bowl.

2. Add whisked eggs to the potato strings, together with salt, chili pepper and wheat flour. Mix well, then spread onto a small baking tray. Bake well, remove and cut into diamonds.

3. Heat oil in a frying pan and fry the baked potato string cakes until both sides are golden yellow. Remove and drain oil, then serve.

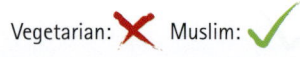

Vegetarian: ✗   Muslim: ✓

Fried potato cake IV
Cui Zha Tudou Bing

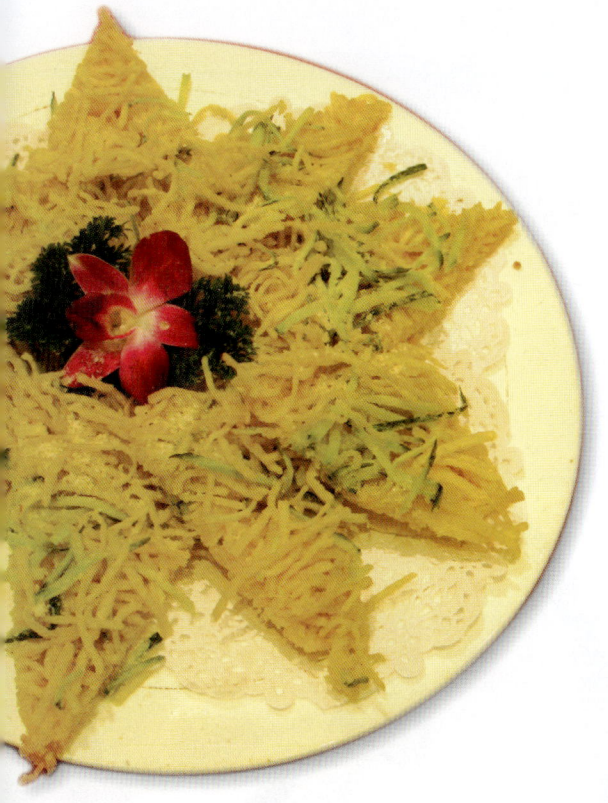

Ingredients:
Potato 500 g, cucumber 500 g, starch, glutinous rice flour

Seasonings:
Oil 250 g, salt to taste

Preparation:
Shred potatoes and cucumbers. Mix with starch and glutinous rice flour then fry in hot oil and serve.

Vegetarian: ✓ Muslim: ✓

Fried potato slices II
Zha Malingshu Pian

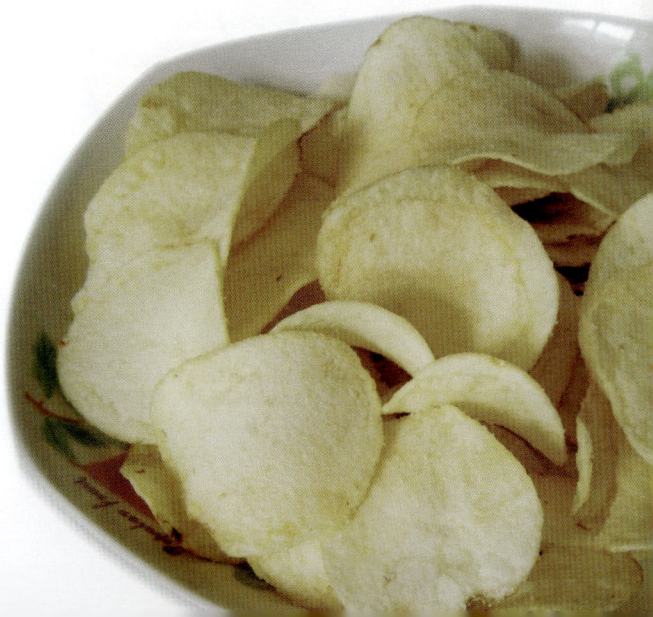

Ingredient:
Potato 500 g

Seasonings:
Vegetable oil 2,000 g (250 g consumed), a little salt

Preparation:
1. Peel potatoes and cut them into about 1.5 mm-thick pieces. Rinse to remove excess starch, then drain.
2. Deep-fry the potato slices in a wok (oil temperature 170°C–180°C) until the potato slices are crisp. Remove, drain oil and sprinkle with salt. Cool the slices, then serve.

Vegetarian: ✓   Muslim: ✓

Fried potato strips
Zha Malingshu Tiao

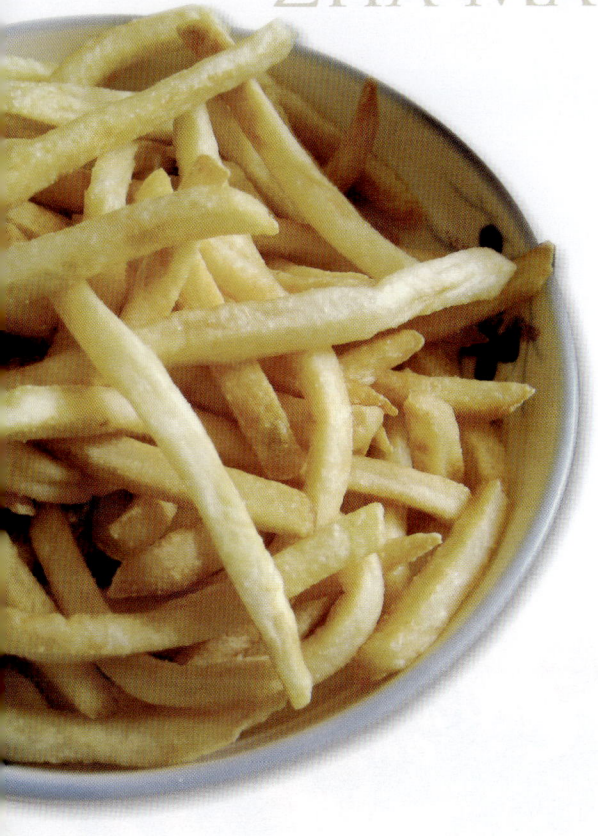

Ingredient:
Potato 500 g

Seasonings:
Vegetable oil 1,500 g (100 g consumed), a little salt, chili pepper

Preparation:
1. Peel the potatoes and cut into strips. Soak in cool water for half an hour, then remove and drain.
2. Deep-fry the potato strips in a wok (oil temperature 170°C–180°C) until golden yellow. Then remove, drain excess oil, sprinkle with salt and chili pepper, then serve.

Vegetarian: ✓   Muslim: ✓

Fried potato strips with spicy peanuts
Xiang Su Shutiao

Ingredients:
Potato 500 g, green and red chili 50 g each, flour 50 g

Seasonings:
Oil 250 g, salt to taste, crispy fried peanuts and chili

Preparation:
Shred potatoes and cover each piece with flour pastry. Fry in hot oil, then stir-fry with green and red chili, crispy fried peanuts, and chili.

Vegetarian: ✓   Muslim: ✓

Fried potato with jellyfish
Tudou Bao Zhetou

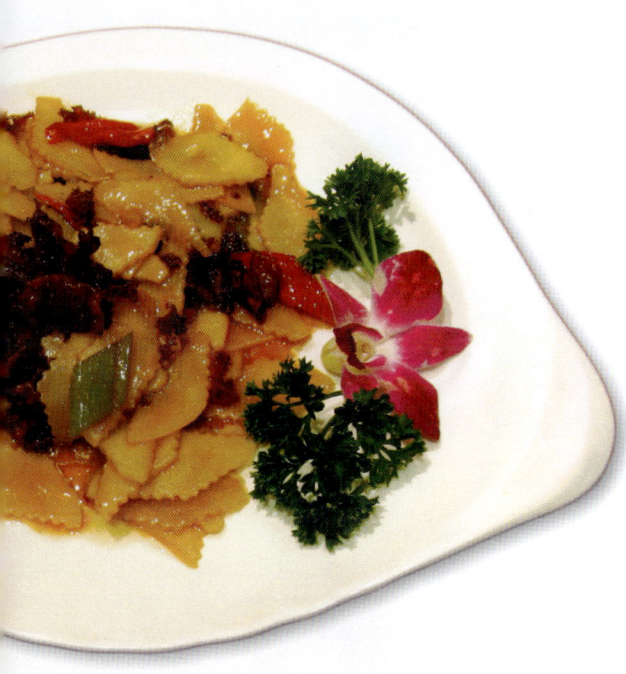

Ingredients:
Potato 300 g, jellyfish 100 g, green and red chili 50g each

Seasonings:
A little oil, vinegar, sugar, salt and gourmet powder

Preparation:
Slice potatoes, then fry with jellyfish and green and red chilis. Add vinegar, sugar, salt and gourmet powder and stew together.

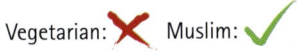

Honey potatoes
Mizhi Malingshu

Ingredient:
Potato 1,000 g

Seasonings:
Honey 75 g, white sugar 80 g

Preparation:
1. Clean potatoes and steam well. Cool the potatoes, then peel and slice.
2. Fry the potato slices in a frying pan.
3. Heat 30 g of white sugar in a small pan and add water. Then add remaining sugar and honey and mix well. Add the sugar mixture into the frying pan with the potatoes.
4. Heat the potatoes and sugar mixture over low heat, then serve.

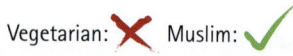
Vegetarian: ✗ Muslim: ✓

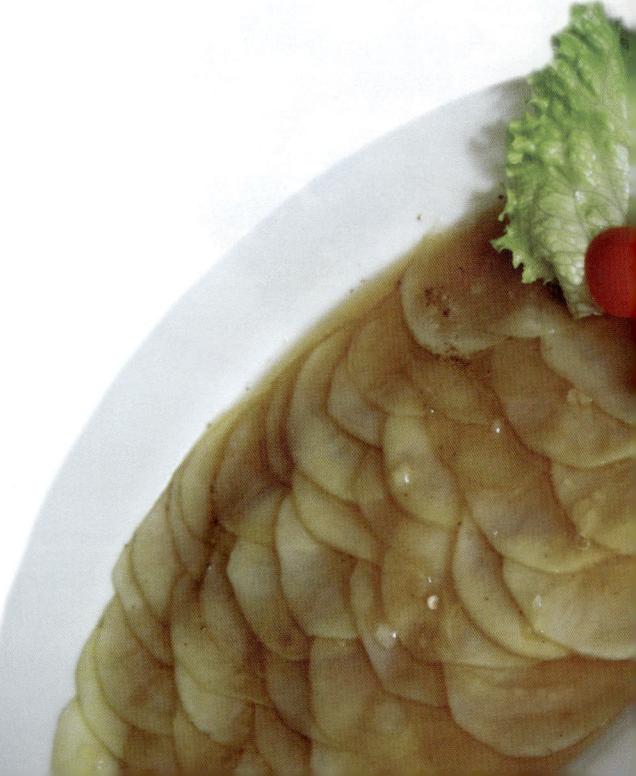

Pagoda-shaped Mashed Potatoes with Shiitake Mushroom
Xianggu Malingshu Ni Ta

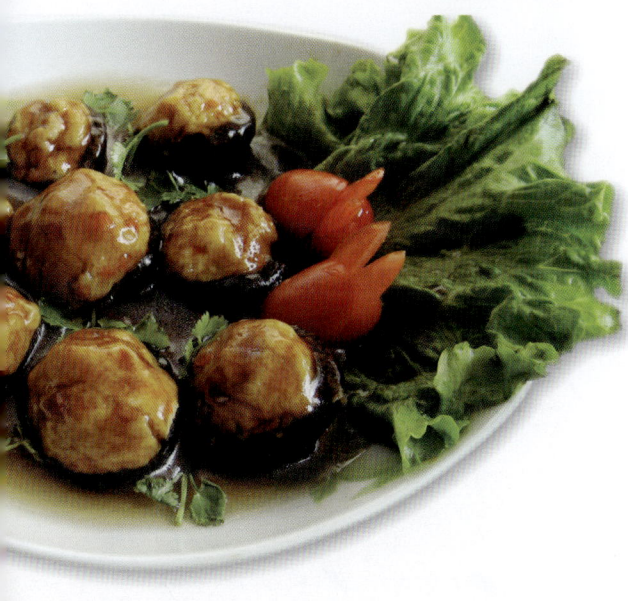

Seasonings:
Salt 5 g, sugar 50 g, soy sauce, a little chili pepper, water starch

Preparation:

1. Peel potatoes and steam well. Mash the potatoes and mix with minced carrots, salt and chili pepper.

2. Soak the shiitake mushroom in water to soften it. Remove the stem and place the cap in a bowl, then add soy sauce, sugar and 1 cup of water. Steam for 10 minutes, then remove the mushroom and cool. Set the excess sauce aside.

3. Sprinkle the mushroom with a little starch, then put the flavored potato paste in the mushroom, forming a pagoda-shape. Steam for 5 minutes.

4. Boil the excess sauce with sugar and water starch, then pour the thickened sauce on the mushroom-potato pagoda and sprinkle with minced cilantro.

Ingredients:
Potato 750 g, shiitake mushroom 250 g, small carrot 50 g, 1 cilantro

Vegetarian: ✓   Muslim: ✓

Potato and egg soup
Tudou Danhua Tang

Ingredients:
Potato 500 g, 1 egg, starch 5 g

Seasonings:
Salt, gourmet powder, sugar to taste

Preparation:
1. Shred and blanch potatoes.
2. Boil water and add starch. Stir eggs in a bowl and slowly add to the boiling water. Then add potatoes, salt, gourmet powder and sugar.

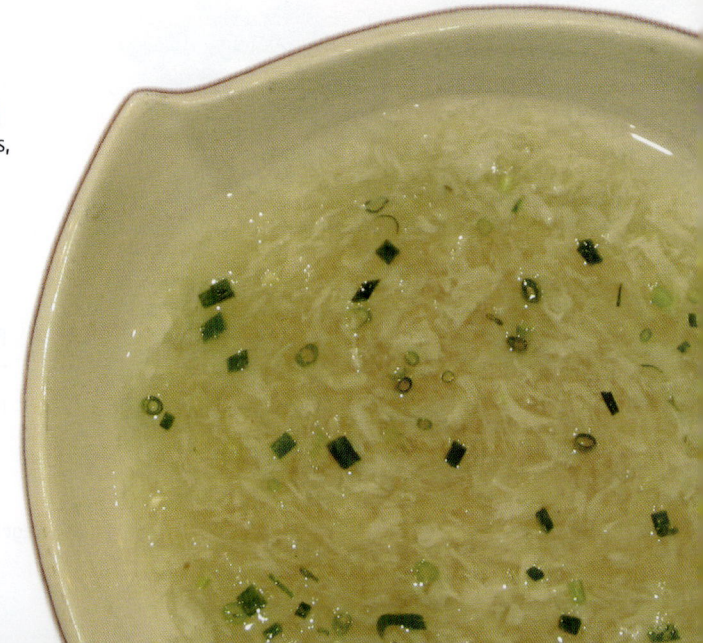

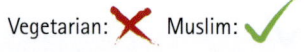

Potato and vegetable salad
Qingcai Malingshu Shalazi

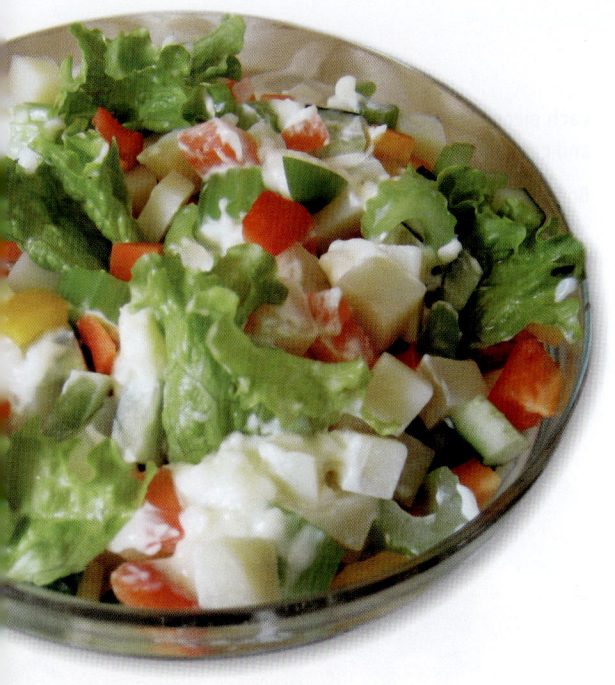

Ingredients:
Potato 400 g, celery 150 g, cucumber 150 g, carrot 100 g, green bell pepper 100 g

Seasonings:
Béarnaise sauce 125 g, vinegar 10 g, chili pepper to taste, salt to taste

Preparation:
1. Peel and boil potatoes.
2. Dice the cooked potatoes, celery, cucumber, carrot and green bell pepper. Mix well with Béarnaise sauce, then serve.

Vegetarian: ✘   Muslim: ✘

Potato balls with ham
Huotui Malingshu Wanz

Ingredients:
Potato 750 g, wheat flour 75 g, 2 eggs, ham 50 g, green pepper 50 g, red pepper 50 g, onion 50 g

Seasonings:
Vegetable oil 25 g, refined salt 5 g

Time:
25 minutes

Preparation:
1. Peel and boil potatoes, then mash into potato paste. Remove to a bowl, add 50 g of flour and 2 eggs, and mix well with salt to make potato dough. Set aside. Remove seeds from the peppers and dice together with the ham.
2. Sprinkle the remaining flour on a rolling board and roll the dough into a big strip. Dice the strip and use each piece to wrap some ham. Knead into small balls and coat evenly with flour.
3. Boil the potato balls, then remove to a dish.
4. Dice onion and fry until golden yellow. Serve potato balls with diced peppers, fried onion and a little salt.

Vegetarian: ✗   Muslim: ✗

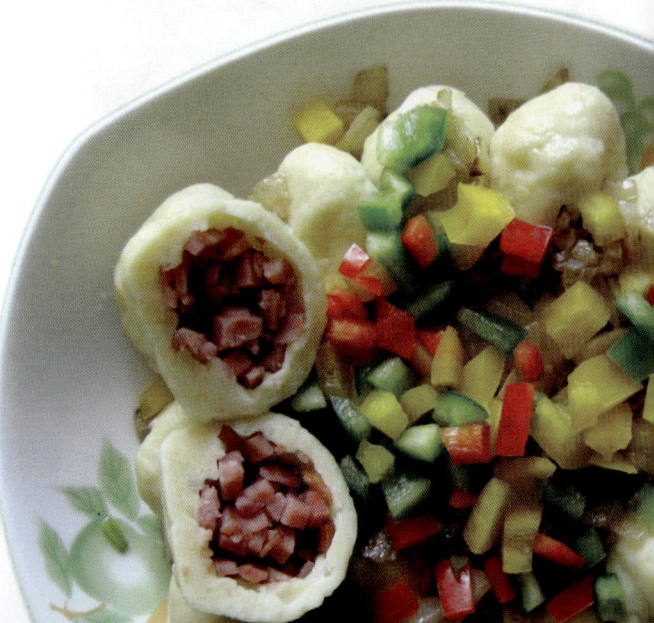

Potato dumplings
Shu Jiao

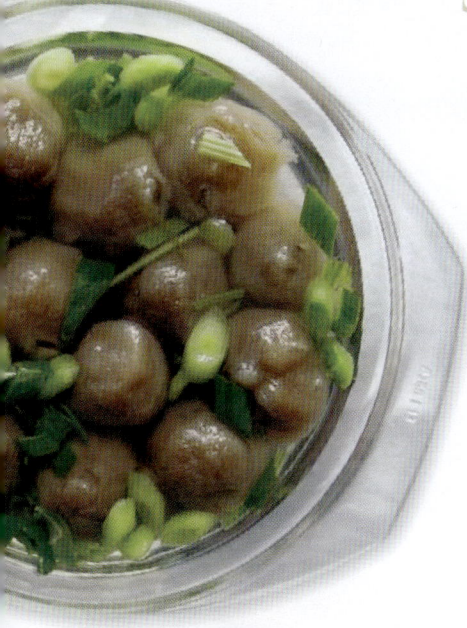

Time:
25 minutes

Preparation:

1. Dumpling wrapper preparation: Peel and dice potatoes into small cubes of about 50 g each. Steam (or stew) the potatoes, then mash, add starch and knead into dough.

2. Filling preparation: Dice pork, mince shiitake mushroom, seaweed and coriander, and mix well with seasonings (gourmet powder, salt and soy sauce).

3. Dumpling making: Divide the dough into small, meatball-sized portions. Roll each ball with a rolling pin to form a dumpling wrapper. Stuff each wrapper with filling and rub into a ball by hand, pinching the edges to seal.

4. Steam (boil) potato dumplings: Steam or boil the potato dumplings, then serve with soup seasoning or freeze for storage.

Ingredients:

Potato 500 g, starch (potato, sweet potato) 250 g, three layer pork 200 g, celery cabbage 200 g, shiitake mushroom 50 g, seaweed 50 g, gourmet powder 50 g, salt 10 g, soy sauce 10 g, coriander 10 g

Seasonings:

Cooking oil 10 g, salt 10 g, garlic sprouts 50 g, coriander 50 g, a little vinegar

Vegetarian: ✗   Muslim: ✗

Potato rolls wrapped in dried tofu
Fupi Malingshu Juan

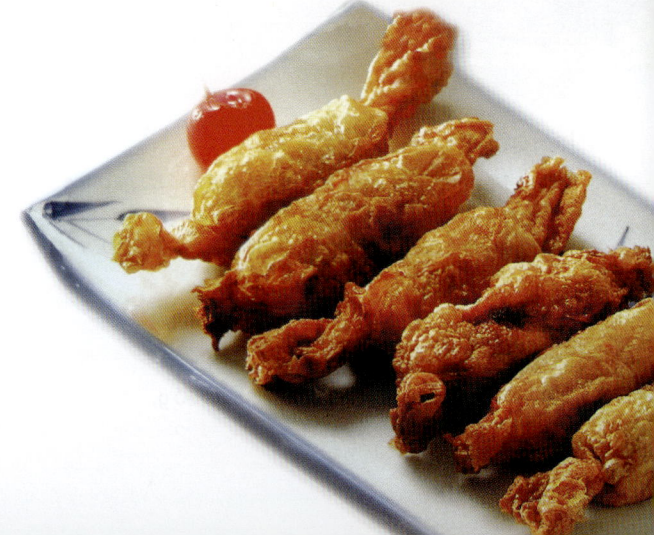

Ingredients:
Potato 375 g, 4 sheets of tofu

Seasonings:
Vegetable oil 500 g, salt 5 g, chili pepper, tomato sauce

Preparation:
1. Peel potatoes and steam well, then mash them. Mix with vegetable oil, salt and chili pepper.

2. Divide the dried tofu crust into small pieces and use them to wrap some of the potato paste. Form into a roll, then tie the two sides of the roll, like candy, sealing the opening with a little paste.

3. Heat oil over high heat and deep-fry the potato rolls until golden yellow. Remove to a dish and serve with tomato sauce.

Vegetarian: ✓ Muslim: ✓

Potato sandwich with pork
You Su Tudou He

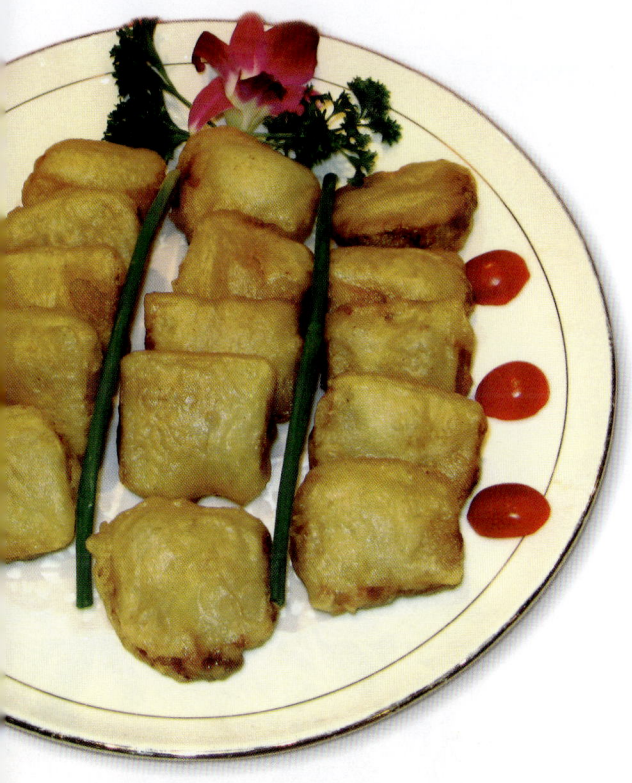

Ingredients:
Potato 750 g, pork 250 g, a little flour

Seasonings:
A little oil, black soy sauce and gourmet powder

Preparation:
1. Finely sliced the potatoes. Mince the pork and season with soy sauce, gourmet powder and a little bit of oil.
2. Stuff two potato slices with some of the pork mixture and coat with a layer of starch pastry, then deep-fry.

Vegetarian: ✗   Muslim: ✗

Potato strings with sea cucumber
Tudou Si Ban Haishen

Ingredients:
Potato 500 g, sea cucumber 125 g

Seasonings:
A little salt, vinegar, sugar, peanut oil and chive oil

Preparation:
Shred potatoes and sea cucumber. Season both with vinegar, a little bit sugar, peanut oil and chive oil, then serve.

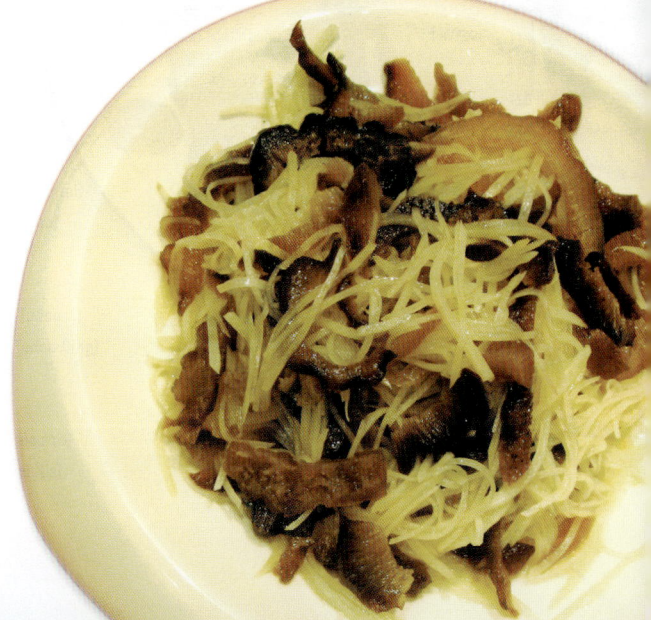

Vegetarian: ✗ Muslim: ✓

Potatoes in Hot Caramel
Basi Tudou

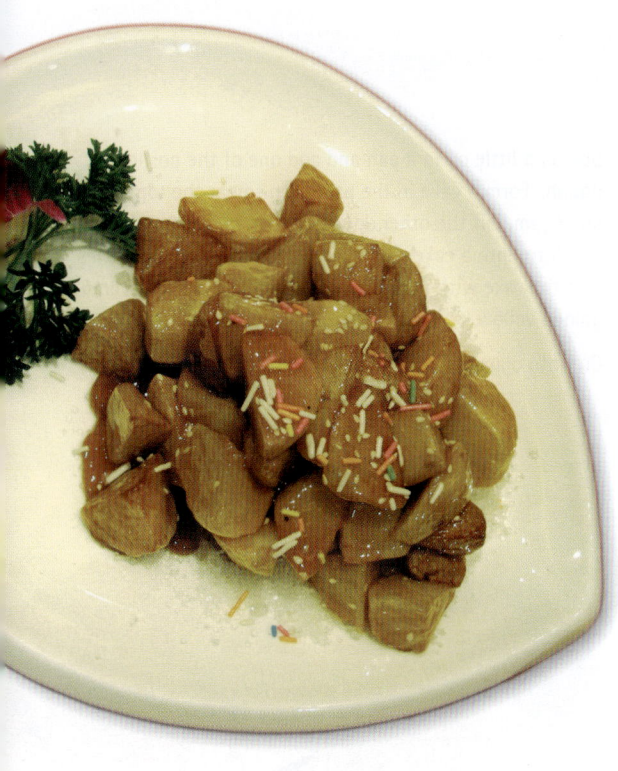

Ingredient:
Potato 500 g

Seasonings:
Oil 500 g, sugar 100 g, sesame seeds to taste

Preparation:
1. Peel potatoes and dice into irregular pieces.
2. Heat oil over medium heat and fry potato pieces, reducing to low heat. Remove from pan when potato pieces turn brown and start to float in the oil.
3. Remove excess oil from the pan and add some water. Add sugar and braise until it turns into syrup.
4. Add fried potato pieces into the syrup, mix evenly, then remove. Garnish with sesame seeds and serve with cold water.

Vegetarian: ✓   Muslim: ✓

Roasted potatoes with jam
Guojiang Malingshu Pai

Ingredients:
Potato 1,000 g, apple jam 250 g, wheat flour 75 g, 2 eggs

Seasonings:
Butter 25 g, a little vegetable oil, salt to taste

Preparation:
1. Peel and boil potatoes, then mash them and remove to a bowl.
2. Put whisked eggs, milk, wheat flour and salt in the bowl with the potato paste and mix well. Knead the mixture into potato dough, then divide it into two portions on a rolling board and set aside.
3. Spread a little oil in a pan and add one of the portions of dough. .Form a cake in the pan, then smear the top with apple jam. Put the other dough portion on the jam layer, and form into a cake. Then coat with egg yolk, carve lines into the cake with a fork, and bake in a preheated oven until golden yellow.
4. Cut into diamonds before serving.

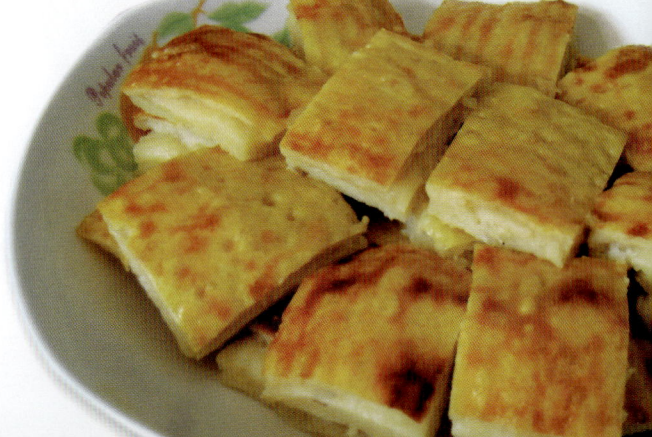

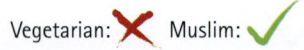

Steamed Potato Strings with Mashed Garlic
Suan Ni Tudou Si

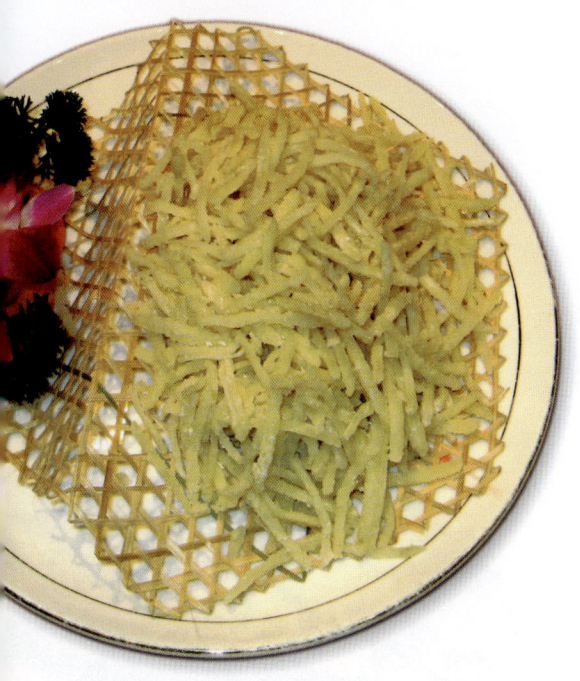

Ingredients:
Shredded potato 500 g, mashed garlic, wheat flour to taste

Seasonings:
Salt, gourmet powder, vinegar, sugar to taste

Preparation:
1. Blanch the shredded potatoes, then mix with flour and steam.
2. Season with mashed garlic, salt, gourmet powder, vinegar and sugar, then serve.

Vegetarian: ✓   Muslim: ✓

Stewed beef with potato
Tudou Shao Niunan

Ingredients:
Potato 500 g, beef sirloin 250 g

Seasonings:
Salt, gourmet powder, hoisin sauce and rice wine to taste

Preparation:
Dice and then fry the potatoes. Season the fried potatoes with hoisin sauce, then stew with rice wine seasoned beef.

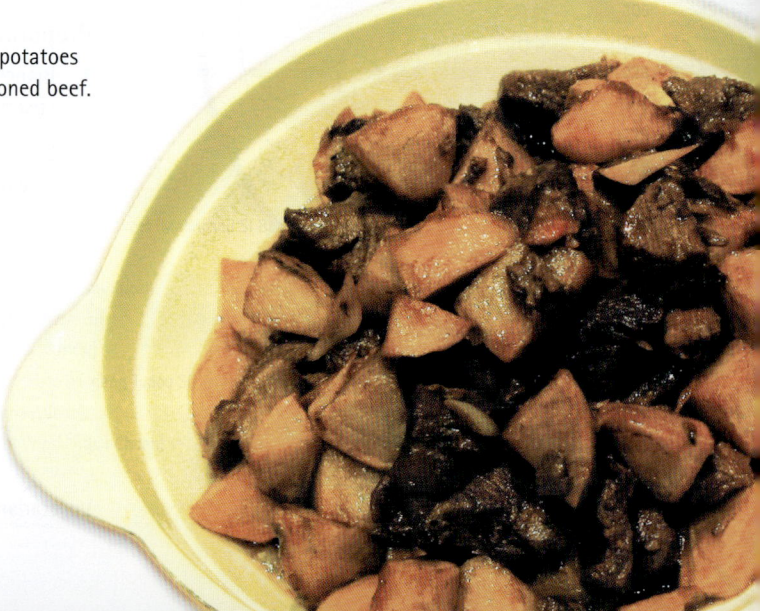

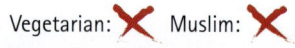

Stir-fried potato strips with celery
Shan Qin Chao Tudou

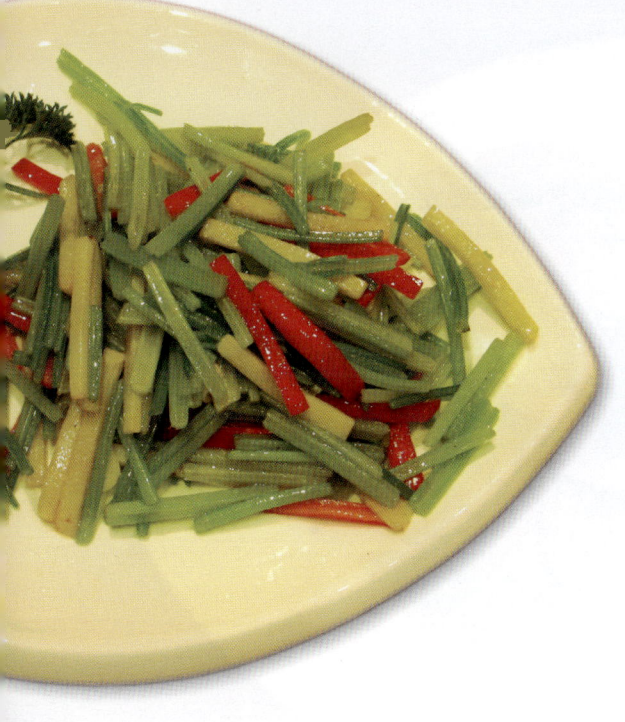

Ingredients:
Shredded potato 500 g, green chili, red chili and celery to taste

Seasonings:
Salt and gourmet powder to taste, oil 50 g

Preparation:
Blanch the shredded potatoes then fry with green and red chili, celery, salt and a little gourmet powder.

Vegetarian: ✓   Muslim: ✓

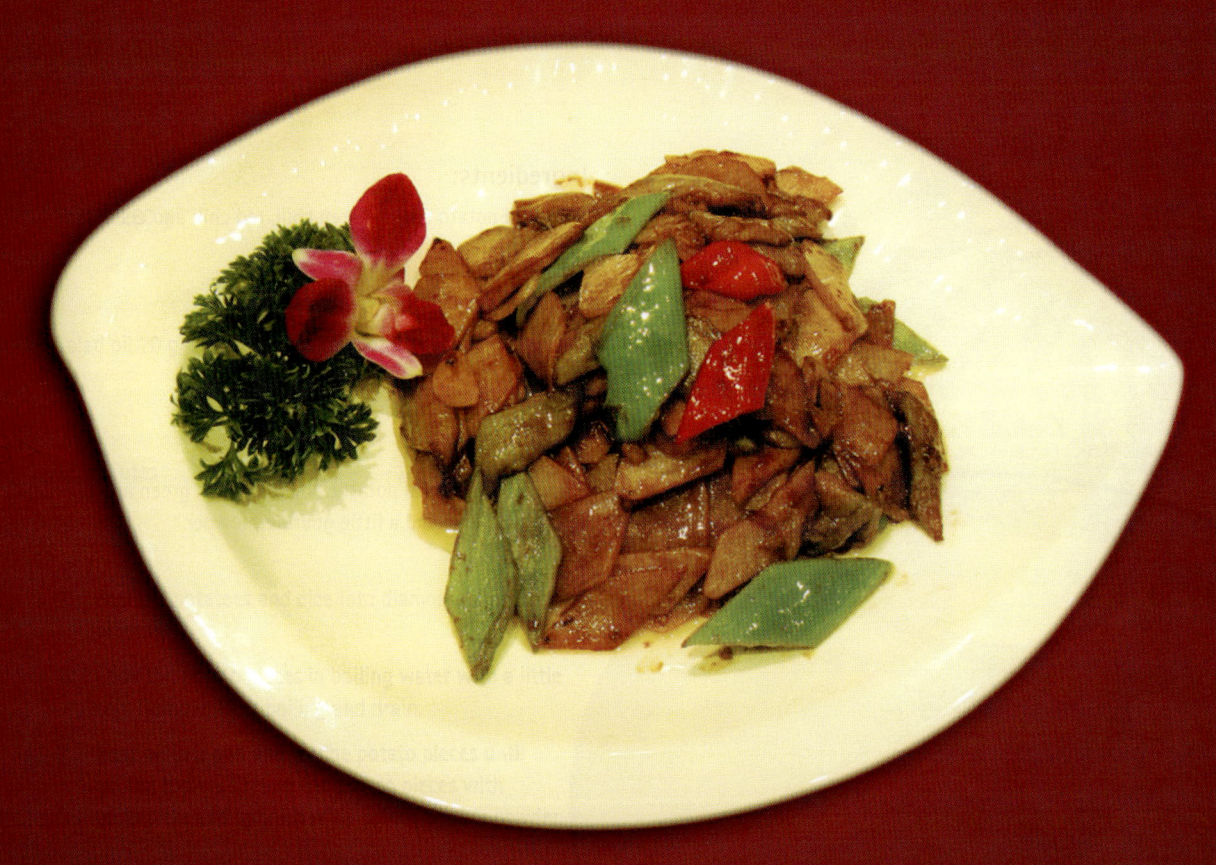

Three Earthly Delights
Jiao Dong Di Sanxian

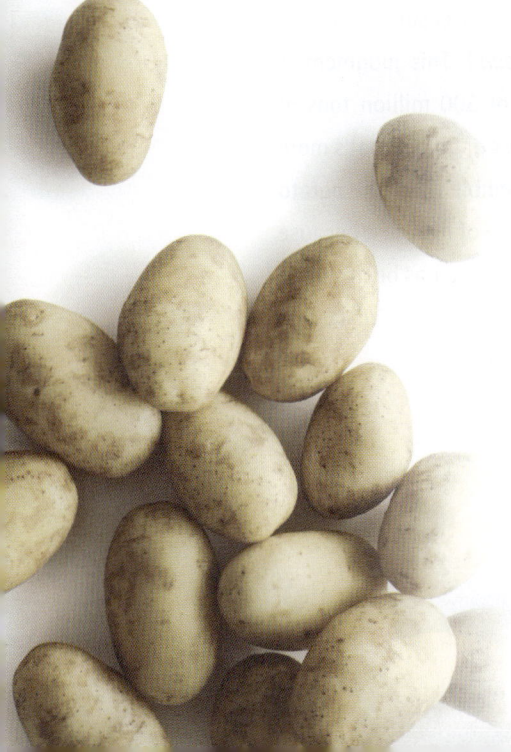

Ingredients:
Potato 250 g, eggplant 125 g, green and red chili

Seasonings:
Sweet sauce, gourmet powder, Weidamei sauce (specific brand of sauce)

Preparation:
Slice potatoes and fry together with eggplant, green and red chili, a little bit of sweet sauce and gourmet powder.

Vegetarian: ✗   Muslim: ✓

The Development and Role of the Potato in China

Although there are various views on the origin of the potato, most people agree that Titicaca Lake, sitting on the border of Peru and Bolivia in South America, is the original home of the potato. In the 16th century, the conquistadores came in search of gold, but the real treasure they took back to Europe was the potato (*Solanum tuberosum*). This judgment is based on the fact that today global annual yield of 300 million tons of potatoes is equal to the value of almost of 1,166 tons of gold. What's more interesting is that before it had been spread as an edible food, the potato had caused near a century of conflict and the sacrifice of lives just because it was not recorded as a food in the Holy Bible. The potato has been spread globally through different routes via Europe and is now the third-largest agricultural crop in the world, only after rice and wheat.

Introduction of the potato to China

It is hard to determine exactly when the potato was introduced to China. However, according to *A summary of the potato history* compiled by Tong Ya-Ping and Zhao Guoqin, it was in the middle of the Ming Dynasty, i.e. 1550. But the actual may be several decades later than that because it is generally agreed that the potato was introduced to China by the Dutch through two routes after it was first introduced Europe by the Spanish in 1565. There is little possibility that potato had been introduced to China before its introduction to Europe.

Figure 3 shows the routes for the spread of the potato based on early European nautical maps. We can see that it is during 1567 to 1593 that the potato was brought to Europe, and then from there to the rest of the world around 1600.

Taking into account the varied evidence and literature, we can conclude that the potato was brought to China about 400 years ago, i.e. after 1600. Furthermore, concerning the routes by which the potato spread, it is most likely that the potato was brought to Taiwan through Southeast Asia from the Netherlands, and then to the coastal regions of Canton and Fujian. This is supported by the fact that between 1622 and 1662, Taiwan was governed by the Netherlands.

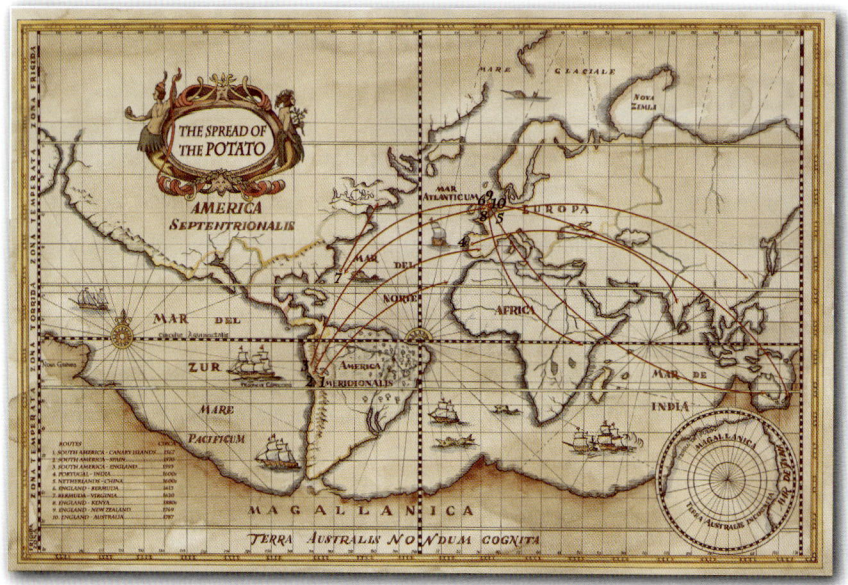

Figure 3: Routes of the spread for the potato around the world (Source: CIP)

An alternative theory suggests that the potato was brought to China by politicians, merchants, and preachers as a royal tribute when they presented themselves before the emperors. An argument against this theory is that is unlikely that any article meant for royal use would be spread out to the larger population. Additionally, the amount of potatoes that might have been introduced in this manner would have been very small, limiting the opportunity for their further spread.

Development of the potato industry in China after the 20th century

In the early 1920s, attempts were made to revitalize farming by persuading farmers to plant potatoes and sweet potatoes. New varieties were introduced, along with new technologies and high-yielding production methods. This greatly increased the planting area of potatoes in China. Foreign preachers and teachers also took the potato to every part of the country, thus speeding up its spread.

On the other hand, the central experimental field of the Department of Agriculture and Commerce of the National Government of the Republic of China carried out potato experiments as early as 1914. They used 25 kg of American white potatoes as seed potatoes for a mu (Chinese measure of area) of land by cutting seeds, and harvested 1,225 kg per mu. Meanwhile, the yield was only 655 kg per mu when the whole tubers were used as seeds. The reasons for this might be that the seed potatoes used in experimental plots were newly introduced varieties with little degradation, whereas the seed potatoes used in the control were old varieties being planted for many years in the fields. The small amount of seed potatoes used in the experiment might be due to the use of small seed tubers (similar to minitubers currently in use).

Efforts to improve the potato varieties in China started in the 1930s. When he was in charge of this effort, Guan Jia-Ji screened out Katahdin, Chippewa, Warba and Golden varieties from 14 varieties imported from Britain and American, of which the Katahdin variety is still used today as a parent in potato breeding. Guan also wrote a paper entitled On China's Potato Improvement, based on the experimental results in four different regions between 1934 and 1936. In this paper, he introduced the advanced breeding methods adopted in other countries and laid out the national potato improvement procedures, including the survey, the introduction of varieties, regional trials, and breeding. This paper was the guide going forward for the efforts to improve the national potato variety. Besides these efforts, there were many other scientists and potato researchers conducting potato research and extensions in Guizhou, Shaanxi and Sichuan provinces.

In order to address the issue of food shortages and meet the military and civilian demand for food during the war with Japan, the Ministry of Agriculture and Forestry of China launched a plan for the improvement of national potato varieties. It invited an American pathologist, T. P. Dyksira, who was the director of the United States Department of Agriculture, Vegetable Production Department, to be the official consultant to assist Chinese experimental stations in carrying out the plan. There were eight tasks for Dyksira: 1 carry out a survey of national potato production; 2 improve local potato varieties; 3 evaluate and multiply foreign varieties;

4 conduct clonal experiments for hybrid crosses; 5 suggest improvements to the potato storage method; 6 inspect seed potatoes; 7 research a potato grading system; and 8 determine and demonstrate superior potato varieties and advanced planting methods.

One of the examples of these efforts was the Potato Training Course held at the Central Farming Experiment Station located in Chengdu in 1944. The course was presided over by Guan Jia-Ji, and included lectures by T. P. Dyksira on potato breeding, potato seed inspection, disease control, and cultivation technology. A field trip to Pengxian County was also arranged.

Meanwhile, in other regions, Mao Zedong (later the first chairman of new China, from October 1949) called for a large-scale production movement under his famous "do-it-yourself, have ample food and clothing" mobilization slogan among borderland armed force and people in 1940. The goal of this movement was to "plant three years then surplus one year" (meaning for every three years of farming there should be one year's worth of surplus produce) and to increase the availability of food and vegetables.

The potato's long storage life and the fact that it could be easily transported made it an important crop, especially in the face of natural disasters. It is worth mentioning that the then Shan Gan Ning borderland government had attached utmost importance to potato production. In 1944, a written statement had been issued by the borderland Government Chairman Li

Boqu, Vice Chairman Li Dingming, Director of the Construction, Gao Zili, and Vice Directors Huo Zile and Gao Changjiu to introduce the potato's high-yield and edibility, and to describe suitable regions for planting, as well as cultivation and storage techniques. All levels of governments were required to make a detailed plan to mobilize the masses, dispense seeds, and increase potato planting area by 300,000 mu, with a yield of 300 to 500 kg per mu.

In areas occupied by the Japanese farmers were forced to expand the planting area of high-yield crops such as potato and sweet potato for military purposes. In northeast China in the late 1930s, the Japanese increased the potato planting area and introduced a number of new potato varieties, including Irish Cobbler and Yanbian Red.

By 1950, the total potato planting area in China reached 23,385,000 mu (1.559 million ha) with an average yield of 375 kg per mu (5.625 t/ha) and a total yield of 8,772,000 tons. During the first five-year plan period (1953–1957) after the founding of new China in 1949, one of the important measures to enhance agricultural yield was to increase the planting areas of high-yield crops, including potato and sweet potato.

In the 1960s, there were about 30 institutions nationwide working on potato research. In 1963, the National Science and Technology Committee and the Ministry of Agriculture officially promulgated the "Scientific and technical development program for 1963–1972," which included

12 scientific potato research projects. As a result, China's potato planting area exceeded 30 million mu (2 million ha) nationwide by 1966.

In the 1970s, a national potato scientific research and production experience exchange workshop was convened in Shandong Province. This workshop summarized and popularized the successful intercropping practice of potato and cotton in a small township of Shandong Province. The township had an average yield over 500 kg per mu (7.5 t/ha) for grain crops and over 5,000 kg per mu (75 t/ha) for potatoes. In 1978 in Enshi, Hubei Province, a national potato scientific research cooperation conference was convened to carry out potato scientific research cooperation projects initiated by the Ministry of Agriculture. The promotion of true potato seeds (TPS) in 1970s broke the traditional concept that growing potatoes required the planting of seed potatoes. The central government's No. 49 document firmly pointed out "we should actively promote the production of TPS and aggressively popularize to ensure the best result." By 1970, China had a steady potato planting area of 30 million mu (2 million ha) per year.

In the 1980s, the national crop variety validation commission was established and the potato and sweet potato variety authorization group was also set up as its subsidiary. The national potato germplasm catalog had been published in 1983, which included 832 germplasms with detailed information on variety, clonal type, allied species and wild species. In line with the practice of opening up to the outside world as a national policy, potato research scientists began to communicate with their international counterparts. This was reinforced by the establishment of International Potato Center Beijing Liaison Office in 1985. By the end of the 1980s, there were four national potato research institutes (centers), 74 scientific institutions and 20 agricultural academies carrying out potato research work. The nation's total potato planting area exceeded 40 million mu by 1988.

Since the 1990s, foreign fast food has flooded into the Chinese market. Typical Western potato food and fast food, such as French fries, mashed potatoes and potato chips, became increasingly popular with Chinese consumers. Along with the setting up of new potato processing branch companies in China by companies such as Simplot and PepsiCo, and the introduction of advanced process equipment (chipping, French frying, refined starch and dehydrated potatoes), China's modern potato manufacturing industry grew strongly.

At the same time, the upstream potato industry also accelerated, especially mini-tuber production. China had been intensifying its financial support to scientific research on potatoes, as well as the whole potato industry. Different kinds of potato processing companies spread quickly and were often an impetus for local economical development. Both national and international potato research activities and exchange became more frequent. Since 1998, The Potato Science Association, under the China Crop Association, has convened an annual national potato conference that attracts an increasing number of participants every year. In 1995, the entire nation's potato planting area exceeded 50 million mu (3.33 million ha) and grew to over 60 million mu (4 million ha) by 1998.

China's potato industry entered a new era from the beginning of 21st century. In 2000, the whole nation's planting area, for the first time in history, exceeded 70 million mu (4.67 million ha). In 2004, the fifth World Potato Congress was held in Yunnan, China. By 2006, the nation's potato planting area was about 80 million mu. In the meantime, modern potato processing capacity was further expanded, which contributed significantly to the enlargement of China's potato planting area. Thanks to modern planting techniques, the national potato yield is now close or equal to that of developed countries. The number of potato researchers and research institutes are also increasing. In 2007, there were over 100 research institutes, universities and colleges carrying out potato research programs. And the number of researchers was over 500 hundred, of which 150 had medium- or high-level technical designations and more than 60 hold doctorate degrees.

Table 2 summarizes China's annual potato planting area, total production and average yield since 1961. It shows that during the past 45 years, between 1961 and 2006, China's potato planting area almost quadrupled from 1.3 million ha to 5.02 million ha, an increase of 285.6%. Total production saw an increase of 476.1% over that of 1961, from 12.907 million tons in 1961 to 74.355 million tons in 2006. And average yield increased from 9.9 tons per ha in 1961 to 14.8 tons per ha in 2006. In

1966 China's potato planting area was over 20 million ha. It took 27 years for an increase of 10 million ha up to 30 million ha in 1993, but only another 5 years for next increase of 10 million ha, achieved in 1998. In 2006, the potato planting area exceeded 50 million ha.

Table 2: China's potato planting area, total production and yield (1961–2006)

Year	Planting area (1000 ha)	Planting area (1000 mu)	Production (1000 ton)	Yield (t/ha)	Yield (kg/mu)
1961	1301	19512	12907	9.9	660
1962	1501	22514	13808	9.2	613.3
1963	1501	22520	12010	8	533.3
1964	1602	24024	14019	8.8	586.7
1965	1701	25519	16016	9.4	626.7
1966	2001	30018	18016	9	600
1967	2002	30028	17923	9	600
1968	2002	30030	17822	8.9	593.3
1969	1902	28535	19328	10.2	680
1970	2002	30036	21524	10.7	713.3
1971	2103	31544	22034	10.5	700
1972	2302	34534	23527	10.2	680
1973	2002	30033	27027	13.5	900
1974	2002	30035	26026	13	866.7
1975	2104	31555	24340	11.6	773.3
1976	2004	30059	22644	11.3	753.3
1977	2020	30294	26730	13.2	880
1978	2243	33637	28585	12.7	846.7
1979	2303	34544	25650	11.1	740
1980	2303	34544	25896	11.2	746.7

Year	Planting area (1000 ha)	Planting area (1000 mu)	Production (1000 ton)	Yield (t/ha)	Yield (kg/mu)
1981	2402	36035	24698	10.3	686.7
1982	2454	36816	23825	9.7	646.7
1983	2562	38432	25275	9.9	660
1984	2562	38424	28400	11.1	740
1985	2478	37163	26750	10.8	720
1986	2510	37649	26520	10.6	706.7
1987	2590	38847	26685	10.3	686.7
1988	2747	41210	31625	11.5	766.7
1989	2823	42338	31055	11	733.3
1990	2865	42978	34550	12.1	806.7
1991	2879	43190	31565	11	733.3
1992	2995	44924	37435	12.5	833.3
1993	3087	46307	46040	14.9	993.3
1994	3208	48114	48735	15.2	1013.3
1995	3434	51512	45735	13.3	886.7
1996	3736	56045	52995	14.2	946.7
1997	3823	57341	57208	13	866.7
1998	4062	60932	56263	13.9	926.7
1999	4418	66266	56096	12.7	846.7
2000	4723	70851	66282	14	933.3
2001	4719	70782	64564	13.7	913.3
2002	4698	70463	70082	14.9	993.3
2003	4522	67836	68100	15.1	1006.7
2004	4597	68951	72080	15.7	1046.7
2005	4881	73214	70865	14.5	966.7
2006	5016	75236	74355	14.8	986.7

Notes: 1 Data for 1961–1981 are from FAO.; 2 Data for 1982-2006 are from China Agriculture Yearbook.; 3) Data were proofed by the authors.; 4 No data for Shandong Province was included after 2003.

Potato production in China

Huge planting area and low yield

Potato is the only crop that can be planted in all the provinces, autonomous regions and municipalities in China. Based on the cropping systems, varieties, biological traits, and geographic and climatic conditions, four potato production zones have been identified. They are:

1) North Single Cropping Zone: including provinces in the northeast China, Inner Mongolia, Hebei, Shanxi, Shaanxi, Ningxia, Gansu, Qinghai and Xinqiang, occupying about 47% of the total planting area in China;

2) Central Double Cropping Zone: including the southern parts of Liaoning, Hebei, Shanxi, and Shaanxi, and most of Hubei, Hunan, Henan, Shandong, Jiangsu, Zhejiang, Anhui and Jiangxi, occupying about 7% of the total planting area in China;

3) South Winter Cropping Zone: including Guangxi, Guangdong, Hainan, Fujian and Taiwan, occupying about 8% of the total planting area in China;

4) Southwest Mixed Cropping Zone: including Yunnan, Guizhou, Sichuan, Tibet and part of Hunan and Hubei, occupying about 38% of the total planting area in China.

The actual potato planting area in 2006 was 5.3424 million ha, but according to official statistics, the area was 5.0175 million ha (see Table 3). According to the FAO's statistics, the potato planting area was 4.9015 ha, which accounted for 26.14% of the global potato planting area. Total production in China was 70.338 million tons and was 22.41% of the global total, while the yield was 14.35 ton/ha—a little bit lower than the world average yield of 16.74 ton/ha.

Table 3: Potato planting area, production and yield in different regions of China in 2006

Region	Area (ha)	Rank	Production (t)	Rank	Yield (t/ha)	Rank
Guizhou	592800	1	7730000	5	13.04	16
Inner Mongolia	589100	2	8795000	2	14.93	13
Gansu	567800	3	9400000	1	16.56	11
Yunnan	539900	4	8610000	3	15.95	12
Sichuan	348200	5	8515000	4	24.45	4
Chongqing	347400	6	4705000	6	13.54	15
Heilongjiang	319300	7	4050000	7	12.68	18
Shanxi	299200	8	2415000	10	8.07	22
Shaanxi	252000	9	2550000	9	10.12	20
Hubei	229800	10	3390000	8	14.75	14
Ningxia	186600	11	1620000	15	8.68	21
Hebei	152900	12	1880000	12	12.30	19

Region	Area (ha)	Rank	Production (t)	Rank	Yield (t/ha)	Rank
Jilin	141900	13	1850000	13	13.04	17
Hunan	113200	14	2085000	11	18.42	9
Liaoning	90000	15	1685000	14	18.72	8
Fujian	87400	16	1510000	17	17.28	10
Qinghai	80100	17	1545000	16	19.29	7
Guangdong	42800	18	940000	18	21.96	6
Xinqiang	22900	19	755000	19	32.97	2
Anhui	7600	20	185000	20	24.34	5
Jiangxi	4200	21	105000	21	25.00	3
Tibet	600	22	35000	22	58.33	1
Total/average	5015700		74355000		14.82	

Notes: 1) The data in the table are from the China Agriculture Yearbook 2007.; 2) The data for Shandong, Guangxi, Zhejiang and Henan are not included.; 3) The data in this table is not the same as the FAO statistics.

There were 10 provinces and autonomous regions with a potato planting area of over 3 million mu (0.2 million ha) in 2006. Of these, the planting areas in Guizhou, Inner Mongolia, Gansu and Yunnan were over 8 million mu (0.533 million ha). The largest province, Guizhou, was close to 9 million mu (0.593 million ha). However, the top four regions were Gansu, Inner Mongolia, Yunnan and Sichuan in terms of total production. Guizhou was ranked 5th in terms of production due to its lower yield. In terms of planting area, each of the top eight regions in China would make a top 10 list of countries in the world, ahead of the 10th ranked country, Germany.

However the potato yield in China has always been low and is increasing only very slowly. In 1973, potato yield reached 13.5 ton/ha, yet the yields in 1997 and in 1999 were 13.0 ton/ha and 12.7 ton/ha, respectively. The highest ever potato yield in China was 15.7 ton/ha in 2004. Besides 2004, the yield exceeded 15 ton/ha only in 1994 and 2003, when it was 15.2 ton/ha and 15.1 ton/ha, respectively.

One important fact is that there are about 30 million ha of winter fallow paddy fields in the southern region around latitude 33°N where many crops can be planted in the winter season, such as rapeseed, winter wheat, potatoes, minor grain crops, forages, melons and vegetables. The harvesting time of winter potato is in what is considered the off-season of potatoes in China, and the farmers can benefit due to the high price. Thus, the planting area of winter potatoes has increased over the years. For example, in Guangxi Autonomous Region, the potato planting area has increased to 130,000 ha from 30,000 in the past few years. Barring competition from other crops, the winter potato's planting area will likely increase in these regions in the coming years.

Achievements in the breeding and extension of new potato varieties

At present, there are a number of institutions in China working on potato breeding, in Heilongjiang, Liaoning, Jilin, Hebei, Inner Mongolia, Shanxi, Gansu, Qinghai, Hubei, Shandong, Henan, Sichuan and Yunnan. As of 2007, about 250 new potato varieties had been released by different institutions, and a number of excellent foreign varieties had been introduced as well. About 90 potato varieties have being used in potato production in China. However, most of them are used for vegetables and few varieties can be used for chips, French fries or flakes. The introduced foreign varieties have accelerated potato production and the potato industry in China. For example, Atlantic and Shepody varieties have advanced the potato processing industry in China, Mira is still a major variety in southwest China, and Favorita is still the most important variety for the Central Double Cropping Zone and South Winter Potato Zone.

Though the newly bred varieties and introduced varieties included all kinds of utilizations, the varieties for specific utilizations were not planted in large areas, and the shortage of the specific raw materials was one of the most important factors limiting the development of the potato industry in China.

Incomplete seed system and the shortage of high-quality seed potatoes

The most important factor leading to a low potato yield is the low quality of seed potatoes in China. Many farmers are still using self-kept seed potatoes from the previous harvest. Though the government has made significant investments in seed potato production, the quality of the seed potatoes has not improved remarkably. The factors limiting the improvement of seed potato quality are:

1) Technical factors. Virus elimination and detection technologies have not been grasped by all the seed multiplication institutions, the quantity and quality of minitubers is not enough to support production, and the practical technical regulations for the seed production and quality control are lacking.

2) Management factors. The seed multiplication institutions are unable to properly manage the different classes of seed potatoes and cannot control seed quality efficiently.

3) Natural factors. Due to the huge potato planting area in China, seed potatoes are often planted next to commercial potatoes, making it very difficult to naturally isolate the different classes of seeds.

4) Economic factors. Farmers have been unwilling to buy more expensive, high-quality seed potatoes when the price of commercial potatoes has been low. At the same time, seed growers have balked at adopting higher-cost quality control measures given that they can't sell the higher-quality seeds at a higher price.

5) Policy factors. There are no effective regulations related to seed potatoes and those that are in place have not been implemented strictly. The existing regulation related to seed potato production, such

as standards for certified seed potatoes, quarantine regulation for seed potato producing areas, and the technical regulations for virus-free seed potato production are, for the most part, not suitable for the situation in China. There are also no special organizations to supervise or implement the regulations. There are two national testing and supervision centers for seed potato quality in China, but they are not authorized by related departments of government and they are not capable of supervising all of China's seed potato production.

The majority of farms are small-scale

Only in some regions in northern China, can potato farms exceed 100 mu (16.7 ha) and few farms can reach 500 mu (33.3 ha). Intensive production can be conducted in these large farms and planting and harvesting are often mechanized. However, these farms occupy less than 5% of the total planting area in China.

Most of the potato farmers in China grow potatoes on land area of less than 15 mu (1 ha) and they mainly use manual and animal power in production. In southwest China, the average potato planting area per family is likely less than 7.5 mu (0.5 ha). This small planting area and steep gradient of the fields make it very difficult for farmers to use machines.

The frequent occurrences of potato pests and diseases

Potato pests and diseases can be biological or non-biological. There are about 300 biological pests and diseases in potato production. Fortunately, not all the pests and diseases will affect potato yield seriously. The major biological potato diseases are fungal diseases, bacterial diseases and virus diseases. Research has shown that there are about 50 biological diseases and pests in China. Of these, there are about 20 fungal diseases, such as late blight, early blight, wart, powdery scab, stem canker, black scurf, dry rot, and wilt; five main bacterial diseases, including bacterial wilt, ring rot, black leg, soft rot and common scab; 20 virus, viroid and mycoplasma-like diseases, such as potato leafroll virus (PLRV), PVX, PVY, PVS, PSTVd, purple top wilt and witch's broom; and 15 pests, including aphids, thrips, leafhoppers, mites, ladybugs, cutworms and wireworms.

Besides the above biological pests and diseases, there are a number of non-biological factors affecting potato growth. Water, fertilizer, air and heat may affect potato growth and development when they are not balanced, and some physiological diseases may occur.

Fortunately, the Colorado potato beetle was only found in a small number of locations in Xinjiang Uyghur Autonomous Region. There are no reports of golden nematodes, cyst nematodes, and the yellow dwarf virus disease in China.

Main roles of the potato in China

Classifying the potato can be difficult, given its diverse uses. It has been called a grain crop, economic crop, vegetable crop, horticultural crop, raw material crop, medicine crop and disaster-relief crop. All these designations are correct, but all of them are incomplete. Besides the universities, the vegetable research institutes, crop research institutes, horticultural research institutes and economic crop research institutes are all studying the potato in China, and there are several potato-specific research institutes as well. The functions of potatoes in food safety, energy security, poverty elimination, value-adding, and response to natural disasters will be discussed in the following sections.

Food safety

Potato is one of the seven major crops in China and has the fourth-largest planting area, behind rice, maize and wheat. With the increase of planting area and total production, the average consumption of potatoes is increasing and has reached 40 kg per capita in recent years, and in some regions exceeds 100 kg per capita. Potatoes play an important role in the Chinese diet and a wide range of potato staple foods and dishes have accelerated their consumption. However, average potato consumption is still relatively low compared to many other countries (see Figure 4).

According to data from Ministry of Land and Resource and the National Statistics Bureau, in 2007, total arable land was 122 million ha, and the average arable land was 0.099 ha per capita—only 39.6% of the global average for arable land per capita. Furthermore, 60% of the arable land is dry land, with the agricultural production in these areas mainly relying on rainfall. Over 6 million ha of arable land are located on slopes with gradients greater than 25 degrees. These arable areas should be return to forestry or grass gradually to ensure water and soil conservation.

With the rapid development of China's economy, more and more arable land has been used as non-agricultural land. According to the data from the Chinese authorities, the net arable land reduction was 933,000 ha (14.44 million mu) in 2000, 627,000 ha (9.41 million mu) in 2001, 1.686 million ha (25.29 million mu) in 2002, 2.537 million ha (38.06 million mu) in 2003, 800,000 ha (12 million ha) in 2004, 361,000 ha (5.42 million mu) in 2005, 307,000 ha (4.6 million mu) in 2006, and 41,000 ha (610,000 mu) in 2007. This meant that between 2000 and 2007 arable land was reduced by a total of 7.292 million ha (109.4 million mu).

Total arable land now stands at 122 million ha (1.826 billion mu) and is close to the "red line," set by Chinese government, of 120 million ha (1.8 billion mu). This situation further aggravates the contradiction between population and arable land and brings much more pressure on food safety in China.

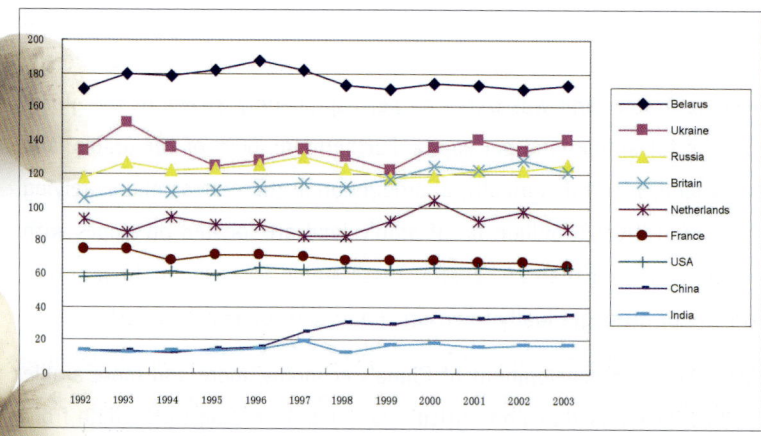

Figure 4: Comparisons of potato consumption between China and other countries (kg/person/year)

In the past 10 years, the planting areas of rice and wheat have both decreased, while maize has seen an increase in planting area (see Table 4).

Table 4: The change in planting area and production of rice, wheat, maize and potato in the past 10 years in China

Crop		1996	2006	2006–1996
Rice	Planting area (1000 ha)	31406.13	29294.80	-2111.33 (-6.72%)
	Production (10000 ton)	19510.20	18257.10	-1253.10 (-6.42%)
Wheat	Planting area (1000 ha)	29610.50	22961.60	-6648.90 (-22.45)
	Production (10000 ton)	11057.00	10446.40	-610.60 (-5.52%)
Maize	Planting area (1000 ha)	24498.30	26970.80	2472.50 (10.1%)
	Production (10000 ton)	12747.00	14548.50	1801.50 (14.1%)
Potato	Planting area (1000 ha)	3736.29	5015.70	1279.41 (34.2%)
	Production (10000 ton)	1059.93	1487.10	427.17 (40.3%)

Note: Potato production is the production of fresh potato divided by 5.

On the other hand, the average yields of the three major crops (rice, wheat and maize) were much higher than those of the world average yields, especially for wheat and rice, which were 58.8% and 52.4% higher than the world average, respectively. This makes it difficult to further increase the yields of the three major crops. However, the average yield for potatoes was lower than the world average—at 85.8% of the world average—so the potential for a potato yield increase is very high (see Table 5).

Table 5: Yield comparison of three major grain crops and potato between China and the world (kg/ha)

Crop	World	China	China - world
Wheat	2804.01	4455.00	1650.99 (58.9%)
Rice	4112.17	6265.15	2152.98 (52.4%)
Maize	4815.39	5365.10	549.71 (11.4%)
Potato	16733.74	14350.3	-2383.44 (-14.2%)

Given that 60% of China's arable land is dry land and most of the potential arable land is in regions with little rainfall, none of the grain crops can get the water utilization efficiency as high as potato under the water stress conditions. The potato yield increases gradually during the growing season and some tubers can be harvested even in the driest conditions. However, nothing may be harvested for other grain crops when there is a serious drought in the later stages of growth.

In the dry and semi-dry regions, potatoes, spring wheat, spring millet, buckwheat and oats are the major crops. Of these, potato has the highest tolerance to drought, the highest yield potential, and the highest photosynthetic efficiency. According to research results, when the yield in a normal year is 100%, then in a dry year, millet can get 55% of the normal yield; oats, 57%; spring wheat, 58%; haricot bean, 63%; pea, 65%; and potato, 76%.

Due to the lack of potential arable land and the reduction of actual arable land; the reduction in planting area of the three major grain crops (rice, wheat and maize) and their low potential for yield increases; and the shortage of water resources, the potential for a production increase for the three major crops is very low. On the other hand, potato can be planted in the winter fallow paddy fields without competition to other crops and the planting area of potatoes could be increased by several million hectares. The potential for yield increases is also significant due to the lower yields and the water utilization efficiency of potatoes relative to other crops. These factors indicate that the potato can play an important role in food safety in China.

Energy security

China's huge population and limited arable land made a secure and sufficient food supply one of the most critical issues. As such, the government has forbidden the production of grain-based energy alcohol from rice, maize and wheat. This has made roots and tubers—including potato, sweet potato and cassava—the main option for energy crops.

Though the alcohol production from potato is lower than that from sweet potato and cassava, based on the same weight, potato has the much wider adaptation than sweet potato and cassava (see Table 6). The planting area of cassava is currently about 400,000 ha (6 million mu), and is only implanted in tropical and sub-tropical regions. Estimates have been made that its planting area could increase to 1 million ha by 2015. Sweet potato can be only planted in warm regions, such as south China, and its planting area stands at 4.71 million ha (70.63 million mu), lower than the potato planting area for the first time.

In some regions in China, such as Tibet and Xinqiang, the potential potato yield is a remarkable 45 to 60 ton/ha (or alcohol production of 4.5 to 6 ton/ha). Given the lack of good transportation infrastructure in these regions, transporting potatoes can be difficult, which may lead to their development as important production bases for fuel alcohol instead. Potato-based fuel alcohol production can increase the value of potatoes, the farmers' employment, and the farmers' incomes, while the volume and weight can be reduced remarkably if the potatoes can be converted into alcohol locally. Normally, 90% of the weight can be reduced if potatoes are converted to alcohol. This could be especially important for Xinqiang, because this method is the most efficient way to control the spread of the Colorado potato beetle, which is found in some counties there.

Table 6: Alcohol production from roots, tubers and grain crops (per 100 kg of raw materials)

Raw material	Starch (%)	Coarse protein (%)	Water (%)	Alcohol production (kg)
Sweet potato (fresh)	15~25	1.1~1.4	70~80	8.5~14.2
Sweet potato (dry)	65~68	1.1~1.5	12~14	36.9~38.6
Potato (fresh)	12~20	1.8~5.5	70~80	6.8~11.4
Potato (dry)	63~70	6~7.4	13	35.8~39.7
Cassava (fresh)	27~33	1~1.5	70~71	15.3~18.7
Cassava (dry)	63~74	2~4	12~16	35.8~42.0
Maize (dry)	65~66	8~9	12	36.9~37.5
Rice	65~72	7~9	11~13	36.9~40.9
Wheat	63~65	10~10.5	12~13	35.8~36.9

Poverty elimination

The majority of China's potato production occurs in the hinterland regions of China, where the crop is a major staple food, feed crop and source of income for the local residents. There are 592 "national poverty counties" in China and, of these, 429 are growing potatoes. Although the proportion of poverty counties is 32.5% of the total potato planting counties (1,330 counties), the total potato planting area in these poverty counties represents 58.13% of the total potato planting area in China (see Figure 5).

The income from potato production accounts for a high proportion of the total average incomes in the western poverty counties in China and most of these incomes are obtained in cash. For example, in Xiji County of Ningxia Hui Autonomous Region, the pure income from potato production is 657 Yuan (US$95) per person and represents 29.7% of the average total income.

Due to the adverse natural conditions in some poverty regions, only a certain few crops can be planted there, such as potatoes, oats, buckwheat, flax, and millet. Fortunately, the weather conditions can be favorable for the production of seed potatoes. As such, the potato can contribute significantly to the elimination of poverty if appropriate varieties can be introduced, seed potato production can be regulated, and seeds are kept sellable.

Potato processing and value-added

While the potato is one of the most important food resources for humans, it has two fatal shortcomings: its volume and a relatively short storage period. How to process potatoes into other products that can be stored for longer periods has been under investigation for many years. The potato industry now has the longest production chain and most abundant products among all the agricultural crops, and potato processing is no longer done only to increase the potato storage period. Processing can now add value to potatoes—potato starch, chips, French fries and flakes (dehydrated potatoes) are the most popular products in the market. Of these, starch and flakes can be used as raw materials to produce many other kinds of products.

Modern potato processing started with potato starch, a process that consumes a large number of potato tubers. The first starch processing plant was founded in the United States in 1831, with more than 100 plants emerging in the following years later. The first chipping plant was established in Ohio in 1895, and there are now about 130 chipping plants that consume about 2.3 million tons of raw materials in the United States. Each year, Americans consume 7.7 kg of potato chips.

Nobody knows the origin of French fries, but it is most likely in France or Belgium. It is very clear that French fries were a product developed during

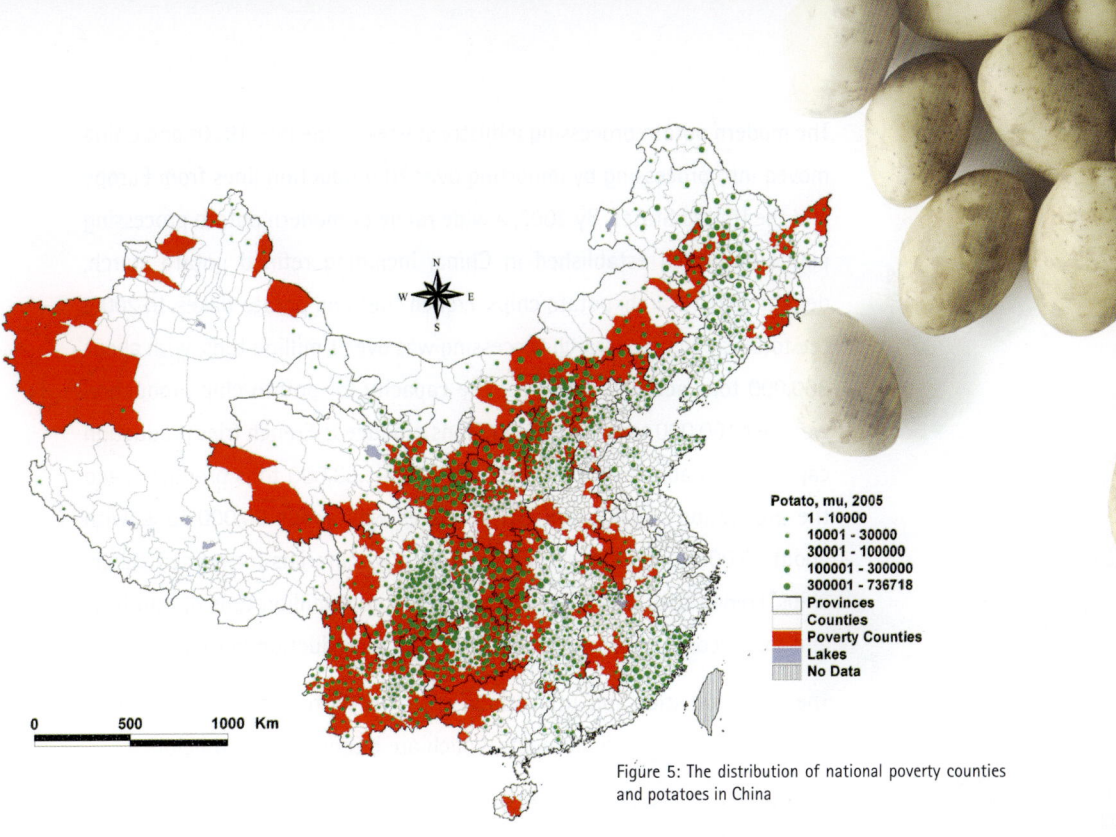

Figure 5: The distribution of national poverty counties and potatoes in China

World War II, and evolved further thereafter. The first French fry plant in the United States was built in Maine in 1947. The processing method was different from modern techniques, and the French fries were stored after being fried twice. Today, French fries are frozen directly after one pre-frying. Frozen French fries are very popular in foreign countries and frozen potato products can consume close to 40% of total potato production every year.

The modern potato processing industry started in the late 1980s and China moved into processing by importing over 20 production lines from Europe and the United States. By 2007, a wide range of modern potato processing plants had been established in China, including refined potato starch, denaturalized starch, potato chips, French fries and potato flakes. In 2006, the total capacity for starch processing was over 1 million tons, with about 300,000 tons actually produced. The capacity for potato chip production was over 160,000 tons with 90,000 tons produced; French fries production capacity was about 100,000 tons, with about 63,000 tons produced; and the production capacity for potato flakes was about 60,000 tons, with about 20,000 tons produced. The annual raw materials for refined starch, chips, French fries and flakes were 3 million to 4 million tons of potatoes, and this accounted for about 5% of the total production in China.

The characteristics and utilizations are quite different among the four major processed potato products, which are briefly described below.

Potato starch: Starch particles are extracted from the potato tuber cells by physical methods and the other components in the tubers are discarded as waste water or waste residues. As with all varieties of starches, potato starch is aggregated by glucose molecules. However, potato starch is considered the best starch for the following characteristics:

1) Potato starch particles are the biggest and give an open structure, high swelling capability, and crispy texture to products. The average diameter of a potato starch particle is 65 um, while maize and sweet potato starch particles are 15 um and rice starch particles are 5 um.

2) The viscosity of potato starch is much higher than other starches. The amylopectin proportion can reach 60% to 80% in potato starch, which is much higher than other starches. Furthermore, the aggregation of amylose in potato starch is very high. The resulting average viscosity peak of potato starch paste can reach 3,000 BU compared to maize starch paste at 600 BU, cassava starch paste at 1,000 BU, and wheat starch paste at 300 BU.

3) The pasting temperature of potato starch is lower and the swelling of potato starch is stronger. The average pasting temperature of potato starch is 56°C, while maize starch pastes at 64°C, wheat starch at 69°C, and sweet potato starch at 79°C. The swelling of potato starch is very strong and potato starch will swell after absorbing water at temperatures over 50°C. Potato starch can absorb 400 to 600 times of water after pasted.

4) The transparency of potato starch paste is high. There are almost no un-swelled and un-pasted particles, which would refract light, in potato paste. The phosphate radical and the lack of fat in potato starch's molecular structure are the main reasons for the higher transparency.

5) Potato starch doesn't have the grain flavor that maize starch and wheat starch have because of its low protein content. The protein residue in potato starch is often less than 0.1%, giving potato starch a very white color and a mild flavor without any stimulation.

6) There is higher phosphorus content in potato starch. A phosphate radical is located in every 200 to 400 glucose molecules and it is balanced by ions such as K^+, Ca^{2+}, and Mg^{2+}. Thus, potato starch is more nutritious when it is used as raw materials for food products.

In conclusion, potato starch and potato denaturalized starch are widely used as raw materials for many industries, such as food, feed, medicine, chemicals, paper-making, architecture and oil extraction because of the above characteristics.

Potato chips:

Potato chips can be classified into natural chips and fabricated chips. Natural chips are produced directly from sliced and fried potato tubers of special varieties. Fabricated chips are the product of dehydrated potatoes, starch and other components after they are mixed, formed and fried. Natural chips can keep the potato flavor perfectly, have a crispy texture and are nutritious. Not all potato varieties can be used for chipping—special varieties have to be used to get a high quality chip. Potato chips are suitable for younger, more active people because they contain 60% dry matter, 35% oil and 5% of water. Fabricated chips can still keep the potato's flavor because they contain dehydrated potatoes. One of their advantages is that they can be produced in a uniform shape to save packing space and carry conveniently.

French fries: The correct name for French fries should be "frozen French fries." Some people translate "French fries" as "potato strips fried in French way," "potato strips," and "fried potato strips." Though they are a very popular potato product in many countries, they have no uniform definition. The French fry in this book means the potato product resulting from the peeling, slicing, rinsing, frying and fast-freezing of fresh tubers. French fries can be eaten directly after taking them from freezer and frying them in the oil. They are also called frozen French fries because they are a half-made product, and need to be stored frozen. Normally, French fries are stored in -18°C to ensure their quality for a long time. Because of their convenience for cooking, French fries have become one of the most popular staple foods in Europe and North America—similar to rice in China. In China, French fries are mainly sold in Western fast food restaurants or hotels, but can be found in some supermarkets in the bigger cities. The advantages of French fries include:

1) It is a convenient fast food for restaurants and families and it can be supplied year-round.

2) It can almost keep the original potato flavor because no other food components are added except oil.

3) It can be fried when still frozen; there is no need to thaw before cooking.

4) French fries can provide abundant nutrition and energy. They are suitable for younger, more active people because they have high oil content.

Potato flakes or granules:

These are also known as mashed potatoes or dehydrated potatoes, and are processed potato products that are quite different from potato starch. The process to produce dehydrated potatoes extracts the carbohydrates that provide energy from potato starch, while the remaining nutritional components, such as vitamins, minerals, amino acids, microelements, and edible fibers, are discharged as waste water and residues. The processing technology for dehydrated potatoes is completely different from that for potato starch processing. According to the processing technologies and the shape of products, dehydrated potatoes can be classified into potato flakes (similar in shape to snowflakes) and granules. Dehydrated potatoes have the following characteristics:

1) Most of the potato cells will be kept unbroken, thus few free starch particles will be produced in flakes, and even less in granules.

2) Most of the nutritional materials remain when potatoes are dehydrated, such as vitamins, minerals, amino acids, microelements and edible fibers.

3) The potato flavor is kept in dehydrated potatoes and can be almost fully recovered after hot water is added.

4) The bulk densities of the two types of dehydrated potatoes are quite different. The bulk density of flakes is very low, from 0.25 kg/liter to 0.55 kg/liter. Because of the different processing technology for granules, the granules are much more compact and the density is between 0.75 kg/liter and 0.85 kg/liter.

Because of their convenient use, long storage period, abundant nutrients, and easy digestion, dehydrated potatoes are widely used as raw materials to produce other kinds of foods, such as mashed potatoes, fabricated French fries, frozen fabricated French fries, fabricated potato chips, many kinds of snack foods, and infant foods. They are also used as an additive for baked foods (bread, cakes and biscuits) and soups. Dehydrated potatoes can also be used in the production of munitions.

The potato and natural disaster relief

Due to their short growing period (especially for the early varieties) and the adaptability to different soils and seasons, potatoes have always played an important role in relief of natural disasters. Normally, after a natural disaster, the suitable planting season for most of the crops is missed, especially for grain crops, and it is difficult to reap a harvest from these crops with the economic organ of seeds. However, potatoes are harvested for the tubers (the nutritional organs), and some tubers can always be harvested, regardless of the situation.

For example, when serious flooding in south China in 1998 damaged many rice fields, the potatoes planted in autumn were one of the most important measures for the relief of the flood disaster. The potato planting area was increased by 200,000 ha (3 million mu) in that year, which was also the first year with the total potato planting area exceeded 4 million ha (60 million mu).

Spring drought is a frequent natural disaster in north China, often resulting in crops missing their suitable planting season by the time the rains come and the soil moisture is sufficient. Potatoes perform well in these conditions, with a harvest still obtainable even when the crop is planted one month later than the normal.

Appendix 1: Indices of all dishes

Bag-shaped oat potato pie (Malingshu Tuntun)	77
Baked potato cake (Lao Malinghshu Yangzi)	78
Baked potato cake with red bean filling (Tudou Dousha Bing)	188
Baked potatoes (Kao Tudou)	187
Baked shredded potatoes (Gan Bei Yangyu Si)	249
Birds nest-shaped shredded potatoes (Niaochao Shu Si)	250
Black beauty potato slices (Hei Meiren Yangyu)	189
Black soy sauce potatoes (Jiangyou Malingshu Tiao)	79
Braised assorted dishes, Yulin style (Yu Lin Da Huicai)	190
Braised beef with potato (Malingshu Shao Niurou)	80
Braised chicken with potato and green pepper (Da Pan Ji)	191
Braised potato balls with black soy sauce (Hongshao Tudouqiu)	251
Braised potato pieces (Hongshao Shukuai)	81
Braised potato with goose (Da E Men Tudou)	47
Braised potato, cabbage and tofu (Malingshu Baicai Tofu)	82
Braised potatoes (Malingshu Dahuicai)	83
Braised potatoes and cabbage (Malingshu Baicai Hui Fenkuai)	84
Braised potatoes and tofu with spareribs (Malingshu tofu Dun Paigu)	85
Braised potatoes with cowpeas and spareribs (Malingshu Doujiao Dun Paigu)	86
Braised potatoes with duck (Tudou Huang Men Ya)	252
Braised potatoes with fish-shaped oat noodles (Malingshu Hui Youmian Yu)	87
Braised potatoes with mutton rack (Tudou Wei Yangpai)	192
Braised potatoes with pumpkin (Dun Nangua Tudou)	193
Braised potatoes with rice (Tudou Men Fan)	253
Braised sheep entrails with noodles (Guozai Fentiao Yangza)	88
Braised side pork and rape with potatoes (Wuhuarou Youcai Hui Malingshu)	89
Braised side pork with potatoes in soy sauce (Tudou Hongshao Rou)	254
Braised sirloin with potatoes (Malingshu Dun Niunan)	90

Braised small potato balls with oxtail (Xiao Tudou Shao Niuwei)	91
Braised spareribs with potatoes (Tudou Dun Paigu)	194
Braised tofu with pakchoi (Xiao Baicai Hui Tofu)	195
Camel palm encircled with shredded potato (Tuozhang Tudou Si)	92
Charcoal-roasted potatoes (Tanhuo Kao Tudou)	255
Chinese chess fun (Qi Qu)	93
Chinese date-filled potato balls with honey (Mizhi Nuoxiang Tudou Zao)	256
Cold potato strings in oil, vinegar and spices (Liangban Malingshu Si)	94
Colorful shredded potatoes (Qicai Tudou Si)	257
Cooked potato chips (Peng Tudou Pian)	48
Countryside tricolor potatoes (Nongjia Tianyuan Sanse)	95
Crisp potato balls coated with sugar (Yinzhuang Suguo)	196
Crisp potato strips I (Xiangsu Shu Tiao I)	258
Crisp potato strips II (Xiangsu Shu Tiao II)	259
Crystal mashed potato roll (Yuni Shuijing Juan)	197
Cucumber with potato noodles (Huanggua Fenpi)	198
Curry potatoes (Gali Malingshu)	343
Dark steamed potato balls (Heilengleng)	199
Deep-fried fat pork and diced potatoes (Cuishao Tudou li)	260
Deep-fried potato balls (Cuizha Tudou Qiu)	344
Deep-fried potato balls covered in sesame seeds (Tudou Matuan)	200
Deep-fried potato chips (Youzha Tudou Pian)	261
Deep-fried potato chips with peanuts and chili (Youzha San Pin)	262
Deep-fried potato doughnuts (Youzha Malingshu Guozi)	96
Deep-fried potato strips with tomato sauce (Mizhi Shasi Tudou Tiao)	97
Diced potatoes with salted egg yolk (Yan Danhuang Tudou Li)	263
Dongxiang county potato chips (Dongxiang Tudou Pian)	201
Drunk potato (Zuijiu Malingshu)	98

Egg, shredded bottle gourd and potato cake (Jidan Hulusi Malingshu Bing)	99
Elegant taste (Ya Qu)	100
Finely shredded potatoes with ginger (Jiangwei Longxu Si)	264
Fish-shaped potato (Malingshu Yu)	101
Fish-shaped potato with fried pork fillet (Guoyourou Malingshu Yu)	102
Fish-shaped potato-oat flour noodles (Tudou Yuzi)	103
Flavored mashed potatoes (Fengwei Tudou Ni)	49
Flavored potato balls (Fengwei Tudou Qiu)	104
French-style mushroom and potato salad (Fashi Xianggu Malingshu Shalazi)	345
Fried chicken-flavored potato (Youzha Malingshu Su Jitui)	105
Fried Chinese sauerkraut and noodles (Suancai Chao Fentiao)	106
Fried Chinese sauerkraut and potato chips (Suancai Malingshu Tiao)	107
Fried Chinese sauerkraut and potato slices (Suancai Malinghsu Ni)	108
Fried country-style potato balls (Shancun Zha Malingshu Wanzi)	346
Fried diced potatoes and lettuce stems (Chao Malingshu Wosunding)	347
Fried dried potato slices (Zha Gan Yangyupian)	265
Fried egg and potato string cake (Jianjidan Malingshusi Bing)	348
Fried green pepper and shredded potato (Qingjiao Tudou Si)	266
Fried lichen and potato chips (Dipi Tudou Pian)	50
Fried mashed potatoes, carrots and mushrooms (Jinsha Fengguang)	109
Fried meatballs (Zha Ge Wanzi)	202
Fried pork liver with potato (Zhugan Tudou Tiao)	203
Fried pork slices with potato (Tudou Chao Rou Pian)	204
Fried potato balls (Youzha Malingshu Wanzi)	110
Fried potato cake I (Jian Tudou Bing)	51
Fried potato cake II (Xiangjian Tudou Bing I)	111
Fried potato cake III (Tudou Jianbing)	205
Fried potato cake IV (Cui Zha Tudou Bing)	349

Fried potato chips (Su Chao Tudou Pian)	267
Fried potato chips with green pepper (Chao Tudou Pian Qingjiao)	52
Fried potato chips with soy sauce (Jiang Bao Tudou Pian)	268
Fried potato chips with spicy cabbage (La Baicai Chao Tudou Pian)	53
Fried potato pancake (Qiaoshou Tuanyuanbing)	269
Fried potato pie (Youzha Shu Bing)	270
Fried potato slices I (Youzha Malingshu Pian)	112
Fried potato slices II (Zha Malingshu Pian)	350
Fried potato slices with dried pickles (Gan Yancai Chao Shu Pian)	271
Fried potato slices with sour bamboo shoots (Suan Sun Chao Shupian)	272
Fried potato strings (Youzha Malingshu Si)	113
Fried potato strings with pickled celery cabbage and mutton fat (Yangyou Suancai Malingshu Si)	114
Fried potato strips (Zha Malingshu Tiao)	351
Fried potato strips coated with sugar (Liuli Shutiao)	115
Fried potato strips coated with yolk (Jinsha Tudou Tiao)	273
Fried potato strips with chili (Ganbian Tudou Tiao)	116
Fried potato strips with garlic bolt (Zha Tudou Tiao Chao Suantai)	54
Fried potato strips with pork (Youbailuo Chao Malingshu Tiao)	117
Fried potato strips with spicy peanuts (Xiang Su Shutiao)	352
Fried potato with jellyfish (Tudou Bao Zhetou)	353
Fried potatoes and chicken with pickled pepper (Paojiao Tudou Ji)	274
Fried potatoes and pork with pickled pepper (Jiang Rou Tudou Ding)	275
Fried potatoes with egg (Tudou Jian Dan)	118
Fried potatoes with four treasures (Jin Shu Hui Sibao)	276
Fried potatoes with soybean sprouts (Tudou Chao Huangdou Ya)	119
Fried prawn coated with fine potato strings (Jinsi Fengwei Xia)	277
Fried shredded potato (Suchao Tudou Si)	55
Fried shredded potato cake I (Xiang Jian Tudou Pai)	120

Fried shredded potato cake II (Tudou Tanbing III)	206
Fried shredded potato with Chinese chives and egg (served with cake) (Malingshu Si Jiucai Jidan Dai Bing)	121
Fried shredded potatoes with vinegar (Culiu Yangyu Si)	207
Fried side pork with potato (Wuhuarou Jian Malingshu)	122
Fried stick-shaped mutton-potato mash (Tu Yang Jiehe Bang)	208
Fried tofu and potatoes with green and red Pepper (Jin Yu Man Tang)	209
Golden fried potato balls (Zha Huangjin Tudou Qiu)	56
Golden potato string cake (Jinhuang Dousi Bing)	278
Golden shredded potato nest (Jin Quechao)	210
Golden thread with lotus (Jinsi Wang Lian)	211
Goulash with potato (Tudou Shao Niurou)	212
Grape-shaped potato dish (Fengshou Putao)	213
Green onion-flavored potato chips (Conghua Shu Pian)	279
Ham-flavored potato strings (Huotui Fengwei Tudou Si)	280
Handmade noodles with potatoes in an earthen pot (Shaguo Malingshu Shouganmian)	123
Honey potatoes (Mizhi Malingshu)	354
Honeycomb-shaped potatoes (Fengwo Tudou)	281
Hot and spicy diced potatoes I (Mala Tudou Ding)	282
Hot and spicy diced potatoes II (Xiangma Tudou Ding)	283
Hotpot potato pieces (Malingshu Huoguo Pian)	124
Hotpot potatoes with preserved ham and radish (Yi Guo Hui)	284
Hunyuan cold potato jelly (Hunyuan Liangfen)	125
Long life shredded potatoes (Changshou Tudou Si)	285
Mashed garlic scallop with potato noodles (Suanrong Fensi Zheng Shanbei)	126
Mashed potatoes fried with fennel (Huixiang Tudou Ni)	286
Mashed potatoes in lotus leaf (Heye Tudou Ni)	287
Mashed potatoes with pakchoi (Hua Cai)	214
Mashed potatoes with pine nuts (Songren Tudou Ni)	288

Mashed potatoes with sauce (Jiaozhi Tudou Ni)	57
Mashed potatoes wrapped in sticky rice pancakes (Zhibao Tudou Ni)	289
Megranate-shaped fried chicken (Fugui Shiliu Ji)	290
Min Bagu (Min Bagu)	127
Minced beef in potato bowls (Yi Wan Chi)	291
Mini embroidered potato balls (Mini Xiuqiu Wan)	128
Mixed shredded potatoes (Ban Tudou Song)	58
Noodles with potato and spinach (Malingshu Bocai Gangsimian)	129
Oat dumplings with potato filling (Malingshu Youmian Jiaozi)	130
Oat flour-wrapped shredded potato (Youmian Tuntun)	131
Pagoda-shaped mashed potatoes with shiitake mushroom (Xianggu Malingshu Ni Ta)	355
Pan-fried potato pastry (Xiangjian Tudou Bing II)	292
Pear-shaped potato (Xiang Sheng Li)	215
Pepper oil-flavored shredded potato (Jiaoyou Tudou Si)	132
Pickled Chinese cabbage with mashed potatoes (Suancai Tudou Ni)	133
Potato and buckwheat pancakes (Malingshu Jianbing)	216
Potato and cabbage soup (Hongcai Tang)	59
Potato and chicken with chili powder (Yangyu Lazi Ji)	293
Potato and egg soup (Tudou Danhua Tang)	356
Potato and millet porridge (Qiangguo Malingshu Xifan)	134
Potato and oat pancake (Tudou Bing II)	135
Potato and oat pancakes (Tudou Bing IV)	217
Potato and pumpkin sandwich (Baihua Tudou He)	218
Potato and shiitake mushroom cake (Tudou Xianggu Bing)	219
Potato and vegetable salad (Qingcai Malingshu Shalazi)	357
Potato balls (Tudou Li Wanzi)	60
Potato balls with ham (Huotui Malingshu Wanzi)	358
Potato bula (Yangyu Bula)	220

Potato cake I (Tudou Bing I)	61
Potato cake II (Malingshu Bing)	136
Potato cake III (Tudou Gao)	221
Potato chicken egg soup (Tudou Jidan Geng)	222
Potato chips served with Yunnan ham (Yuntui Tudou Pian)	294
Potato chips with fried pork fillet (Guoyourou Malingshu Pian)	137
Potato dumplings (Shu Jiao)	359
Potato egg cake with sesame seeds (Malingshu Jidan Zhima Bing)	138
Potato Kuilei (Tudou Kuilei)	139
Potato lambsquarter goosefoot salad in vinegar sauce (Malingshu Ban Huicai)	140
Potato noodles (Yangyu Mian)	223
Potato noodles mixed with sauce (Jiachang Ban Fen)	141
Potato noodles with needle mushrooms (Malingshu Fensi Jinzhengu)	142
Potato nut cake (Malingshu Ganguo Gao)	224
Potato pancake with salted vegetables (Xuecai Tudou Bing)	295
Potato pie (Malingshu Gao)	143
Potato pot-stickers (Malingshu Guotie)	144
Potato rolls wrapped in dried tofu (Fupi Malingshu Juan)	360
Potato salad (Tudou Shala)	225
Potato salad with green vegetables (Qingcai Tudou Shala)	62
Potato sandwich with pork (You Su Tudou He)	361
Potato shoot salad in vinegar (Liangban Shumiao)	296
Potato shoot soup with sour bamboo shoots (Suan Sun Shumiao Tang)	297
Potato soup with pickled cabbage (Suancai Tudoupian Tang)	298
Potato starch jelly (Malingshu Liangfen)	226
Potato string cake with five spices (Wuxiang Tudou Si Bing)	299
Potato strings with lichen (Dipicai Malingshu Si)	145
Potato strings with sea cucumber (Tudou Si Ban Haishen)	362

Potato strips with Japanese rhodea (Wannianqing malingshu Tiao)	146
Potato with laver (Zi Cai Tudou Bing)	300
Potato with twice-cooked pork (Tudou Huiguo Rou)	301
Potatoes cooked in tin foil (Xizhi Tudou)	302
Potatoes in hot caramel (Basi Tudou)	363
Potatoes in soy sauce (Jiang Xiang Tudou)	303
Potatoes in soybean milk (Hezha Yangyu)	304
Potato-oat flour made fishlike noodles (Xiangjian Tudou Roujuan)	147
Potato-wrapped beef rolls (Tudou Niurou Juan)	227
Roasted potato (Kao Malingshu)	148
Roasted potato slices (Kao Malingshu Pian)	149
Roasted potatoes (Kang Yangyu)	305
Roasted potatoes with jam (Guojiang Malingshu Pai)	364
Rolls with potato and beef filling (Tudou Niurou Bing)	228
Salted meat with colored potatoes (Yanrou Caiyangyu)	306
San zha wu pin (San Zha Wu Pin)	229
Seasoned potato strings and noodles (Qiang Tudou Si, Fensi)	63
Shredded potato and bean salad (San Si Bao Dou)	64
Shredded potato and wild vegetables in vinegar and spices (Malingshu Si Ban Yan Kucai)	150
Shredded potato salad in vinegar (Liangban Shu Si)	307
Shredded potato with sow thistle (Malingshu Si Ban Kucai)	151
Shredded potatoes with beef jerky (Ganba Yanyu Si)	308
Shredded potatoes with pickles (Yangyu Si Xiancai)	309
Shredded potatoes with sweet and sour sauce (Yuxiang Tudou Si)	230
Silver boat carries the valuables (Yinzhou Zaibao)	152
Silver thread noodles and potato strings (Yinsi Tudou Chuan)	310
Sizzling Potato (Tieban Tudou)	311
Soft potato cake (Yangyu Langao)	231

Soft-fried sliced potatoes (Ruanzha Tudoupian)	312
Soft-shell turtle encircled with small potatoes (Xiao Tudou Jiayu)	153
Sour and spicy potato chips (Suanla Tudou Pian)	313
Sour and spicy shredded potato soup (Suanla Tudou Si Tang)	314
Sour diced potato soup (Shu Kuai Suan Tang)	315
Sour pickle and chive flower potato soup (Suanyancai Tudou Tang)	316
Sour pickle and potato chip soup (Suanyancai Tudou Pian Tang)	317
Spareribs with Chinese sauerkraut and mashed potatoes (Paigu Suancai Malingshu Ni)	154
Spicy and hot potatoes (Xiangla Tudou)	318
Spicy diced potatoes I (Xiangla Malingshu Ding)	155
Spicy diced potatoes II (Xiangla Shu Kuai)	319
Spicy potato chips (Xiangla Tudou Pian II)	320
Spicy potato slices (Xiangla Tudou Pian I)	321
Spicy shredded potatoes (Xiangla Tudou Si)	156
Spicy Sichuan-style potato strings (Ganbian Tudou Si)	322
Steamed abalone-shaped potato pie (Su Bao Pai Fan)	157
Steamed buns with potato and Chinese chive filling (Tudou Jiucai Baozi)	158
Steamed dumplings (Zheng Jiao)	159
Steamed fish-shaped oat noodles (Youmian zheng Yu)	160
Steamed fish-shaped potatoes with Chinese sauerkraut (Suancai Malingshu Yu)	161
Steamed oat rolls with potato and eggplant (Malingshu Men Qiezi)	162
Steamed potato and eggplant served with soy sauce (Nongjia Dajiang Zheng Tudou Qiezi)	65
Steamed potato and lichen dumplings (Tudou Diruan Baozi)	232
Steamed potato balls (Tudou Wanzi)	163
Steamed potato cake (Zheng Malingshu Yangzi)	164
Steamed potato flakes mixed with flour (Yangyu Caca)	233
Steamed potato jelly (Yangyu Jinjin)	234
Steamed potato strings with mashed garlic (Suan Ni Tudou Si)	365

Steamed potatoes and pork balls (Jing Wan Wan)	165
Steamed potatoes and spareribs (Fen Zheng Tudou Paigu)	323
Steamed potatoes I (Zheng Malingshu)	166
Steamed potatoes II (Zheng Tudou)	235
Steamed potatoes with chicken (Tudou Zheng Ji)	236
Steamed potatoes with pickled chili (Culajiao Zheng Tudou)	324
Stewed beef with potato (Tudou Shao Niunan)	366
Stewed chicken with potato (Malingshu Dun Xiaoji)	167
Stewed chicken with potato and tofu (Malingshu Tofu Dun Jiaji)	168
Stewed pork bones with potato and squash (Malingshu Wogua Dun Gutou)	169
Stewed pork ribs with potato and squash (Malingshu Wogua Dun Paigu)	170
Stewed potato chips with goose (Tudou Gan Dun Da E)	66
Stewed potatoes (Men Tudou)	237
Stewed potatoes and pork ribs with spices (Xiangla Paigu Men Tudou)	325
Stewed potatoes served in wok (Ganguo Tudou)	326
Stewed potatoes with chicken (Xiaoji Dun Tudou)	171
Stewed potatoes with cowpeas (Tudou dun Doujiao)	67
Stewed potatoes with cucurbit (Xiao Gua Men Yangyu)	327
Stewed potatoes with curry chicken (Tudou Dun Gali Ji Kuai)	68
Stewed potatoes with eggplant (Malingshu Men Qiezi)	172
Stewed potatoes with eggplant in thick sauce (Tudou Jiang Dun Qiezi)	69
Stewed potatoes with pumpkin I (Malingshu Dun Wogua)	173
Stewed potatoes with pumpkin II (Nangua Dun Tudou)	328
Stewed potatoes with rice (Yangyu Kongganfan)	329
Stewed potatoes with yellow sturgeon (Xunhuangyu Men Tudou)	70
Stewed sheep entrails with potato noodles (Yu Lin Yang Zasui)	238
Stewed silver carp soup (Guiyu Zahui Tang)	330
Stewed small potatoes I (Youmen Xiao Tudou I)	71

Stewed small potatoes II (Youmen Xiao Tudou II)	331
Stewed spareribs with potato and frozen tofu (Malingshu Paigu Dong Tofu)	174
Stir-fried beef with potato noodles (Niurou Chao Fen)	239
Stir-fried knife-sliced noodles with potato chips and fried pork fillet (Guoyourou Malingshu Pian Chao Daoxiaomian)	175
Stir-fried mashed potatoes (Chao Malingshu Kuailei)	176
Stir-fried pork with potato noodles (Zhurou Qiao Ban Fen)	240
Stir-fried potato shoots (Su Chao Shumiao)	332
Stir-fried potato strips and shredded carrot (Malingshu Tiao Chao Huluobo Si)	177
Stir-fried potato strips with celery (Shan Qin Chao Tudou)	367
Stir-fried potato, green pepper and eggplant (Di Sanxian)	73
Stir-fried shredded vegetables (Chao San Si)	333
Strawberry-filled mashed potato cake (Caomei Yuni Su)	241
Street potato snacks from Yunnan (Jie Bian Xiao Chi)	334
Swan playing with water (Tian E Xishui)	178
Sweet and sour potato sandwiches (Tangcu Tudou Jia)	335
Sweet fried potato chips (Huanying Tudou Pian)	242
Three earthly delights (JiaoDong Di Sanxian)	369
Three kinds of stewed vegetable balls (Shao San Yuan)	243
Tired bird returns to the nest (Juan Niao Gui Chao)	179
Tofu soup with potato and cabbage (Malingshu Baicai Tofu Tang)	180
Toothpick potato diamonds (Yaqian Tudoukuai)	336
Translucent dumplings (Boli Jiaozi)	181
Tree tomato-flavored potatoes (Shu Fanqie Fenwei Tudou Si)	337
Tricolor mashed potatoes (Sanse Tudou Ni)	183
Western-style mashed potatoes (Xi Shi Tudou Ni)	339
Xinjiang chicken and potato dish (Xinjiang Da Pan Ji)	244
Yulin three fresh delicacies (Yulin Pin Sanxian)	245

Appendix 2: Indices of the dishes for vegetarians

Bag-shaped oat potato pie (Malingshu Tuntun)	77
Baked potato cake (Lao Malinghshu Yangzi)	78
Baked potato cake with red bean filling (Tudou Dousha Bing)	188
Baked potatoes (Kao Tudou)	187
Baked shredded potatoes (Gan Bei Yangyu Si)	249
Braised potato pieces (Hongshao Shukuai)	81
Braised potatoes with pumpkin (Dun Nangua Tudou)	193
Braised tofu with pakchoi (Xiao Baicai Hui Tofu)	195
Charcoal-roasted potatoes (Tanhuo Kao Tudou)	255
Cold potato strings in oil, vinegar and spices (Liangban Malingshu Si)	94
Colorful shredded potatoes (Qicai Tudou Si)	257
Crisp potato balls coated with sugar (Yinzhuang Suguo)	196
Crisp potato strips I (Xiangsu Shu Tiao I)	258
Crystal mashed potato roll (Yuni Shuijing Juan)	197
Cucumber with potato noodles (Huanggua Fenpi)	198
Dark steamed potato balls (Heilengleng)	199
Deep-fried potato balls (Cuizha Tudou Qiu)	344
Deep-fried potato balls covered in sesame seeds (Tudou Matuan)	200
Deep-fried potato chips (Youzha Tudou Pian)	261
Deep-fried potato chips with peanuts and chili (Youzha San Pin)	262
Deep-fried potato doughnuts (Youzha Malingshu Guozi)	96
Deep-fried potato strips with tomato sauce (Mizhi Shasi Tudou Tiao)	97
Drunk potato (Zuijiu Malingshu)	98
Finely shredded potatoes with ginger (Jiangwei Longxu Si)	264
Fish-shaped potato (Malingshu Yu)	101
Flavored potato balls (Fengwei Tudou Qiu)	104
French-style mushroom and potato salad (Fashi Xianggu Malingshu Shalazi)	345

Fried chicken-flavored potato (Youzha Malingshu Su Jitui)	105
Fried country-style potato balls (Shancun Zha Malingshu Wanzi)	346
Fried diced potatoes and lettuce stems (Chao Malingshu Wosunding)	347
Fried dried potato slices (Zha Gan Yangyupian)	265
Fried green pepper and shredded potato (Qingjiao Tudou Si)	266
Fried lichen and potato chips (Dipi Tudou Pian)	50
Fried potato balls (Youzha Malingshu Wanzi)	110
Fried potato cake I (Jian Tudou Bing)	51
Fried potato cake IV (Cui Zha Tudou Bing)	349
Fried potato chips (Su Chao Tudou Pian)	267
Fried potato chips with soy sauce (Jiang Bao Tudou Pian)	268
Fried potato chips with spicy cabbage (La Baicai Chao Tudou Pian)	53
Fried potato pie (Youzha Shu Bing)	270
Fried potato slices I (Youzha Malingshu Pian)	112
Fried potato slices II (Zha Malingshu Pian)	350
Fried potato slices with dried pickles (Gan Yancai Chao Shu Pian)	271
Fried potato slices with sour bamboo shoots (Suan Sun Chao Shupian)	272
Fried potato strings (Youzha Malingshu Si)	113
Fried potato strips (Zha Malingshu Tiao)	351
Fried potato strips coated with sugar (Liuli Shutiao)	115
Fried potato strips with garlic bolt (Zha Tudou Tiao Chao Suantai)	54
Fried potato strips with spicy peanuts (Xiang Su Shutiao)	352
Fried potatoes with soybean sprouts (Tudou Chao Huangdou Ya)	119
Fried shredded potato (Suchao Tudou Si)	55
Fried shredded potato cake I (Xiang Jian Tudou Pai)	120
Fried shredded potato cake II (Tudou Tanbing III)	206

Fried tofu and potatoes with green and red Pepper (Jin Yu Man Tang)	209
Golden fried potato balls (Zha Huangjin Tudou Qiu)	56
Grape-shaped potato dish (Fengshou Putao)	213
Green onion-flavored potato chips (Conghua Shu Pian)	279
Hot and spicy diced potatoes I (Mala Tudou Ding)	282
Hot and spicy diced potatoes II (Xiangma Tudou Ding)	283
Hotpot potato pieces (Malingshu Huoguo Pian)	124
Hunyuan cold potato jelly (Hunyuan Liangfen)	125
Mashed potatoes fried with fennel (Huixiang Tudou Ni)	286
Mashed potatoes in lotus leaf (Heye Tudou Ni)	287
Mashed potatoes with pakchoi (Hua Cai)	214
Mixed shredded potatoes (Ban Tudou Song)	58
Oat flour-wrapped shredded potato (Youmian Tuntun)	131
Pagoda-shaped mashed potatoes with shiitake mushroom (Xianggu Malingshu Ni Ta)	355
Pear-shaped potato (Xiang Sheng Li)	215
Pepper oil-flavored shredded potato (Jiaoyou Tudou Si)	132
Potato and millet porridge (Qiangguo Malingshu Xifan)	134
Potato and oat pancake (Tudou Bing II)	135
Potato and oat pancakes (Tudou Bing IV)	217
Potato and shiitake mushroom cake (Tudou Xianggu Bing)	219
Potato cake II (Malingshu Bing)	136
Potato cake III (Tudou Gao)	221
Potato Kuilei (Tudou Kuilei)	139
Potato lambsquarter goosefoot salad in vinegar sauce (Malingshu Ban Huicai)	140
Potato noodles (Yangyu Mian)	223
Potato noodles mixed with sauce (Jiachang Ban Fen)	141
Potato pie (Malingshu Gao)	143

Potato rolls wrapped in dried tofu (Fupi Malingshu Juan)	360
Potato shoot salad in vinegar (Liangban Shumiao)	296
Potato shoot soup with sour bamboo shoots (Suan Sun Shumiao Tang)	297
Potato soup with pickled cabbage (Suancai Tudoupian Tang)	298
Potato starch jelly (Malingshu Liangfen)	226
Potato string cake with five spices (Wuxiang Tudou Si Bing)	299
Potato strings with lichen (Dipicai Malingshu Si)	145
Potato strips with Japanese rhodea (Wannianqing malingshu Tiao)	146
Potatoes cooked in tin foil (Xizhi Tudou)	302
Potatoes in hot caramel (Basi Tudou)	363
Potatoes in soy sauce (Jiang Xiang Tudou)	303
Potatoes in soybean milk (Hezha Yangyu)	304
Roasted potato (Kao Malingshu)	148
Roasted potato slices (Kao Malingshu Pian)	149
Roasted potatoes (Kang Yangyu)	305
Seasoned potato strings and noodles (Qiang Tudou Si, Fensi)	63
Shredded potato and bean salad (San Si Bao Dou)	64
Shredded potato and wild vegetables in vinegar and spices (Malingshu Si Ban Yan Kucai)	150
Shredded potato salad in vinegar (Liangban Shu Si)	307
Shredded potato with sow thistle (Malingshu Si Ban Kucai)	151
Shredded potatoes with pickles (Yangyu Si Xiancai)	309
Silver boat carries the valuables (Yinzhou Zaibao)	152
Soft potato cake (Yangyu Langao)	231
Soft-fried sliced potatoes (Ruanzha Tudoupian)	312
Sour and spicy potato chips (Suanla Tudou Pian)	313
Sour and spicy shredded potato soup (Suanla Tudou Si Tang)	314
Sour diced potato soup (Shu Kuai Suan Tang)	315

Sour pickle and chive flower potato soup (Suanyancai Tudou Tang)	316
Sour pickle and potato chip soup (Suanyancai Tudou Pian Tang)	317
Spicy and hot potatoes (Xiangla Tudou)	318
Spicy diced potatoes I (Xiangla Malingshu Ding)	155
Spicy diced potatoes II (Xiangla Shu Kuai)	319
Spicy potato chips (Xiangla Tudou Pian II)	320
Spicy potato slices (Xiangla Tudou Pian I)	321
Spicy shredded potatoes (Xiangla Tudou Si)	156
Spicy Sichuan-style potato strings (Ganbian Tudou Si)	322
Steamed buns with potato and Chinese chive filling (Tudou Jiucai Baozi)	158
Steamed fish-shaped oat noodles (Youmian zheng Yu)	160
Steamed potato and eggplant served with soy sauce (Nongjia Dajiang Zheng Tudou Qiezi)	65
Steamed potato and lichen dumplings (Tudou Diruan Baozi)	232
Steamed potato balls (Tudou Wanzi)	163
Steamed potato cake (Zheng Malingshu Yangzi)	164
Steamed potato flakes mixed with flour (Yangyu Caca)	233
Steamed potato strings with mashed garlic (Suan Ni Tudou Si)	365
Steamed potatoes I (Zheng Malingshu)	166
Steamed potatoes II (Zheng Tudou)	235
Stewed potatoes (Men Tudou)	237
Stewed potatoes served in wok (Ganguo Tudou)	326
Stewed potatoes with cucurbit (Xiao Gua Men Yangyu)	327
Stewed potatoes with pumpkin I (Malingshu Dun Wogua)	173
Stewed potatoes with pumpkin II (Nangua Dun Tudou)	328
Stewed potatoes with rice (Yangyu Kongganfan)	329
Stewed small potatoes II (Youmen Xiao Tudou II)	331
Stir-fried mashed potatoes (Chao Malingshu Kuailei)	176

Stir-fried potato shoots (Su Chao Shumiao)	332
Stir-fried potato strips with celery (Shan Qin Chao Tudou)	367
Stir-fried potato, green pepper and eggplant (Di Sanxian)	73
Stir-fried shredded vegetables (Chao San Si)	333
Strawberry-filled mashed potato cake (Caomei Yuni Su)	241
Sweet fried potato chips (Huanying Tudou Pian)	242
Toothpick potato diamonds (Yaqian Tudoukuai)	336
Tree tomato-flavored potatoes (Shu Fanqie Fenwei Tudou Si)	337
Tricolor mashed potatoes (Sanse Tudou Ni)	183
Western-style mashed potatoes (Xi Shi Tudou Ni)	339

Appendix 3: Indices of the dishes for Muslims

Bag-shaped oat potato pie (Malingshu Tuntun)	77
Baked potato cake (Lao Malinghshu Yangzi)	78
Baked potato cake with red bean filling (Tudou Dousha Bing)	188
Baked potatoes (Kao Tudou)	187
Baked shredded potatoes (Gan Bei Yangyu Si)	249
Birds nest-shaped shredded potatoes (Niaochao Shu Si)	250
Black beauty potato slices (Hei Meiren Yangyu)	189
Black soy sauce potatoes (Jiangyou Malingshu Tiao)	79
Braised potato with goose (Da E Men Tudou)	47
Braised potatoes with duck (Tudou Huang Men Ya)	252
Braised potatoes with mutton rack (Tudou Wei Yangpai)	192
Braised potatoes with pumpkin (Dun Nangua Tudou)	193
Braised sheep entrails with noodles (Guozai Fentiao Yangza)	88
Braised tofu with pakchoi (Xiao Baicai Hui Tofu)	195
Camel palm encircled with shredded potato (Tuozhang Tudou Si)	92
Charcoal-roasted potatoes (Tanhuo Kao Tudou)	255
Chinese date-filled potato balls with honey (Mizhi Nuoxiang Tudou Zao)	256
Cold potato strings in oil, vinegar and spices (Liangban Malingshu Si)	94
Colorful shredded potatoes (Qicai Tudou Si)	257
Cooked potato chips (Peng Tudou Pian)	48
Crisp potato balls coated with sugar (Yinzhuang Suguo)	196
Crisp potato strips I (Xiangsu Shu Tiao I)	258
Crisp potato strips II (Xiangsu Shu Tiao II)	259
Crystal mashed potato roll (Yuni Shuijing Juan)	197
Cucumber with potato noodles (Huanggua Fenpi)	198
Curry potatoes (Gali Malingshu)	343
Dark steamed potato balls (Heilengleng)	199

Deep-fried potato balls (Cuizha Tudou Qiu)	344
Deep-fried potato balls covered in sesame seeds (Tudou Matuan)	200
Deep-fried potato chips (Youzha Tudou Pian)	261
Deep-fried potato chips with peanuts and chili (Youzha San Pin)	262
Deep-fried potato doughnuts (Youzha Malingshu Guozi)	96
Deep-fried potato strips with tomato sauce (Mizhi Shasi Tudou Tiao)	97
Diced potatoes with salted egg yolk (Yan Danhuang Tudou Li)	263
Dongxiang county potato chips (Dongxiang Tudou Pian)	201
Egg, shredded bottle gourd and potato cake (Jidan Hulusi Malingshu Bing)	99
Fish-shaped potato (Malingshu Yu)	101
Flavored potato balls (Fengwei Tudou Qiu)	104
French-style mushroom and potato salad (Fashi Xianggu Malingshu Shalazi)	345
Fried chicken-flavored potato (Youzha Malingshu Su Jitui)	105
Fried Chinese sauerkraut and noodles (Suancai Chao Fentiao)	106
Fried Chinese sauerkraut and potato chips (Suancai Malingshu Tiao)	107
Fried Chinese sauerkraut and potato slices (Suancai Malinghsu Ni)	108
Fried country-style potato balls (Shancun Zha Malingshu Wanzi)	346
Fried diced potatoes and lettuce stems (Chao Malingshu Wosunding)	347
Fried dried potato slices (Zha Gan Yangyupian)	265
Fried egg and potato string cake (Jianjidan Malingshusi Bing)	348
Fried green pepper and shredded potato (Qingjiao Tudou Si)	266
Fried lichen and potato chips (Dipi Tudou Pian)	50
Fried mashed potatoes, carrots and mushrooms (Jinsha Fengguang)	109
Fried potato balls (Youzha Malingshu Wanzi)	110
Fried potato cake I (Jian Tudou Bing)	51
Fried potato cake III (Tudou Jianbing)	205
Fried potato cake IV (Cui Zha Tudou Bing)	349

Fried potato chips (Su Chao Tudou Pian)	267
Fried potato chips with soy sauce (Jiang Bao Tudou Pian)	268
Fried potato chips with spicy cabbage (La Baicai Chao Tudou Pian)	53
Fried potato pancake (Qiaoshou Tuanyuanbing)	269
Fried potato pie (Youzha Shu Bing)	270
Fried potato slices I (Youzha Malingshu Pian)	112
Fried potato slices II (Zha Malingshu Pian)	350
Fried potato slices with dried pickles (Gan Yancai Chao Shu Pian)	271
Fried potato slices with sour bamboo shoots (Suan Sun Chao Shupian)	272
Fried potato strings (Youzha Malingshu Si)	113
Fried potato strips (Zha Malingshu Tiao)	351
Fried potato strips coated with sugar (Liuli Shutiao)	115
Fried potato strips coated with yolk (Jinsha Tudou Tiao)	273
Fried potato strips with garlic bolt (Zha Tudou Tiao Chao Suantai)	54
Fried potato strips with spicy peanuts (Xiang Su Shutiao)	352
Fried potato with jellyfish (Tudou Bao Zhetou)	353
Fried potatoes with egg (Tudou Jian Dan)	118
Fried potatoes with four treasures (Jin Shu Hui Sibao)	276
Fried potatoes with soybean sprouts (Tudou Chao Huangdou Ya)	119
Fried shredded potato (Suchao Tudou Si)	55
Fried shredded potato cake I (Xiang Jian Tudou Pai)	120
Fried shredded potato cake II (Tudou Tanbing III)	206
Fried shredded potato with Chinese chives and egg (served with cake) (Malingshu Si Jiucai Jidan Dai Bing)	121
Fried shredded potatoes with vinegar (Culiu Yangyu Si)	207
Fried stick-shaped mutton-potato mash (Tu Yang Jiehe Bang)	208
Fried tofu and potatoes with green and red Pepper (Jin Yu Man Tang)	209
Golden fried potato balls (Zha Huangjin Tudou Qiu)	56

Golden potato string cake (Jinhuang Dousi Bing)	278
Golden shredded potato nest (Jin Quechao)	210
Goulash with potato (Tudou Shao Niurou)	212
Grape-shaped potato dish (Fengshou Putao)	213
Green onion-flavored potato chips (Conghua Shu Pian)	279
Handmade noodles with potatoes in an earthen pot (Shaguo Malingshu Shouganmian)	123
Honey potatoes (Mizhi Malingshu)	354
Honeycomb-shaped potatoes (Fengwo Tudou)	281
Hot and spicy diced potatoes I (Mala Tudou Ding)	282
Hot and spicy diced potatoes II (Xiangma Tudou Ding)	283
Hotpot potato pieces (Malingshu Huoguo Pian)	124
Hunyuan cold potato jelly (Hunyuan Liangfen)	125
Long life shredded potatoes (Changshou Tudou Si)	285
Mashed potatoes fried with fennel (Huixiang Tudou Ni)	286
Mashed potatoes in lotus leaf (Heye Tudou Ni)	287
Mashed potatoes with pakchoi (Hua Cai)	214
Mashed potatoes with pine nuts (Songren Tudou Ni)	288
Mashed potatoes wrapped in sticky rice pancakes (Zhibao Tudou Ni)	289
Megranate-shaped fried chicken (Fugui Shiliu Ji)	290
Minced beef in potato bowls (Yi Wan Chi)	291
Mini embroidered potato balls (Mini Xiuqiu Wan)	128
Mixed shredded potatoes (Ban Tudou Song)	58
Oat dumplings with potato filling (Malingshu Youmian Jiaozi)	130
Oat flour-wrapped shredded potato (Youmian Tuntun)	131
Pagoda-shaped mashed potatoes with shiitake mushroom (Xianggu Malingshu Ni Ta)	355
Pear-shaped potato (Xiang Sheng Li)	215
Pepper oil-flavored shredded potato (Jiaoyou Tudou Si)	132

Potato and cabbage soup (Hongcai Tang)	59
Potato and egg soup (Tudou Danhua Tang)	356
Potato and millet porridge (Qiangguo Malingshu Xifan)	134
Potato and oat pancake (Tudou Bing II)	135
Potato and oat pancakes (Tudou Bing IV)	217
Potato and pumpkin sandwich (Baihua Tudou He)	218
Potato and shiitake mushroom cake (Tudou Xianggu Bing)	219
Potato cake I (Tudou Bing I)	61
Potato cake II (Malingshu Bing)	136
Potato cake III (Tudou Gao)	221
Potato chicken egg soup (Tudou Jidan Geng)	222
Potato egg cake with sesame seeds (Malingshu Jidan Zhima Bing)	138
Potato Kuilei (Tudou Kuilei)	139
Potato lambsquarter goosefoot salad in vinegar sauce (Malingshu Ban Huicai)	140
Potato noodles (Yangyu Mian)	223
Potato noodles mixed with sauce (Jiachang Ban Fen)	141
Potato noodles with needle mushrooms (Malingshu Fensi Jinzhengu)	142
Potato nut cake (Malingshu Ganguo Gao)	224
Potato pie (Malingshu Gao)	143
Potato pot-stickers (Malingshu Guotie)	144
Potato rolls wrapped in dried tofu (Fupi Malingshu Juan)	360
Potato salad (Tudou Shala)	225
Potato salad with green vegetables (Qingcai Tudou Shala)	62
Potato shoot salad in vinegar (Liangban Shumiao)	296
Potato shoot soup with sour bamboo shoots (Suan Sun Shumiao Tang)	297
Potato soup with pickled cabbage (Suancai Tudoupian Tang)	298
Potato starch jelly (Malingshu Liangfen)	226

Potato string cake with five spices (Wuxiang Tudou Si Bing)	299
Potato strings with lichen (Dipicai Malingshu Si)	145
Potato strings with sea cucumber (Tudou Si Ban Haishen)	362
Potato strips with Japanese rhodea (Wannianqing malingshu Tiao)	146
Potatoes cooked in tin foil (Xizhi Tudou)	302
Potatoes in hot caramel (Basi Tudou)	363
Potatoes in soy sauce (Jiang Xiang Tudou)	303
Potatoes in soybean milk (Hezha Yangyu)	304
Potato-wrapped beef rolls (Tudou Niurou Juan)	227
Roasted potato (Kao Malingshu)	148
Roasted potato slices (Kao Malingshu Pian)	149
Roasted potatoes (Kang Yangyu)	305
Roasted potatoes with jam (Guojiang Malingshu Pai)	364
Rolls with potato and beef filling (Tudou Niurou Bing)	228
Seasoned potato strings and noodles (Qiang Tudou Si, Fensi)	63
Shredded potato and bean salad (San Si Bao Dou)	64
Shredded potato and wild vegetables in vinegar and spices (Malingshu Si Ban Yan Kucai)	150
Shredded potato salad in vinegar (Liangban Shu Si)	307
Shredded potato with sow thistle (Malingshu Si Ban Kucai)	151
Shredded potatoes with beef jerky (Ganba Yanyu Si)	308
Shredded potatoes with pickles (Yangyu Si Xiancai)	309
Shredded potatoes with sweet and sour sauce (Yuxiang Tudou Si)	230
Silver boat carries the valuables (Yinzhou Zaibao)	152
Soft potato cake (Yangyu Langao)	231
Soft-fried sliced potatoes (Ruanzha Tudoupian)	312
Sour and spicy potato chips (Suanla Tudou Pian)	313
Sour and spicy shredded potato soup (Suanla Tudou Si Tang)	314

Sour diced potato soup (Shu Kuai Suan Tang)	315
Sour pickle and chive flower potato soup (Suanyancai Tudou Tang)	316
Sour pickle and potato chip soup (Suanyancai Tudou Pian Tang)	317
Spicy and hot potatoes (Xiangla Tudou)	318
Spicy diced potatoes I (Xiangla Malingshu Ding)	155
Spicy diced potatoes II (Xiangla Shu Kuai)	319
Spicy potato chips (Xiangla Tudou Pian II)	320
Spicy potato slices (Xiangla Tudou Pian I)	321
Spicy shredded potatoes (Xiangla Tudou Si)	156
Spicy Sichuan-style potato strings (Ganbian Tudou Si)	322
Steamed abalone-shaped potato pie (Su Bao Pai Fan)	157
Steamed buns with potato and Chinese chive filling (Tudou Jiucai Baozi)	158
Steamed fish-shaped oat noodles (Youmian zheng Yu)	160
Steamed fish-shaped potatoes with Chinese sauerkraut (Suancai Malingshu Yu)	161
Steamed potato and eggplant served with soy sauce (Nongjia Dajiang Zheng Tudou Qiezi)	65
Steamed potato and lichen dumplings (Tudou Diruan Baozi)	232
Steamed potato balls (Tudou Wanzi)	163
Steamed potato cake (Zheng Malingshu Yangzi)	164
Steamed potato flakes mixed with flour (Yangyu Caca)	233
Steamed potato strings with mashed garlic (Suan Ni Tudou Si)	365
Steamed potatoes I (Zheng Malingshu)	166
Steamed potatoes II (Zheng Tudou)	235
Steamed potatoes with chicken (Tudou Zheng Ji)	236
Stewed potatoes (Men Tudou)	237
Stewed potatoes served in wok (Ganguo Tudou)	326
Stewed potatoes with cucurbit (Xiao Gua Men Yangyu)	327
Stewed potatoes with curry chicken (Tudou Dun Gali Ji Kuai)	68

Stewed potatoes with eggplant (Malingshu Men Qiezi)	172
Stewed potatoes with eggplant in thick sauce (Tudou Jiang Dun Qiezi)	69
Stewed potatoes with pumpkin I (Malingshu Dun Wogua)	173
Stewed potatoes with pumpkin II (Nangua Dun Tudou)	328
Stewed potatoes with rice (Yangyu Kongganfan)	329
Stewed sheep entrails with potato noodles (Yu Lin Yang Zasui)	238
Stewed silver carp soup (Guiyu Zahui Tang)	330
Stewed small potatoes II (Youmen Xiao Tudou II)	331
Stir-fried beef with potato noodles (Niurou Chao Fen)	239
Stir-fried mashed potatoes (Chao Malingshu Kuailei)	176
Stir-fried potato shoots (Su Chao Shumiao)	332
Stir-fried potato strips and shredded carrot (Malingshu Tiao Chao Huluobo Si)	177
Stir-fried potato strips with celery (Shan Qin Chao Tudou)	367
Stir-fried potato, green pepper and eggplant (Di Sanxian)	73
Stir-fried shredded vegetables (Chao San Si)	333
Strawberry-filled mashed potato cake (Caomei Yuni Su)	241
Swan playing with water (Tian E Xishui)	178
Sweet and sour potato sandwiches (Tangcu Tudou Jia)	335
Sweet fried potato chips (Huanying Tudou Pian)	242
Three earthly delights (JiaoDong Di Sanxian)	369
Toothpick potato diamonds (Yaqian Tudoukuai)	336
Translucent dumplings (Boli Jiaozi)	181
Tree tomato-flavored potatoes (Shu Fanqie Fenwei Tudou Si)	337
Tricolor mashed potatoes (Sanse Tudou Ni)	183
Western-style mashed potatoes (Xi Shi Tudou Ni)	339